Too Small To See, Too Big To Ignore: Child Health and Well-being in British Columbia

TOO SMALL TO SEE, TOO BIG TO IGNORE: CHILD HEALTH AND WELL-BEING IN BRITISH COLUMBIA

edited by

Michael V. Hayes and Leslie T. Foster

Canadian Western Geographical Series

Volume 35

Copyright 2002

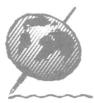

Western Geographical Press

DEPARTMENT OF GEOGRAPHY, UNIVERSITY OF VICTORIA
P.O. BOX 3050, VICTORIA, BC, CANADA V8W 3P5
PHONE: (250)721-7331 FAX: (250)721-6216
EMAIL: HFOSTER@OFFICE.GEOG.UVIC.CA

Canadian Western Geographical Series

editorial address

Harold D. Foster, Ph.D.
Department of Geography
University of Victoria
Victoria, British Columbia
Canada

Since publication began in 1970 the Western Geographical Series (now the Canadian and the International Western Geographical Series) has been generously supported by the Leon and Thea Koerner Foundation, the Social Science Federation of Canada, the National Centre for Atmospheric Research, the International Geographical Union Congress, the University of Victoria, the Natural Sciences Engineering Research Council of Canada, the Institute of the North American West, the University of Regina, the Potash and Phosphate Institute of Canada, and the Saskatchewan Agriculture and Food Department. This volume received generous support from the BC Ministry of Health and Ministry Responsible for Seniors.

TOO SMALL TO SEE, TOO BIG TO IGNORE

(Canadian western geographical series; 1203-1178; v. 35)
ISBN 0-919838-25-1

1. Child health services—British Columbia. 2. Child welfare—British Columbia. I. Foster, Leslie T., 1947- II. Hayes, Michael V. III. Series.

RJ103.C3T66 2002   362.1'9892'0009711   C2002-910819-5

SERIES EDITOR'S ACKNOWLEDGEMENTS

Several members of the Department of Geography, University of Victoria co-operated to ensure the successful publication of this volume of the Canadian Western Geographical Series. Special thanks are due to the Technical Services Division. Diane Braithwaite undertook the very demanding tasks of typesetting and layout, while cartography and cover design was in the expert hands of Ken Josephson. Their dedication and hard work is greatly appreciated.

University of Victoria   Harold D. Foster
Victoria, British Columbia   *Series Editor*
July, 2002

ACKNOWLEDGEMENTS

This volume has been a "work in progress" for some time. We would like to thank all of the authors for their contributions and for their patience. The staff in the Department of Geography, especially Diane Braithwaite, Ken Josephson, and Harry Foster, deserve a big thanks for suggestions and for putting together the volume. Thanks, too, to Ron Danderfer and the BC Vital Statistics Agency for providing the incentive to take on this work, and to Brian McKee who worked with and supported the editors throughout the project.

We would like to acknowledge the perseverance of our partners, Lillian Bayne and Mary Virtue, who allowed us to use those scarce and precious hours in the evenings and the weekends to complete this volume.

We dedicate the volume to all children, but especially to our own—Eliot, Oliver, Dylan, Christopher, Stefan, and Noelle.

Michael V. Hayes   Leslie T. Foster
Simon Fraser University   *University of Victoria*

Contents

4   Sudden Infant Death Syndrome: A Literature Review and a Summary of BC Trends 51

L.T. Foster, W.J. Kierans, and J. Macdonald

5   Quality Child Care and Community Development: What is the Connection? 75

Jessica Ball, Alan Pence, and Allison Benner

LIST OF FIGURES

LIST OF TABLES

xiv

List of Plates

Plate 1   Race to the future ⬧

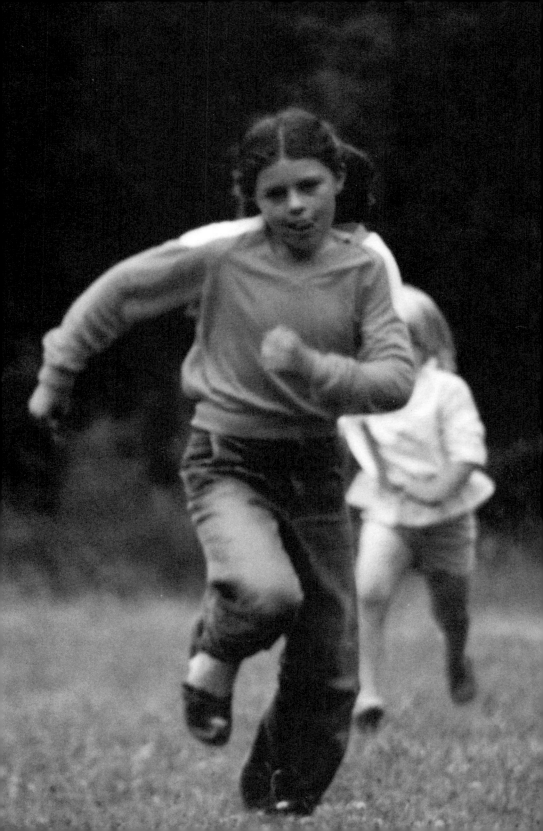

Introduction

Michael V. Hayes

Department of Geography and Institute for
Health Research and Education, Simon Fraser University

CHILDREN IN VIEW

Politically and economically, children are too small to see. Children can't vote, rarely protest, don't make financial contributions to parties of any stripe, and they are not as a group highly organized. Their political influence is indirect and fragmented. They are represented in political arenas by adult groups pursuing various interests and agendas on their behalf. Relative to other demographic groups, children have the least amount of political power and their wheels seldom squeak.

Children are out of place in the work place, though a considerable breadth of workplaces are formed around them—schools, crèches, paediatric wards, juvenile corrections, manufacturers of toys, games, and clothing, large sectors of the advertisement and entertainment industry, ... In the market, children are a terrific stimulus for consumption but are dependent upon the incomes of others to satisfy their needs. While their labour may be used in making goods found in our marketplaces, they are not managers, executives, or board members of firms or corporations. They don't make executive investment decisions.[1]

Children don't set the news agenda. When featured, they appear somewhat paradoxically as victims (of disease, disaster, depravity, destruction, dysfunctional public administration, family discord, or adult depression) and as villains (perpetrators of violence of astonishing proportion)—as both songs of innocence *and* experience. Of course, they feature prominently in human interest stories at the conclusion of newscasts, where they are always portrayed positively. A very high social value is placed upon childhood. A great deal is done by the state, by non-governmental organizations, and by individual contributors in support of nurturing child well-being, above and beyond the nurture provided by families, caregivers, and communities. We obviously care a great deal about children within our cultural ethos. They may be small, but they are neither unimportant nor invisible. It behoves us as guardians of children to be mindful of seeing them, and of how we see them, within the organization of social policy given their inherent lack of competitive political advantage. This responsibility is too big to ignore.

The increasing percentage of children living in poverty in BC and in Canada over the last two decades indicates that we can and should do more to fulfil our obligation toward future generations. The present volume is offered in support of our responsibilities toward children, and in particular toward the continued development of cultural attitudes and social policies that nurture healthy human development.

The stimulus for this collection of essays and research papers comes from two sources. The BC Provincial Health Officer's Annual Report of 1997 (BC, 1998) contained a feature report on the health and well-being of BC's children, and made recommendations on 122 specific actions that should be taken to improve their life chances. That report provides the 'big picture' population health backdrop for this volume. Coincidentally, health and social services for children were extensively reorganized with the advent of the BC Ministry for Children and Families in 1996 (recently renamed the Ministry of Child and Family Development by the new Liberal government). The essays in this volume engage the main issues arising from these two policy sources—nurturing healthy human development and providing effective services, particularly for the most vulnerable children.

Too small to see, too big to ignore also describes the fundamental dilemma that a population health approach to public policy creates in relation to children. By definition, population health involves a life-course perspective. From this vantage, health status, however measured, is clearly influenced more by the quality of the day to day encounters of our routine, often unremarkable lives than by the high moments of drama associated with health care emergencies (heart attacks, violence, injury, or systemic crisis). The lack of high drama associated with the most profound health influences disadvantages population health in political arenas, which tend to focus on immediate concerns—as there is never a shortage of fires to fight, the hottest gets the quickest attention. The impact of life chances upon health does not register greatly in traditional health status measurements of children. After age one, deaths of children are extremely rare events, and most often caused by violence, misadventure, or congenital anomalies. Only a small percentage of children have chronic illnesses. Thus, the health consequences arising from the conditions of daily life children experience are too small to see. It is as adults that the cumulative effects life chances have upon health and the need for health care and social services become most apparent. This evidence, which clearly supports the case for investing early in human development to improve health outcomes throughout the life course, is too big to ignore. The greatest cost driver in health care is our fundamental inability to get upstream—to create conditions conducive to the long-term development of people, ensuring the healthiest possible start in life. Failure to invest wisely and fully in human development threatens the fabric of civil society, because it helps to facilitate processes of social disintegration— exclusion, marginalization, violence, fear, anxiety, and social fragmentation.

Health outcomes are not, in the aggregate, randomly distributed within populations. They systematically correspond to gradients of social and economic power (measured, for example, as income, occupational status, educational attainment, or sense of control over events of daily life) that cut across major disease groups. Gradients in school achievement, in social and behavioural skills, and ability to reason appear among children in elementary school. Life chances of childhood profoundly shape adult experiences of disease, of job satisfaction, of stability in intimate relations, and other important dimensions of human well-being. Studies have shown that relative equity in the ability to participate meaningfully and materially in the routines of everyday life improves the health status of everyone (Wilkinson, 1996; Lynch et al., 1998; Kawachi, Kennedy, and Wilkinson, 1999). Societies with relatively high levels of equity (typically measured in terms of income distributions) have the highest levels of overall health status, and the shallowest gradients. People in the lowest economic groups in societies with high levels of equity have better health outcomes than the highest income groups in societies with low levels of equity.

Enlightened self interest dictates that the health and well-being of children is far too big to ignore. The challenges arising from the twin issues of making children more visible within political and economic spheres, and of making long-term investments in human health and well-being in the face of the short-term pressures in the political arena, are considerable and operate on many fronts. Yet while they are great, they are not insurmountable. There are many groups and individuals operating locally, provincially, nationally, and internationally, determined to bring about changes to public policies to improve the health and well-being of children. This volume seeks to make a positive, if modest, contribution to this end.

THIS VOLUME IN VIEW

Contributors to this volume were asked to write about issues of child health and well-being based upon their knowledge of experiences in BC. The list of authors includes public servants, academics, and representatives of non-governmental agencies. Topics cover a range of issues; rights, protection, violence, labour force participation, service organization and provision, and policy evaluation. The list of contributions does not cover all issues related to child health, but it does explore many important ones, particularly in relation to children who are extremely vulnerable.

In Chapter 2, Philip Cook makes the link between population health and children's rights. One way to increase the relative power of children is to formally recognize their rights as human beings. A review of the development of the UN's Convention on the Rights of the Child is followed by discussion of how rights contribute to improved health outcomes.

Michael Guralnick discusses the effectiveness of early intervention upon future life chances in Chapter 3. The purpose of his analysis is to provide a basis for a 'best practice' approach to public policy. The framework he presents is family centred, and involves assessment of external stressors, family patterns of interaction, and developmental outcomes.

Foster, Kierans, and Macdonald discuss recent trends in sudden infant death syndrome (SIDS) in BC in Chapter 4. Death rates from SIDS have fallen remarkably over the last 15 years, from a high of 2.14 per 1,000 in 1987 to a rate of 0.35 per 1,000 in 1998 (the last year for which data are available). Although the protocol governing attribution of SIDS deaths has changed over this period, the decline is not due to artefact. Reasons for declining rates of SIDS are discussed.

In Chapter 5, Ball, Pence, and Benner discuss the connection between quality child care and community development. They review the findings of program evaluations, anecdotal commentaries, and interpretive analyses of program models from around the world in their discussion of the reciprocal links between child care services of high quality and processes of community development. Lessons learned from other jurisdictions could be put to great use in BC to the benefit of children and communities alike.

The next three chapters deal with the issue of child protection. In Chapter 6, Foster and Wright provide a historical overview of the number of, and reasons for, children being in various forms of state care in BC. The number of children in care has varied considerably over the past two decades, with the introduction of changes to legislation, the introduction of new programs, and the influence of high profile cases involving child abuse—especially in the aftermath of the 1992 death of Matthew Vaudreuil, a 5 year old boy murdered by his mother despite the well documented history of concern in the caseload files of the then Ministry of Social Services.

Weller and Wharf discuss the process of reporting child neglect and consider the consequences for mothers of being so reported in Chapter 7. Ministry officials dismiss three out of four cases of reported neglect upon examination, but this does little to reduce feelings of anxiety, guilt, and inadequacy experienced by the mothers being investigated. As reporting of possible neglect is both mandatory and anonymous, and most reports concern children living in low income, single parent families and are based upon the norms of people with much greater affluence, Weller and Wharf argue that the present system severely punishes women for being relatively powerless. Interviews with women falsely reported for neglect are used to illustrate the contradiction between what is sought from the legislation and what is experienced as its consequence.

In Chapter 8, Cynthia Morton, the former Children's Commissioner of BC, provides an historical overview of attempts to restructure children's services following the release of the Gove Report in 1995. Judge Thomas Gove was commissioned to investigate the death of Matthew Vaudreuil in the face of what appeared to be a severe systemic failure on the part of government protection and child-serving services. In addition to documenting the process of reform of government services (particularly the establishment of the Ministry for Children and Families), Morton provides a number of recommendations for improving services for children.

Policies to improve the health and well-being of children is also the focus of Chapter 9. Rebecca and William Warburton discuss issues encountered in trying to establish evidence of the effectiveness of specific public policies upon positive outcomes for children. Based on a review of available evidence, they identify a number of specific policy options that are likely to be good investments in child well-being.

Tonkin and Murphy discuss issues relating to youth in Chapter 10, based primarily on two surveys of youth conducted by the McCreary Centre Society. The Adolescent Health Survey (HCS), initially administered in 1992 and again in 1998, is representative of all youth enrolled in grades 7 through 12 in BC. Tonkin and Murphy report on a number of health behaviours and beliefs, and analyse regional, gender, and ethnic differences in reported behaviours.

In Chapter 11, Moretti, Holland, and Moore focus on high-risk youth who repeatedly appear on case loads of social workers and who often require emergency intervention (often through the corrections system). They discuss the need for an integrated understanding of the life conditions and psychological development of such high-risk adolescents, and present a transactional-ecological model of development rooted in attachment theory as a way of achieving this integrated understanding.

In Chapter 12, Joe Michalski draws attention to the interplay between 'at risk' children, family dynamics, and labour market attachment in shaping family experiences of life satisfaction and life stress. Michalski analyses data generated from a study of 25 families living in Surrey, BC, to tease out factors related to family resilience, or their ability to cope with life stressors and bounce back from adversity.

Chapter 13, the last in this volume, provides a summary of recent changes in service provision announced by the new Liberal government taken from a review of core service reports announced in February, 2002 (as this volume was going to press). The purpose is to reflect on the recent changes in policy and program funding in light of what has been written by authors of this volume.

These are uncertain times in BC. Our hope is that the information contained in this volume, and the lessons learned in BC and elsewhere concerning policies to promote the health and well-being of children, will not be lost in the dramatic reorganization and re-profiling of priorities currently underway in the province. Of course, time will tell.

REFERENCES

BC (1998). *A report on the health of British Columbians: Provincial Health Officer's annual report 1997. Feature report: The health and well-being of British Columbia's children.* Victoria, BC: Ministry of Health and Ministry Responsible for Seniors.

Kawachi, I., Kennedy, B., and Wilkinson, R.G. (Eds.) (1999). Income inequality and health. *The Society and Population Health Reader,* Vol. 1. New York: New Press.

Lynch, J.W., Kaplan, G.A., Pamuk, E.R., Cohen, R.D., Heck, K.E., Balfour, J.L., and Yen, I.H. (1998). Income inequality and mortality in metropolitan areas of the United States. *American Journal of Public Health,* 88(7), 1074-1080.

Wilkinson, R.G. (1996). *Unhealthy societies.* London: Routledge.

ENDNOTE

[1] Comedy in the popular movie "Big" turns on this point.

Developing an Ecology of Children's Health: Recent International Trends Linking Children's Rights to Determinants of Health

2

Dr. Philip Cook
School of Child and Youth Care, University of Victoria

CHILDREN'S HEALTH, CHILDREN'S RIGHTS

Large disparities in health and well-being between children around the world remain today despite the bold intentions and promises of the World Health Organization's "Health for All by the Year 2000," made at Alma Ata in 1978. This chapter argues that children's health needs (including provision of basic health services) must be more closely tied to the rights approach arising from the 1990 World Summit for Children and global ratification of the UN Convention on the Rights of the Child. A global rights approach significantly shifts the way children's health and well-being is conceived. It implicates a global collectively in addressing issues of inequalities in health status and the distribution of life chances, and focuses attention on the physical and social environment surrounding a child's development. Global rights of children transcend state boundaries (Canadian Council on Social Development, 1996).

According to UNICEF (2000), two thirds of deaths among children worldwide are caused by pneumonia, diarrhoea, measles, and malaria. Malnutrition is a major contributor to these deaths. Half of Asia's children are malnourished and in Africa one in three children is underweight (UNICEF, 1998). Some 35,000 children die in every day in the worlds' less developed countries—about 12 million deaths annually. To be sure, significant progress has been achieved during the last decade in protecting more children through immunization and greatly reducing the number of cases of polio, tetanus, and whooping cough. A great challenge still remains, however, in improving conditions for children, particularly the poorest and most marginalized—wherever they live. Adequate nutrition, safe water, sanitation, access to primary health care, and opportunities for physical, mental and emotional growth and development will contribute enormously to improvements in the health and well-being of children everywhere. Special measures need to be introduced to safeguard the security and healthy development of children at risk from political and social neglect, upheaval, and discrimination.

While the rate of child mortality and morbidity is currently much lower in the developed world, the relatively favourable status of children's health in industrialized countries cannot be taken for granted. The collapse of the communist state health infrastructure in the Eastern Block countries and subsequent decline in health status of children living there, and the increase in child poverty and homelessness in North America and related health risks of abuse, malnutrition, and reduced access to supportive environments, provide clear evidence of the fragility of children's health promotion and prevention in industrialized nations (UNICEF, 1998).

A number of recent developments have provided new approaches and opportunities to address global inequalities in children's health. These include: the international development of child health goals established at the World Summit for Children and resulting Plan of Action (UNICEF, 1991); subsequent international Summits for social action such as the World Summit for Social Development; and the near universal ratification of the Convention on the Rights of the Child (CRC). When taken as a whole these frameworks provide an ecology, or socially supportive system, of children's rights to survival and healthy development.

Finally, there is growing support among governments, researchers and other sectors of civil society for a population health approach that situates the importance of children's health in the context of a life course. Through this lens, the powerful influence of the social environment upon overall health and well-being highlights the fundamental importance of providing stable, secure and nurturing environments for children. (Keating and Hertzman, 1999; Provincial Health Officer, 1998; Marmot and Wilkinson, 1999). The impact of childhood developmental experiences cast long shadows across our entire lifetimes.

THE WORLD SUMMIT FOR CHILDREN, DECLARATION AND PLAN OF ACTION

The World Summit for Children, which took place in September 1990, resulted in a number of goals for children in the 1990s and established health targets for the year 2000. These goals have provided clear and measurable markers for monitoring children's well-being in relation to malnutrition, preventable disease, and literacy. Of equal importance has been the unparalleled success in creating an enabling environment to implement these goals through a global advocacy process supported by UN agencies, governments, non-governmental organizations (NGO's), and community members.

At the 1990 Children's Summit, 71 Heads of State attended this historic meeting co-chaired by then Canadian Prime Minister, Brian Mulroney, and the Prime Minister of Nigeria. The timing of the Summit was opportune as, 10 years after the International Year of the Child, children's issues had reached a global high point on the international agenda. The Summit goals, outlined in the World Declaration and Plan of Action on the Survival, Protection, and Development of Children (UNICEF, 1991), include targeted reductions in infant and maternal mortality, child malnutrition and illiteracy, as well as improved levels of access to basic services for health and family planning, education, water, and sanitation.

Specific decade goals were set for the year 2000, and intermediate goals were established for 1995. Within 3 years of the Summit, 105 industrialized and developing nations, covering a total of 88% of the world's children, had prepared national programmes of action (NPAs) for meeting the World Summit goals. Canada's NPA was the Brighter Futures initiative announced in 1992 (Health Canada, 1993). While many Canadians held great promise for the bold objectives of this program, there has been a great deal of disappointment Canada's failure to support the rights of all children. This is particularly troubling with regards to the still large numbers of children living in poverty, the high rate of Aboriginal suicide and substance abuse, and the decreased services to children resulting from the cuts to Federal transfer payments to provinces. Cuts to international programming (including children's programming) during the past decade have also reflected poorly on Canada's commitment to children's rights, although the Canadian International Development Agency's (CIDA) recent Child Protection strategy offers some promise for future support for children's rights.

The World Summit goals represent a significant global commitment to improve children's basic survival and development requirements. A major focus is placed on children's health and education, with an emphasis on early intervention strategies to reduce childhood morbidity and mortality.

The 10th Summit goal addresses child protection issues through the target of achieving universal ratification of the CRC, including improved protection for children in especially difficult circumstances. However, the major Summit success lies in its setting specific and measurable primary health and education goals, and in creating a framework through the national programmes of action, to mobilize resources to achieve these goals.

UNICEF estimates that, due to countries' success in implementing the Decade goals, roughly three quarters of a million fewer children each year will be blinded, crippled, or mentally retarded (UNICEF, 1996). Particular success stories include the eradication of polio in the western hemisphere and the significant reduction of polio in East Asia and the Middle East and North Africa, as well as the reduction in childhood blindness caused by Vitamin A deficiency, and the retreat of measles.

In North America, "aid fatigue" has set in as rich nations feel increasingly poorer, and popular support for international programming wanes. Interestingly, a 1993 poll found that most Canadians believed their Aid budget was

5 times larger than was the case, and Americans thought their aid budget was 20 times higher than it actually was (UNICEF, 1995). In fact, in comparison with other industrialized countries Canada is ranked 9th, behind Belgium, Finland, and France, providing 0.32% of the GNP to overseas developmental assistance (ODA) (UNICEF, 1998). Denmark and Sweden lead the industrialized nations with ODA levels of 1.05% and 0.88% of GNP—three times as much per person as in Canada.

A recent strategy to help raise and better direct ODA is the 20/20 formula. The 20/20 strategy was introduced by Norway and launched at the World Summit for Social Development in Copenhagen in 1995. The formula suggests an allocation of 20% of the recipient governments' national budget and 20% of the donor countries' AID budget to basic social services. The 20/20 formula has been jointly adopted by the UNDP, UNESCO, UNICEF, and WHO. If accepted, this proposed strategy could have a significant impact in reaching societies' poorest and most vulnerable, in particular children.

Recent statistics through the Organization for Economic Cooperation and Development (OECD) are now available on the percent of ODA that is being targeted at basic education and basic health services. Among countries providing data in 1999 the US gave the highest portion of bilateral aid to basic health care: 5.5%. Germany provided 4.2% of its bilateral aid for basic education, the highest for reporting countries. Of Canada's total bilateral aid, 0.1% was provided for basic education and 4.1% was directed at health care, a small percentage of the 20/20 strategy (UNICEF, 2000).

While the World Summit for children has been undeniably successful from a global perspective, some of the Summit goals have been more difficult to achieve, most notably the reduction of maternal mortality (UNICEF, 1996). In addition, the impact of HIV/AIDS and social instability, particularly in Africa, has wiped out many of the initial child survival gains of the 1980s and early 1990s. Rwanda, for example, once had one of the highest rate of immunization and child survival in Africa and now is experiencing staggering increases in both areas (UNICEF, 1996). Increasingly, the realization of Health for All is being tied to programs targeting poverty and resource reallocation. Similarly, the more difficult goal of supporting children in especially difficult circumstances will likely never be reached unless the fundamental problem of economic marginalization of the poorest nations and the poorest people, including children and youth, is addressed. The primary obstacle to achieving adequate health care and education is poverty—a barrier both against contributing to, or benefiting from, the processes of economic and social development. This was acknowledged globally in the Copenhagen Summit goals of 1995 which specifically attempt to address issues relating to the distribution of economic growth, discrimination against women and children, particularly girls, and the deterioration of the environment.

The three broad objectives underlining the Copenhagen Summit include: reduction of the proportion of people living in absolute poverty; creation of necessary jobs and sustainable livelihoods; and the significant reduction in disparities among various income classes, sexes, age groups, ethnic groups, geographical regions, and nations. For children, these goals reflect a broadening of focus from basic child survival and development mirrored in the children's Summit goals to more widespread social reform. The challenge of the remainder of this decade will be to apply the ingredient for success from the children's Summit goals and implementing mechanisms and apply them to the deeper and more challenging social issues impacting on children's health.

Specific strategies include the breaking down of broad goals and objectives into "doable" and measurable propositions; the securing and sustaining of the greatest possible political commitment at the highest possible political level, and the simultaneous mobilization of the media and public support; the mobilization of a much wider range of social resources than is conventionally associated with social development efforts, including educational systems, mass media, schools, religious groups, the business community, and non-governmental organizations; the demystification of knowledge and technology in order to empower individuals and families; the reduction of procedures and techniques to relatively simple and reliable formulas, allowing large scale operations and the widespread use of large numbers of professionals; and the deployment of the expertise and resources of the UN and its agencies, and of bilateral assistance programmes, in close support of agreed goals. This should include the close monitoring of progress, followed up when necessary by increased support (UNICEF, 1995).

Richard Jolly, former UNICEF Deputy Executive Director for Programmes at UNICEF, describes these expanded Children's Summit strategies as follows (UNICEF, 1995):

> *This mixture—which I term a new paradigm for development action—is I believe of widespread applicability. Just as the success of immunization over the 1980's has led to a broader agenda of goals for improving the health and welfare of children, so this model could also be applied to other areas of international action; to new approaches to peacemaking and conflict prevention; to human development focused on the eradication of poverty; to strengthening of human rights and democratic processes; to environmental protection and sustainable development; to managing of global economic and financial relationships* (p. 41).

The CRC, by protecting all the rights of children and not only those targeted in the World Summit goals, allows for an holistic approach to promoting the well-being of all children in both developing and developed nations. It provides, for the first time, a language supporting children's well-being that is global. All children now have human rights, and while the specific issues facing a child in Cambodia may differ from a child in Canada, their civil, political, social, economic, and cultural rights are the same.

The Summit goals are presently being re-assessed, and will be reformulated and commitments renewed at the UN Special Session for Children in 2002. While many of the original Summit health priorities will likely remain in the new goals being drafted (e.g., the importance of providing clean drinking water), a number of new priorities have emerged. Primary amongst these from a global perspective is the threat to children's life survival and healthy development posed by HIV/AIDS. Many of the new goals for children will attempt to address these and other threats to children and childhood through the lens of the CRC and the application of a "rights" approach to children's health and well-being.

A "Rights" Approach to Children's Health

The CRC, adopted by the UN General Assembly in 1989, and entered into force on September 2, 1990, has now become a human rights landmark by reaching near universal ratification in record time. As of 2001, it has been ratified by 191 out of 193 nation states (Somalia, which at that time had no government, and the US, which has signed but yet to ratify the CRC are the exceptions). In its preamble and 54 articles, the CRC provides a comprehensive paradigm for supporting the totality of children's healthy development, drawing on the support of governments and non-governmental organizations alike, and is revolutionary in promoting children's participation in reaching minimum standards of care and protection including standards of health care, education, and child protection. The CRC for the first time recognizes the child as a full human being with his or her own unique identity, distinct from that of their parents and community. The CRC follows in the footsteps of the Universal Declaration of Human Rights, the Covenants on Civil and Political Rights and Economic, Social, and Cultural Rights. It establishes social and economic rights for children -the right to survival and early development, education, health care and social assistance. It also covers civil and political rights. These include the right of a child to a name and a nationality, to freedom of expression, to participation in decisions affecting his or her well-being, and to protection from discrimination on the grounds of race, gender, or minority status, as well as protection from sexual and other forms of abuse and exploitation.

Countries ratifying the CRC must submit periodic reports to a committee of ten experts making up the UN Committee on the Rights of the Child. In these reports, governments must report on the steps taken to change national laws and formulate policies and programs supporting children's rights. UNICEF and non-governmental organizations play an important role in helping the Committee assess the accuracy and completeness of country reports through the submission of alternative reports and supplementary information. Article 24 of the Convention is devoted to the health rights of the child. It builds on and develops the right to life, survival, and development as set out in Article 6.

The key provisions of Article 24 reflect a broad based definition of health with the overall goal of reducing infant and child mortality through "the enjoyment of the highest attainable standard of health."

Specific actions are also laid out to address health promotion and prevention through the principles of primary health care, specifically by combining health knowledge with social action on specific goals (i.e., basic knowledge of child health and nutrition, promoting breast feeding, hygiene, and environmental sanitation). Article 24 also targets the right of the child to protection from traditional practices prejudicial to the health of the child. Finally, Article 24 encourages countries to undertake international cooperation in promoting children' health, especially in developing countries. Other articles in the CRC that complement Article 24 are: Article 2 (non-discrimination); Article 23 (rights of a child with a disability); Articles 26 (the right to social assistance) and 27 (right to an adequate standard of living); and Articles 28 (right to education) and 29 (the aims of education). Article 24 thus holistically links the promotion of child health to equity and the role of the state in ensuring social support and assistance. It also suggests a close relationship between a child's health and "the development of the child's personality, talents and mental and physical abilities to their full potential" (Article 29.1.a).

The Committee on the Rights of the Child places significant emphasis on Article 24 in country reports. State parties are requested to provide information including: the status and indicators of children's health (i.e., incidence of HIV/AIDS); current legislation and responsible agencies; distribution of services (i.e., rural/urban); persistent gaps and measures adopted to reduce existing disparities; prevalence of educational campaigns; as well as specific information on women and children's health.

While the reporting process has been constructive and has resulted in significant and important improvements for children's health, problems remain. Some countries have been surprisingly progressive in addressing the reporting guidelines on health. For example, Panama's initial report discussed the disproportionately high incidence of disease amongst indigenous children (Panama, Initial Report, paras. 153 and 155). Many countries, however, have missed their reporting deadlines, and implementing the CRC beyond ratification is still in its infancy.

One of the conceptual tensions being played out in the debate on international children's health is the discussion about "basic needs" and "basic services" and the rift between "human rights" specialists and "human development." Parker and Sepulveda (1995) rightly describe both philosophical approaches as "tilling the same land." The fundamental difference lies in the human development community emphasizing the need to position the technologies and services needed to provide "basic services" to satisfy the "basic needs" of the population. The human rights community instead focuses on identifying and developing legal instruments and the enforcement mechanisms needed to support human development activities (Parker and Sepulveda, 1995). Indeed, one of the aims of a rights approach is to build on the success of the technological advances of child health made during the last 20 years, for example immunization programs. This offers a much needed avenue for furthering the success of the Summit and goals in order to more effectively and ethically address issues of equity with regard to economic and social mobilization for all children irrespective of a child's gender, race or minority status, and age.

Promoting an Ecology of Children's Well-being: Combining Population Health and Children's Rights

The CRC can help strengthen the links between social policy and health policy when combined with a population health approach. This approach requires "that we consider why it is that some people are healthier than others, why these differences are systematically distributed across identifiable social characteristics, and how public expenditures ought to be deployed to maximize the health status of the general population" (Hayes, 1994, p. l). "Determinants of health" comprise a set of significant health factors that influence the health of children and adults. A growing body of research indicate key determinants for children's healthy development include factors such as: income and social status; social support and networks; education; employment and working conditions; social environments; physical environments; biological and genetic inheritance; health services; gender; and culture (Health Canada, 1997; Keating and Hertzman, 1999).

The synthesis of the CRC and population health has two positive outcomes. First, principles of population health targeting children grounded in research on determinants of children's health can help guide strategic implementation of children's rights. Second, a rights approach can provide an ethical and legal framework for health policy. Primary foundations from both perspectives include: 1) the key determinants of children's health—the social and economic environment, the physical environment, personal health practices, individual capacity and coping skills, and existing health services; and 2) the 4 "pillars" of the CRC (non-discrimination (CRC Article 2); best interests (CRC Article 3); life, survival, and development (CRC Article 6); and participation (CRC Article 12).

When combined they become a powerful advocacy model of an "ecology" for children's health. This "ecology" refers to the systems of support required by a child to develop to the maximum of his or her abilities. This notion builds on Uri Bonfenbrenner's theory of the social ecology of human development (1979, 1990). In this framework, Bronfenbrenner places the child at the centre of a series of socially nested systems. This begins with the *mesosystem,* or those people immediately in contact with the child (family, peers, teachers, other caretakers, etc.), and continues out to the *macrosystem* or wider society and socio-cultural norms and values of the child's social environment. The effective functioning of child rearing processes in the family and other child settings requires public policies and practices that provide place, time, stability, status, recognition, belief systems, customs, and actions in support of child-rearing activities not only on the parts of the parents, caregivers, teachers, and other professional personnel, but also relatives, friends, neighbours, co-workers, communities, and major economic, social, and political institutions of the entire society (Bronfenbrenner, 1990).

Bronfenbrenner's social ecology of child development proposes a theory for children's well-being that provides a common ground for both the comprehensive social ethic of a child rights approach, and the population approach to children's health determinants. This then becomes a framework for establishing an empirical and moral minimum for child-related development. While the specific issues affecting children in developing countries and in industrial nations may differ in character (e.g., maternal and child survival, and provision of basic services versus child abuse, injury, and teen pregnancy), such a framework provides a common ground for promoting a "first call" demanding children's rights and well-being be given precedence, especially in times of economic hardship. Research based on an ecology of children's rights would require an examination of areas where family, community, or socio-cultural support of the child is not functioning or under pressure from external forces (e.g., social breakdown due to rapid economic change) and where there is a lack of integrated child-focused policy at the local, national, or international level.

When examining gaps in the current global social ecology of children's healthy development some specific areas for research and program development emerge. Three areas are particularly important:

1) Better understanding of children and childhood

If health researchers and children's advocates are serious about children's well-being and child rights, greater attention needs to be focused on understanding children's lives and the ways in which childhood is constructed in various social settings. As Qvortrup (1993) explains, childhood is a framework for the organization and the location of the various social spaces in which children participate and through which they pass. Childhood is therefore a "permanent social category" (1993) that varies across time and cultural context. The CRC is itself a framework based on certain concepts of childhood promoting the right of a child to a quality of life during this time of a person's life. For example, the preamble to the CRC describes childhood as a human condition during which the individual is entitled to "special care and assistance." Furthermore, Article 1 defines childhood as every human being below the age of 18 years (the rights of the foetus are not specifically addressed in the Convention). Knutson (1997) eloquently describes the importance of better understanding the various social perspectives on childhood (including children's own perceptions of their lives). This is especially important in order to untangle the rhetoric of a "child saving" society based on uninformed and arbitrary notions of welfare, from a society whose social attitudes are more oriented towards notions of "children first" and a rights approach. Research building on the work of Qvortrup and others (Hardy, Qvortrup, Sgritta, and Wintersberger, 1990; Knutson, 1997; Qvortrup, 1993) is needed to better understand how social policy promoting children's health development is itself based on unacknowledged assumptions regarding the role of children in society and the value placed on childhood.

2) Deconstructing economic security and children's rights

In both the developing and developed world, great gains have been made in child survival. The greatest challenge in both contexts is to address the right to a healthy development for children falling between the cracks of current economic policy and service programming. In addressing the needs of economic equity for children, the CRC through the lens of Article 2, non-discrimination, provides guidelines for the equitable distribution of resources in two other articles. These are Article 4 (implementation of the CRC) targeting general measures of implementation, including appropriate legislative administrative measures, participation of civil society, and international cooperation; and Article 27 (child's right to an adequate standard of living) which identifies a standard of living adequate for physical, mental, spiritual, moral, and social development, parent's primary responsibilities, the state's duty to support the child and family relative to national conditions and means, nutrition and housing, and the child's rights to maintenance. Addressing issues of economic, social, and political discrimination of groups of children is critical to children's health. Population health research has shown that regions with large disparities in wealth between rich and poor also have large disparities in health status, and overall levels of health status for both rich and poor tend to be lower than regions with less severe disparities (Wilkinson, 1996; Lynch et al., 1997). Mothers and children from lower socio-economic groups are thus at higher risk than other sectors of the population to low birth weight, chronic health problems, and premature death (Avard, 1994; Provincial Health Officer, 1998). Children and youth who are marginalized from the wider civil society (e.g., children living in poverty, girls, street children, children who are sexually exploited, and children from certain ethnic minorities) are also more prone to injury and illness than other sectors of society with greater access to resources and information (Canadian Council on Social Development, 1996). Therefore, child protection strategies need to be better understood within the context of social and cultural marginalization and economic disparity.

3) Better understand the social and physical environmental factors affecting children

One of the key findings of research on the health determinants is that the social environment in which children live, from conception through early adulthood, has long lasting effects over their entire life course. Mustard and Frank (1991) point out that how children are cared for at an early age can influence their coping skills for the rest of their lives. Keating and Mustard (1993) and Keating and Hertzman (1999) similarly note the strong evidence of the relationship between development of competency and coping skills, the social context of everyday life, and individual health and well-being.

The focus on children's perceptions of their lives supports the growing literature on children's coping styles and resiliency (Fraser, 1997; Werner and Smith, 1992; Keating and Hertzman, 1999). An important question for policy makers and human service practitioners is 'what kind of intervention may help individuals overcome barriers to health development encountered in early life'? For example, high risk children who do well despite the odds typically have found at least one significant person who cares about them (parent, grandparent, other relative, or non-family mentor) in the community in which they live (Goulet, 1994; Werner and Smith, 1992). This kind of buffering notion is supported in the CRC's focus on respect and support for the rights of parents, the extended family, and the community in Article 5. Similarly, Article 18 supports the responsibilities of parents for children's well-being, with the best interests of the child being their primary concern. Article 18 also acknowledges the importance of day care as a buffering factor for children of working parents.

While the importance of the social environment is critical to a child's life, survival, and health development (Article 6), there is a growing realization that many children's psychosocial well-being is partially related to a sense of interconnectedness with their physical environment. This relationship, while difficult to prove quantitatively, is becoming more apparent in studies linking indigenous children's health to self identity in terms of a personal sense of connectedness with traditional indigenous lands and knowledge of their tribal language (ECOSOC, 1996; Pepper and Henry, 1992). In this regard, it is important to find ways of linking the various international treaties that speak to children's health and the environment. The most important of these treaties is the Rio Declaration on the Environment and Development (including Agenda 21) ratified in 1992. The Rio Declaration emphasizes the need to educate children on the need for sustainable development and care for the natural environment. Specifically, Principle 10 states: "Environmental issues are best handled with the concerns of all concerned citizens, at the relevant level". Principle 21 strengthens the role of youth in this process by stating "the creativity, ideals, and courage of the youth of the world should be mobilized to forge a global partnership in order to achieve sustainable development for all."

Hodgekin and Newell (1998) suggest a number of measures for implementing an ecology of children's rights to health. These include general measures of implementation and specific measures in implementing Article 24. With regard to general measures, responsible departments and agencies for children's health should be identified at all levels of government. Similarly, non-governmental agencies and civil society partners should be identified. Other general measures include: a review of the relevant legislation, policy, and practice; the adoption of a strategy to secure full implementation including rights-based indicators and relevant standards; making the implications of Article 24 widely known to adults and children; and development of appropriate training of all relevant human service professionals involved in children's health.

Specific measures associated with implementing Article 24 include: identifying the extent to which the state has implemented Article 24 to the maximum extent of available resources; promoting the participation and views of the child in decisions affecting him or her (e.g., planning and developing health care and decision making in relation to individual health treatment of the child); assessing the accessibility and quality of services for children with a disability, girls and other marginalized children; measuring success or failure in attaining the World Summit goals for health; and identifying the degree to which the state supports social and environmental health through health education, health promotion, and support to public health especially for parents and children.

These measurements provide a useful assessment tool for measuring state support for children's health that include perspectives of rights and population health. They also provide a starting place for moving from implementation of rights through ratification of the CRC setting goals and developing health strategies for children that build on global initiatives such as the World Summit and are supported by research on determinants of children's health. This success will be measured by the commitment of civil society to heed the growing knowledge on determinants linking healthy children's development to social equity and respect for the environment, while fostering a rights awareness that sees all children as full human beings with a right to full physical, mental, spiritual, moral and social development within the context of a healthy family, community, and culture.

REFERENCES

Avard, D. (1994). *Povery and child health.* Ottawa: Human Rights and Education Centre. Unpublished report.

Bronfenbrenner, U. (1979). *The ecology of human development: Experiments by nature and design.* Cambridge, MA: Harvard University Press.

Bronfenbrenner, U. (1990). Discovering what families do. In D. Blankenhorn, D. Bayme, and J.B. Elshtain (Eds.), *Rebuilding the nest: A new commitment to the American family* (pp. 27-38). Milwaukee, WI: Family Service America.

Canadian Council on Social Development (CCSD) (1996). *The progress of Canada's children 1996.* Ottawa: CCSD.

Economic and Social Council (ECOSOC) (1996). *Health and Indigenous peoples.* 11 June. Geneva: ECOSOC.

Fraser, M. (1997). *Risk and resilience in childhood: An ecological perspective.* Washington, DC: NASW Press.

Goulet, L. (1994). *The UN Convention on the Rights of the Child: Giving voice.* University of Victoria: Unpublished Curriculum.

Hayes, M. (1994). Introduction. In M. Hayes, L.T. Foster, and H.D. Foster (1994). *The determinants of population health: A critical assessment* (pp. 1-5). Victoria, BC: University of Victoria, Department of Geography, Western Geographical Series, Vol. 29.

Health Canada (1993). *A vision of health for children and youth in Canada*. Health Promotion Directorate, Government of Canada, Ottawa, Ontario.

Health Canada (1997). *Towards a common understanding: Clarifying the core concepts of population health*. A discussion paper. Ottawa: Government of Canada.

Hodgekin, R., and Newell, P. (1998). *Implementation handbook for the Convention on the Rights of the Child*. New York: UNICEF.

Keating, D., and Mustard, J.F. (1993). *Social economic factors and human development*. Ottawa: CCSD.

Keating, D., and Hertzman, C. (1999). *Developmental health and the wealth of nations*. New York: Guilford.

Knutson, E. (1997). *Children: Noble causes or worthy citizens*. Aldershot, UK: Arena.

Lynch, J.W., Kaplan, G.A., Pamuk, E.R., Cohen, R.D. Heck, K.E., Balfour, J.L., and Yen, I.H. (1998). Income inequality and mortality in metropolitan areas of the United States. *American Journal of Public Health*, 88(7), 1074-1080.

Marmot, M., and Wilkinson, R. (1999). *Social determinants of health*. Oxford: Oxford University Press.

Mustard, J.F., and Frank, J. (1991). *The determinants of health*. Toronto: Canadian Institute for Advanced Research, Publication 5.

Parker, D., and Sepulveda, C. (1995). Children's rights to survival and healthy development. In J. Himes (Ed.), *Implementing the Convention on the Rights of the Child: Resource mobilization in low-income countries*. The Hague: Matinus Nijhoff Publishers.

Pepper, F., and Henry, S. (1992). *An Indian perspective on self-esteem*. Vancouver, BC: Mowachat Education and Research Association.

Provincial Health Officer, BC (1998). *1997 Annual report on the heath of British Columbians*. Victoria, BC: Ministry of Health and Ministry Responsible for Seniors.

Qvortrup, I. (1993). *Childhood as a social phenomenon: Lessons from an international project*. Eurosocial reports, 47, Vienna: European Centre for Social Welfare Policy and Research.

Qvortrup, I., Bardy, M., Sgritta, G., and Wintersberger, H. (Eds.). *Childhood matters: Social theory, practice, and politics*. Aldershot, UK: Avebury.

United Nations Children's Fund (UNICEF) (1991). *The World Summit for Children: The World Declaration and Plan of Action*. New York: United Nations Children's Fund.

UNICEF (1995). *The state of the world's children 1995*. New York: UNICEF.

UNICEF (1996). *The state of the world's children 1996*. New York: UNICEF.

UNICEF (1998). *The state of the world's children 1998*. New York: UNICEF.

UNICEF (2000). *The state of the world's children 2000*. New York: UNICEF.

Werner, E., and Smith, R. (1992). *Overcoming the odds: High risk children from birth to adulthood*. Ithaca, NY: Cornell University Press.

Wilkinson, RG. (1996). Unhealthy societies:

Plate 2 Future possibilities ▶

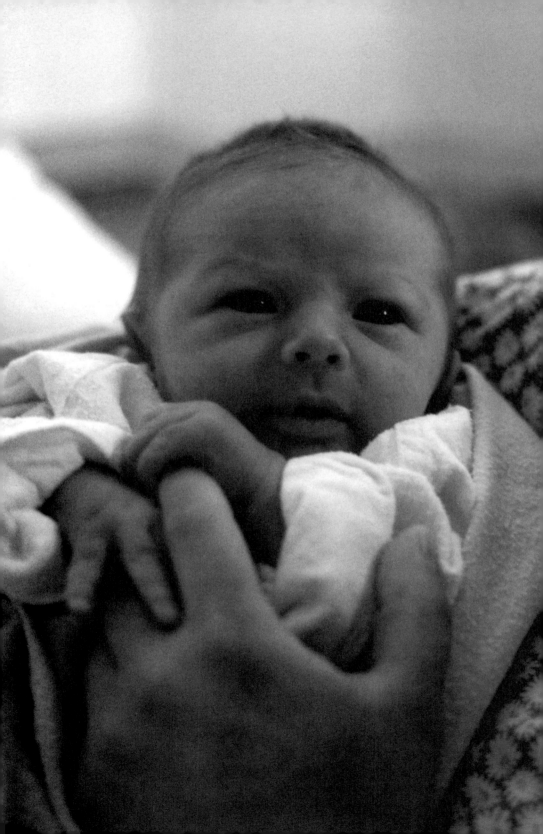

Contemporary Issues in Early Intervention

3

Michael J. Guralnick
University of Washington

INTRODUCTION

During the past few years there has been a remarkable surge of interest in providing early intervention services and supports to vulnerable children and their families. Political leaders are according high priority to early intervention, at least in rhetoric; research on early brain development has captured the attention of the public; and new information is emerging that can further improve the quality of existing early intervention practices. With regard to the latter issue, recent large-scale longitudinal studies as well as more focused investigations have provided new insights into the mechanisms through which early intervention produces its effects.

In so doing, more thorough and comprehensive models of development related to early intervention have evolved helping us understand "why" early intervention works and providing a basis for guiding the development and implementation of best practices. As will be seen, these advances are relevant to critical systems design issues including organizing child and family assessments, facilitating the process of individualizing and optimizing interventions, helping to set priorities, maximizing cost effectiveness, and evaluating outcomes.

The purpose of this chapter is to highlight recent conceptual and empirical advances related to the effectiveness of early intervention and to apply this information to best practice approaches.

To do so, a model linking early childhood development and early intervention will be presented and best practice information will be embedded within that framework. Where appropriate, consideration will be given to definable groups of children, particularly those at risk due to biological factors, those at risk due to environmental factors, and those children with established developmental disabilities.

FAMILY CENTRED PRACTICE AS A CORE PRINCIPLE

The concept of family-centred practice has emerged in recent years not simply as a best practice, but rather as a core principle in the field of early intervention. Developmental and ecological models that have been postulated over the years such as Belsky's (1994) parenting model, Sameroff's (1993) transactional model, Ramey's biosocial model (Ramey, Bryant, Wasik, Sparling, Fendt, and LaVange, 1992), Dunst's (1985) social support model, and Bronfenbrenner's (1979) ecological model are now seen as providing a basis for a common framework that has firmly established family-centred practice as a core principle in the field of early intervention (Guralnick, 1998).

The centrality of the family's influence on child development is now well understood and can be organized within three forms of Family Patterns of Interaction: (1) the quality of parent-child transactions; (2) family-orchestrated child experiences; and (3) health and safety provided by the family. The second and third columns of Figure 3.1 illustrate these straightforward connections between family patterns of interaction and child development.

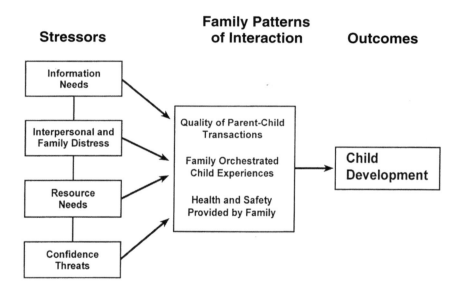

Figure 3.1   The relationships among potential stressors, family patterns of interaction, and child developmental outcomes for children at biological risk or those with established disabilities (Guralnick, 2000)

As far as the quality of parent-child transactions or, more generally, caregiver-child interactions is concerned, a number of important constructs have been identified that define this relationship. Prior and ongoing research has clearly revealed that the following relationship constructs correlate, both independently and jointly, with children's developing intellectual and social competence (Baumrind, 1993; Clarke-Stewart, 1988; Hart and Risley, 1995; Wachs, 1992):

- respond contingently;
- be sensitive to child developmental levels and patterns;
- create effectively warm social exchanges;
- remain non-intrusive;
- appropriately structure and scaffold the environment; and
- be discourse-based.

Importantly, each of these relationship constructs have well developed, research-based systems of measurement, and some have been incorporated into assessment instruments that are of clinical value (Elardo, Bradley, and Caldwell, 1977).

The second family pattern of interaction is equally important as it represents the myriad of activities that parents orchestrate and organize for their children that can substantially influence child development. Given the dependent nature of young children, it is unquestionably the family's role to orchestrate a range of intellectual and social experiences for their child. These experiences include deciding upon and selecting day care, providing developmentally appropriate toys and materials in the home, arranging for non-day care or nursery school experiences with peers, and seeking out and organizing activities that are responsive to their child's special interests or special needs. Although not as well developed as the relationship constructs for the quality of parent-child transactions, evidence continues to mount that these family-orchestrated child experiences can have a substantial impact on child developmental outcomes (NICHD Early Child Care Research Network, 1999; Ladd, Profilet, and Hart, 1992). This is particularly the case for vulnerable children.

Finally, families, of course, have an essential obligation to provide for the child's health and safety. Ensuring proper immunizations, providing adequate nutrition, minimizing environmental toxins, and protecting the child from neglectful or violent environments are all aspects of family patterns of interaction that govern child outcomes (Gorman, 1995; Osofsky, 1995; Taylor, Zuckerman, Harik, and Groves, 1994). Although parents may have limited control over some of these factors, they nevertheless must be considered a critical dimension of family influences on child development and therefore as a consideration in developing a comprehensive early intervention program.

STRESSORS: CHILDREN AT BIOLOGICAL RISK AND WITH ESTABLISHED DISABILITIES

In the general population, threats to the three family patterns of interaction are usually minimal. Even if a threat does arise in one area, the more optimal nature of the other dimensions of family patterns of interaction can serve as buffers and therefore not compromise a child's development. However, when a number of family patterns of interaction appear to be non-optimal, the collective evidence suggests that children's cognitive and social competence will be compromised. The prospect of this occurring increases substantially for a child at significant biological risk, and is of special concern for a child with an established disability. From the very outset, a series of *stressors* are created which threaten the quality of all three major family patterns of interaction (see left-hand column of Figure 3.1).

Information Needs

Four categories of stressors are well documented for children at biological risk or those with established developmental disabilities. First, information needs are created and perhaps constitute the most pervasive and persistent set of stressors for families (Mahoney and Filer, 1996). Early on, issues of highly technical medical procedures that can influence their child's future development arise (Meyer, Garcia Coll, Seifer, Ramos, Kilis, and Oh, 1995) and the active pursuit of a diagnosis or an explanation for their child's developmental problems are driving forces (Holm and Dinno, in press). Indeed, failure to resolve the diagnostic issue can be a disruptive force for subsequent family interaction patterns (Marvin and Pianta, 1996). As development proceeds, literally hundreds of studies have documented the unexpected and often challenging developmental patterns parents must confront that make it far more difficult to provide optimal family patterns of interaction. For example, particularly for children with established disabilities, parents face unusual problems in forming attachments with their child, establishing joint attention, recognizing the meaning of their child's frequently ambiguous social cues, and appropriately adapting their language to their child's cognitive and linguistic levels (Guralnick and Bricker, 1987; Cicchetti and Beeghly, 1990; Shonkoff, Hauser-Cram, Krauss, and Upshur, 1992). At each new developmental period new issues arise challenging parents and requiring information that can help support them in their parenting role. Relatedly, as parents begin to focus on therapeutic services, inevitable questions arise with respect to the effectiveness of specific services, gaining access to those services, and finding programs and clinicians with which parents are most comfortable (Sontag and Schacht, 1994).

It is this stressor—this information need—that requires that an effective service system have available an array of knowledgeable specialists. This is not an easy task given parents' diverse responses to these challenges. Most parents exhibit a reasonable degree of motivation and actually seek out answers, while others are reluctant to do so because of stressors related to environmental factors (see below), or due to their own reticence. Still others may not be aware of the non-optimal family patterns of interaction created by a child's disability or biological risk. A service system that is sensitive to this diversity, yet one that is proactive and vigorous in its provision of information, is essential. The challenge is to both assess the level of the information needs of caregivers at the proper developmental periods and have a responsive system available.

Interpersonal and Family Distress

The second stressor captures the interpersonal and family distress that often arises as a consequence of a child's biological risk or disability. The range of reaction for families is quite extensive, but at minimum it demands reassessment of family expectations and numerous adjustments that together constitute a major challenge for most families (Gallimore, Coots, Weisner, Garnier, and Guthrie, 1996; Gallimore, Keogh, and Bernheimer, 1999). Clearly, parent distress and threats to family harmony appear at various points during the early childhood years (Beckman and Pokorni, 1988; Hodapp, Dykens, Evans, and Merighi, 1992; Roach, Orsmond, and Barratt, 1999; Wikler, 1986). Such threats to family harmony, especially early on, can be especially damaging to a child's emerging adaptive and particularly social competence (Hauser-Cram, Warfield, Shonkoff, Krauss, Upshur, and Sayer, 1999). Compounding these issues is the increased stress associated with sometimes self-imposed social isolation and associated "shared stigma" that too easily occurs despite substantial improvements in societal attitudes towards individuals with disabilities (Bailey, Jr. and Winton, 1989; Goffman, 1963; Guralnick, 1999b; Stoneman, 1993). Evidence from social network research (Emery and Kitzmann, 1995) clearly suggests the potential for stressors related to interpersonal and family distress to adversely influence family patterns of interaction, especially family-orchestrated child experiences. Accordingly, this indicates that a system sensitive to these stressors and their varying appearance at different points during the early childhood years, integrated with a service and support network that can mitigate as many stressors as possible, should be an essential component of any comprehensive early intervention system.

Resource Needs

Families frequently report that substantial additional resources are needed to meet the needs of a child with a disability or one at biological risk, a circumstance that defines the third category of stressor—resource needs. Adjustments to routines noted earlier create increased and often unwelcome demands on all family members (Bristol, 1987; Gallimore et al., 1996; Dyson, 1993). Trying to organize and coordinate the array of services likely to be needed by their child serves to further heighten stress, particularly for those who are most conscientious (Rubin and Quinn-Curran, 1985). Many parents sense as well that they must set into motion a support system for their child and other family members that will be both least disruptive and maximize their vulnerable child's development.

Moreover, despite the availability of many publicly supported services for early intervention, financial burdens related to the health of their child, the need for respite care, and providing additional therapies can increase substantially (Birenbaum, Guyot, and Cohen, 1990). Furthermore, many mothers of children with disabilities choose to return to work later than mothers of typically developing children, thereby creating additional financial stress (Booth and Kelly, 1999; Thyen, Kuhlthau, and Perrin, 1999).

Of importance, stressors related to resource needs can be quite subtle and difficult to assess—particularly disturbances that occur in family routines. Nevertheless, a service system sensitive to this important issue and that can provide the necessary resource supports for families can help prevent disruptions in family patterns of interaction.

Confidence Threats

Finally, as suggested in Figure 3.1, this entire set of stressors can serve to threaten the very core of parental confidence in their ability to appropriately parent their child. The existence of information needs, the presence of interpersonal and family distress, and the need for additional resources can easily create a situation in which the parenting role is displaced by specialist advice and service system activities. It is with respect to this stressor—a growing lack of confidence and sense of competence in relation to the parenting role—that early intervention systems must be designed to truly establish a partnership with parents. Avoiding dependency is certainly one goal. However, developing respectful relationships and organizing a supportive system of services to literally empower families to ensure they retain control and decision-making, is a goal with far reaching consequences.

SHORT-TERM EFFECTIVENESS OF EARLY INTERVENTION: BIOLOGICAL RISK AND ESTABLISH DISABILITY

Accordingly, the model described above suggests that less than optimal developmental outcomes will result for children at biological risk and those with established disabilities as a consequence of the four categories of stressors. Available evidence does indeed suggest that, at least for cognitive development, in the absence of early intervention children at biological risk and those with established disabilities generally experience a decline over the first 5 years of life (Liaw and Brooks-Gunn, 1993; Guralnick, 1988; Guralnick, 1998; Guralnick and Bricker, 1987; Infant Health and Development Program, 1990; Rauh, Achenbach, Nurcombe, Howell, and Teti, 1988).

The primary mechanisms for the delays in development appear to be perturbations in one or more of the three family interaction patterns that govern child development (Guralnick, 1998).

It is equally clear that comprehensive early intervention programs exhibiting state-of-the art practices can prevent these declines in intellectual development. Numerous studies have now documented that effect sizes of 0.50 to 0.75 SDs are common and are of considerable clinical significance

(Berry, Gunn, and Andrews, 1984; Blair and Ramey, 1997; Infant Health and Development Program, 1990; Rauh et al., 1988; Guralnick, 1998). Although the development of children with disabilities remains well below that of their typically developing counterparts, these effects of comprehensive early intervention programs are extremely important and easily replicable. In contrast, the preventive-type interventions for children at biological risk have the potential to completely prevent delays for major groups of children. As discussed shortly, the components of these successful interventions are highly compatible with the conceptual framework presented in this chapter. However, it must be emphasized that these effects are observed while intervention is being provided or shortly thereafter. A subsequent discussion will address long-term effects.

BEST PRACTICE PRINCIPLES

With this background, and anticipating subsequent discussions of children at environmental risk, it is now possible to put forward an overarching set of Best Practice Principles that can serve as a developmental framework for the design of a system of supports and services in early intervention.

- A developmental model linking family patterns of interaction and child developmental outcomes is an appropriate framework for *all* children.
- A family-centred approach constitutes a core principle of early childhood development and early intervention.
- Stressors due to a child's disability or risk status can adversely affect family interaction patterns and, consequently, child development.
- A comprehensive assessment of potential stressors must be included in the design of an early intervention system

The next step is to go beyond these principles and see how they translate to specific components of best practice that are carried out on a day-to-day level.

BEST PRACTICE COMPONENTS

Based on the four best practice principles, it would be expected that best practice components would constitute a system of supports and services that are responsive to the stressors identified above. Indeed when an analysis of the components of the comprehensive and effective early intervention programs reported in the literature is carried out, that is exactly what appears to be the case (Guralnick, 1997b; Guralnick, 1998).

As indicated in Figure 3.2, it is suggested that comprehensive and effective early intervention programs are organized within three components that are

uniquely suited to respond appropriately to stressors. These components are
the provision of: (1) resource supports; (2) social supports; and (3) information
and services. Within each of these major components, specific services and
supports can be identified which, taken together, constitute the key features of
best practices.

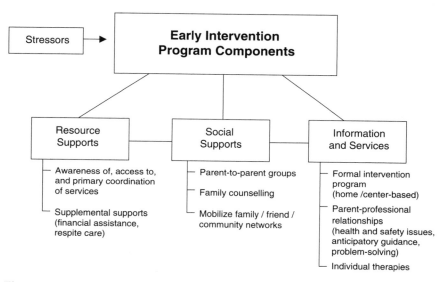

Figure 3.2   Components of early intervention programs as a response to
stressors (Guralnick, 1997b, p. 9)

Resource Supports

In many respects, resource supports collectively functions as a unifying component of an early intervention program. It serves as a central mechanism that
informs families about service availability and how to gain access, and facilitates the coordination of services. The intent of this component is to go beyond
the practice of service coordination or case management and to seek the complete integration of services and supports.

The notion of the "whole child" and a developmental perspective must be
established at the earliest point of contact with the family. Although the practice of coordinating the activities of discipline specialists and services is important, children and families appear to be best served when a true *integration*
exists. This best practice of integration occurs at four levels. First, integration
of relevant disciplines must occur at the level of early identification in conjunction with corresponding assessments to establish eligibility for services and to
obtain a general profile of child and family functioning. A process for interdisciplinary assessment that can achieve a high level of integration has been well

developed, and a set of principles guiding interdisciplinary team assessments articulated (Guralnick, in press-c). The second level of integration occurs at the stage when individualized child and family plans are developed following an initial assessment of potential stressors. The intensity and form of any formal intervention program would be addressed here. Maintaining a focus on the integration of services and supports is critical at this stage, as the involvement of numerous agencies and disciplines is needed in many instances. Care must be taken to maintain a focus on all stressors related to family interaction patterns, not only those that can be addressed as part of a formal intervention program (for example, centre-based activities). Principles and processes to achieve this level of integration have been identified elsewhere (Bruder and Bologna, 1993).

The third level of integration is a more recent phenomenon and focuses on the models of service integration that occur when specialists from different disciplines interact with one another, usually in the context of the formal intervention program.

Termed "integrated therapy," strong rationales and thoughtful models are now available that suggest that *collaborative consultation* is a best practice approach, one that maximizes the integration of discipline specific services through naturalistic activity routines both at the formal intervention program level (McWilliam, 1996a) and in other environments. There remain many practical and professional problems to solve before integrated therapy models become common practice. However, a strong conceptual rationale, including that consistent with inclusion (see later discussion), can be established along with the limited empirical data available (McWilliam, 1996b) which fails to indicate any adverse effects of this approach on child outcomes in comparison to more traditional non-integrated models of services.

The fourth and final level of integration occurs at the level of the system itself. To fully achieve integration at the three levels discussed, an integrated system governing the various agencies and professionals involved must be in place (Bruder, 1996; Bruder and Bologna, 1993). In some instances, this may require an entire restructuring of the multiple systems of supports and service. In other cases, communities can accomplish the same ends through collaborative agreements. Barriers to this level of integration are substantial, including administrative and financial concerns, legal issues, differing professional philosophies, and efforts to maintain a clear discipline identity. Nevertheless, the information available indicates that integration at all levels is best practice in early intervention.

Supplemental supports such as obtaining financial assistance where appropriate, helping to identify respite care agencies or personnel, and recommending appropriate day care options are also key elements of the component of resource supports. Together, these resource supports provide the essential foundation for the remaining two components: social supports and information and services.

Social Supports

As noted earlier, one of the most insidious effects on families of adapting to a child with a disability in particular is the impact on interpersonal and family distress. Because isolation and distress can be so debilitating, virtually all three family interaction patterns can be severely affected. This fact has been recognized by the spontaneous growth of numerous parent-to-parent groups that have gradually become critical aspects of the social support component of early intervention programs (Santelli, Turnbull, Marquis, and Lerner, 1995). The functions of these parent-to-parent groups are diverse, including providing emotional backing and helping to build a network of natural supports for families (Cooley, 1994). Moreover, parent-to-parent groups are an excellent source of information about most matters including the credibility of professionals, emerging therapies, and parental rights. Connecting with families whose children have already been through early childhood/early intervention systems provides a vital perspective for families new to the issues. Finally, should the interpersonal distress prove to be overwhelming, referrals by the early intervention program for family counselling may be needed.

Information and Services

The third and final component of the early intervention system is the complex array of information and services available to families. The formal early intervention program provided by most communities in the form of home and/or centre-based activities is the most visible and the most expensive part of the system. It is here that individualized plans are developed and interventions implemented based on the assessments that have occurred earlier. Moreover, it is in this context that parents are provided with information and strategies to ensure parent-child transactions that best match the skills and abilities of their child. These "parent education" activities (Mahoney et al., 1999) must be carried out in a balanced manner, maintaining the essence of the parent-professional partnership. This is particularly important because the formal intervention aspect often contains most of the child-focused features of the early intervention program supported by specific curricula (Bailey Jr., 1997; Bruder, 1997). Discipline specialists generally participate as well. The danger is that by immersing the child in formal curricula, the larger aspects of family-centred practice can be lost. Indeed, there exists a tendency of qualified, earnest, and caring professionals to lose sight of this larger picture and to focus almost exclusively on child-centred activities (McBride and Peterson, 1997).

The issue of the intensity of the services and supports needed generally arises in the context of the formal intervention program. Surprisingly, research has indicated that program intensity for children with disabilities, particularly measured in terms of service hours, is quite low averaging around 7 hours per month (Shonkoff et al., 1992). The intensity increases as children move into the preschool years, but generally remains at modest levels. Equally surprising, however, is the range of service intensity. At the extreme, services for both children at biological risk and those with established disabilities have been provided for more than 40 hours per week for a period of 2 to 3 years (Infant Health and Development Program, 1990; Lovaas, 1987).

In fact, service intensity is one of the most contentious issues in the early intervention field today. The costs for highly intensive services can be extraordinary, as can the burdens on the children and families who participate. Questions such as how much speech or physical therapy is adequate, how many home visits are needed to support a particular family, or whether a 40 hour per week program for a child recently identified with autism is warranted confront early interventionists and families on a regular basis. Indeed, intensity is also related to expectations for long-term benefits and will be discussed in a subsequent section of this chapter.

To help with decisions about intensity as well as the type of intervention to provide, more and more early intervention systems are relying on "evidence-based" approaches (Kennell, 1999). By carefully analysing available scientific research on the effectiveness of specific interventions, evidence-based guidelines are now being developed for specific populations of children. Recommendations are put forward based on the supporting evidence in a format accessible to administrators, practitioners, and families (New York State Department of Health, undated). It must be recognized that even with these guidelines, considerable uncertainty remains as research can be contradictory and incomplete. Nor do evidence-based recommendations address the issue of whether the gains expected from a particular intensity or type of intervention justify the expense. Nevertheless, research linking specific child and family characteristics and early intervention program features is now being conducted that addresses these concerns and is part of a shift toward "second generation" research in the field of early intervention (Guralnick, 1993; Guralnick, 1997a). Consequently, an evidence-based approach constitutes a major advance in the field of early intervention and must be considered as best practice.

The formal intervention program is often the focal point for many of the components of the longer early intervention program. It is a continuous source of information and connections to other support systems, and is a "place" that families recognize. At the same time, however, parents build other parent-professional relationships, such as with their primary care physician or health specialist, and seek out other conventional and unconventional therapies for their child that go beyond the formal intervention program (Shonkoff et al., 1992). These relationships provide useful sources of information and help families to grapple with health and safety issues and to anticipate and solve child-related problems that may arise in specific developmental domains. The availability of quality professionals to supplement the formal aspects of early intervention is important to many families and must be coordinated as part of the more comprehensive early intervention program.

It is important to recognize that the nature and extent of participation of children as part of the formal intervention system is a decision made by the families themselves; that is, it is a family-orchestrated child experience (see Figure 3.1). Families may press for more or less service, and they vary substantially in terms of their motivation to actively participate at all. This is especially true for aspects of the program that focus on family rather than child issues. Sometimes family participation in specific components can be increased by addressing family concerns such as locating high quality day care. However, many families may view going beyond a child focus as an intrusion on their privacy.

To be sure, care must be taken by professionals to respect these views. Yet it is also important that professionals express their positions and their rationales for recommendations. A meaningful partnership between families and professionals will require a continuous process of negotiation, taking into consideration the differing priorities, values, and perspectives of all concerned (Bailey, 1987; Duwa, Wells, and Lalinde, 1993). Again, however, final decisions rest with the families.

Taken together, a well-designed and coordinated set of early intervention components organized within the framework presented in Figure 3.1, in which family-centredness is a core principle, may well be able to minimize stressors, including threats to a families' perceptions of their ability to carry out their parenting roles effectively. By providing the network of ongoing services and supports that consider all three major early intervention components (resource supporter/social supporter/information and services), the confidence of families will likely continue to increase.

FAMILY CHARACTERISTICS: POTENTIAL SOURCE OF ENVIRONMENTAL STRESSORS

To this point, it has been assumed that families would normally be capable of providing optimal patterns of interaction with their children, but that stressors associated with a child with a disability or one at biological risk create perturbations in these patterns. However there are, of course, many *family characteristics* that can perturb the three family patterns of interaction even in the absence of stressors caused by a child's biological risk or disability status. These include personal characteristics of the parents, such as inappropriate beliefs and attitudes related to child rearing, usually transmitted through the generations (Murphey, 1992). Other family characteristics of major significance are maternal mental health difficulties, especially depression (Cicchetti and Toth, 1992; Heneghan, Silver, Bauman, Westbrook, and Stein, 1998), limited parental intellectual abilities (Feldman, 1997), and parents who are substance abusers (Olsen and Burgess, 1997). The nature of the relationships among family members matters as well. The absence of adequate social support networks (Melson,

Ladd, and Hsu, 1993) and difficult marital relationships (Emery and Kitzmann, 1995) are important. Of course, chronic poverty creates a circumstance that can negatively influence virtually all relationships and interaction patterns (Duncan, Brooks-Gunn, and Klebanov, 1994). Finally, child characteristics such as a difficult temperament (here, unrelated to a child's biological risk or disability) can also perturb family patterns of interaction (Sameroff, 1993).

As suggested in Figure 3.3, just as in the case of stressors related to a child's biological risk or disability, these adverse family characteristics constitute stressors and operate by affecting one or more of the three family patterns of interaction. Ample evidence is available to indicate that, when this occurs, children's cognitive and social competence are compromised. Similar to children at biological risk or those with established disabilities, in the absence of intervention to address these adverse family characteristics, a gradual decline in development occurs over the course of the first few years of life (Bryant and Maxwell, 1997; Ramey and Campbell, 1984).

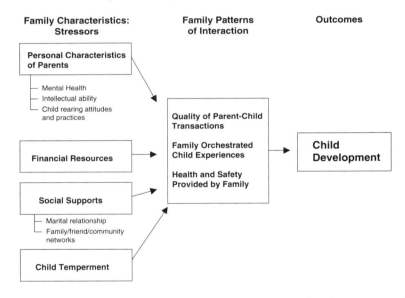

Figure 3.3 The relationship among potential stressors, family patterns of interaction, and child developmental outcomes for children at environmental risk

These non-optimal family characteristics which function as stressors are similar to a cluster of dimensions normally referred to as "environmental risk" factors. Research has clearly indicated that the cumulative number of risk factors, rather than any single or small number of risk factors, is associated with adverse developmental outcomes (Sameroff, Seifer, Barocas, Zax, and Greenspan, 1987; Keating and Hertzman, 1999). The cumulative risk model is understandable in relation to Figure 3.3, as a larger number of stressors is likely to create more of a negative impact on family interaction patterns and, therefore, child development. Similarly, so-called doubly vulnerable children, (that is, those at both environmental and biological risk or those with established disabilities also at environmental risk) would be expected to fare most poorly, as stressors from both sources combine to perturb the same three family interaction patterns. Indeed, data are available to indicate that children at both environmental and biological risk suffer a far greater developmental lag than children without such double vulnerabilities, and that it is difficult to find any factors that would protect them from experiencing substantial developmental delays and related problems in the absence of intervention (Bradley, Whiteside, Mudfrom, Casey, Kelleher, and Pope, 1994).

The fact that family characteristics and stressors created by a child's biological risk or disability interact with one another at the level of family patterns of interaction also suggests the potential protective nature of non-stressor forms (non-risk) of family characteristics. Indeed, available evidence indicates that low environmental risk families can mitigate many of the stressors confronting families of children at biological risk and those with established disabilities (Bradley, Rock, Whiteside, Caldwell, and Brisby, 1991; Dunst, Trivette, and Cross, 1986). This would suggest that only modest interventions may be needed for families who can mitigate stressors through their own strengths to ensure a favourable outcome for their child. Research focusing on children at biological risk suggests that this is indeed the case (Blair, Ramey, and Hardin, 1995; Brooks-Gunn, Gross, Kraemer, Spiker, and Shapiro, 1992; Rauh et al., 1988). Consequently, and as discussed shortly, even for children at biological risk or those with established disabilities, a careful assessment of stressors associated with family characteristics has important implications for both the type and intensity of the intervention program.

SHORT-TERM EFFECTIVENESS OF PREVENTIVE INTERVENTIONS: ENVIRONMENTAL STRESSORS

How, then, is it possible to minimize the declines in cognitive and social competence that are due to non-optimal family characteristics? It appears that the same early intervention program components described earlier are applicable (see Figure 3.2), although the nature of the stressors and, therefore, the profile of program components would differ accordingly. In a real sense, components are best characterized as *preventive interventions*. As Sameroff et al. (1987) have clearly pointed out, the fact is that, at least over a reasonable period of time, some stressors associated with family characteristics are highly resistant to change. Affecting a parent's mental health or addressing marital conflicts, for example, pose unusual challenges for any early intervention system. Nevertheless, as will be seen, much can be accomplished.

Stressors associated with limited resources that result in health and safety concerns can be addressed in a variety of ways by providing supplemental nutrition, arranging for visits by public health services, and through other forms of public assistance. As might be expected, however, the quality of parent-child transactions is difficult to alter due to the chronic and highly personal nature of the stressors that influence this family pattern of interaction. Home visiting, family support, and parent education programs carried out by well-trained and highly qualified providers have not, for the most part, been able to overcome these stressors to alter parent-child transactions and, consequently, child development (Behrman, 1993; Guralnick, in press-a; Scarr and McCartney, 1988; Wasik, Ramey, Bryant, and Sparling, 1990).

Perhaps the intensity of these programs is inadequate. Yet, even with substantial variations in intensity and approach, the field has not yet produced consistent evidence that programs of this type can independently influence the quality of parent-child transactions for families at high environmental risk (Black, Dubowitz, Hutcheson, Berenson-Howard, and Starr, 1995; Burchinal, Campbell, Bryant, Wasik, and Ramey, 1997).

In contrast, considerable success in fostering child development has been achieved when interventionists have been able to alter the patterns of family-orchestrated child experience by having families agree to place their child in intervention-oriented child care (Bryant and Maxwell, 1997; Ramey et al., 1992). Although the decline in cognitive development in particular is not completely eliminated through these formal intervention programs, the effect sizes are of a similar order of magnitude as those found for children at biological risk and those with established disabilities (approximately 0.50 to 0.75 SDs).

These effective programs are clearly child-focused and are of considerable intensity. What appears to happen is that through the efforts of trained professionals on a daily basis working within the framework of a developmentally oriented but clearly structured curriculum, more advanced child development and more engaging positive child characteristics result (specifically, more responsiveness to adults and greater task orientation). These advances are directly correlated with the intensity of child-focused activities (Ramey et al., 1992; Sparling, Lewis, Ramey, Wasik, Bryant, and LaVange, 1991). In turn, these child characteristics appear to elicit more positive responses from parents and teachers (Burchinal et al., 1997). Accordingly, strong consideration should be given to intervention-oriented day care programs for children at risk due to environmental factors—particularly those at extremely high risk.

SUMMARY OF BEST PRACTICE COMPONENTS

Based on the conceptual model and related evidence presented to this point, a number of best practices specific to the early intervention program components can be identified and serve to supplement the best practice principles discussed earlier. These are as follows.

- Systems must be comprehensive and flexible, addressing the three early intervention program components of resource supports, social supports, and information and services.

- For each of the program components, interventions must be carefully individualized based on assessments of stressors.

- Family characteristics should be evaluated to determine potential stressors or protective factors, to evaluate the possibility of double vulnerability, as well as to assist in selecting an intervention approach.

- Program intensity, curriculum approaches, and specific therapeutic procedures must be evidence-based.

- Integration of services and supports must occur at all levels.

RELATED BEST PRACTICE DOMAINS

A number of important best practice domains extend beyond the best practice principles and best practice components identified above and also must be considered in the development of a comprehensive early intervention system. Each of these best practice domains influences the nature of specific interventions or serves as a guide for larger scale systems factors.

LONG-TERM EFFECTIVENESS

Early intervention is certainly not believed by most to constitute an inoculation against future threats to child development, but the expectation nevertheless exists that long-term gains will result. Unfortunately, however, there have been many disappointments when children demonstrating positive short-term effects of early intervention have been followed over time, as most positive effects simply dissipate (Barnett, 1995; Brooks-Gunn et al., 1994; Gibson and Harris, 1988; McCarton et al., 1997). Despite these disappointments, further research and analyses have revealed that long-term effects can in fact be achieved for many groups of children, but that attention must be given to issues of *intensity* and *specificity* (Guralnick, 1993; Guralnick, 1997b; Guralnick, 1998).

As noted earlier, intensity is a complex and controversial issue. Changes in the intensity of early intervention services and supports can be achieved by varying the same types of services within a specific time period, altering their comprehensiveness (for example, add a parent education dimension to a child-focused component), or changing the duration of the intervention (for example, increase the number of years of the program). Specificity refers to the characteristics of families (that is, the nature and extent of environmental stressors) and to child characteristics (the type and severity of risk or disability).

Together, as the research described next indicates, these family and child characteristics can serve as a useful framework for determining both the form and intensity of interventions likely to yield long-term effects.

For children at biological risk but with minor environmental stressors, programs of only low intensity in the first year of life are needed in order to produce substantial long-term benefits (Achenbach, Howell, Aoki, and Rauh, 1993; Als, Lawhon, Duffy, McAnulty, Gibes-Grossman, and Blickman, 1994). Once the stressors associated with a child's biological risk are addressed, families are able to move forward and maintain an effective set of family interaction patterns. However, periodic monitoring should continue for these high-risk children.

In contrast, to achieve long-term effects for children at risk due to family characteristics (high environmental risk), far more intensive programs are needed. In particular, long-term success has only been achieved when interventions have been unusually intensive (participation on a daily basis), such that the child is engaged at a high rate by the program's activities and that the program extends for the first 5 years of the child's life (Campbell and Ramey, 1994; Burchinal et al., 1997). As noted earlier, most of the effects of these interventions have been attributed to participation in intervention-oriented day care (Burchinal et al., 1997). Whether or not intervention is needed all 5 years is unclear, but programs that fail to extend beyond the first 3 years have produced primarily short-term effects for children (Guralnick, 1998). Of note, these empirical findings can be understood with the model presented in this chapter, as stressors for high environmental risk families are likely to persist or at least reoccur throughout the entire early childhood period.

These stressors, even at child ages 4 and 5 years, are certainly likely to adversely affect family patterns of interaction and lead to poorer developmental outcomes (Guralnick, in press-a). Intervention-oriented day care functions as a protective factor, particularly in connection with child responsiveness and task orientation.

Circumstances that can produce long-term outcomes for children with established disabilities are more uncertain, however. The remarkable heterogeneity of the population in conjunction with co-occurring environmental risk factors has made this research difficult to conduct. Nevertheless, some important evidence is available within the specificity/intensity framework. For children with autism, highly intensive interventions appear to produce unusually positive long-term effects, at least for a subgroup of that population (McEachin, Smith, and Lovaas, 1993). Replication of these findings is desperately needed, as is a more careful definition of children in the studies. As that occurs, specificity will increase further as subgroups emerge that can be linked to different forms and intensities of early intervention program components. In the next decade, this second generation research should begin to generate valuable information for interventionists (Guralnick, 1997a).

Only limited information is available for children from other etiologic subgroups, as no controlled longitudinal studies have been carried out. However, the developmental knowledge base, particularly the stressors, for children with Down Syndrome is most complete (Guralnick and Bricker, 1987; Guralnick, 1996; Guralnick, 1999a; Spiker and Hopmann, 1997). It indicates that substantial information is needed by families of children with Down Syndrome at various developmental periods across the child's first 5 years of life to address a range of issues—particularly those related to expressive language development, health concerns, and peer relationships. Developmental information patterns regarding other etiological subgroups as well as children with general (unspecified) developmental delays is also available (Gallimore et al., 1999). Consequently, long-term benefits are more likely to result through a program of continuous support through the early childhood period but varying in accordance with the waxing and waning of individual stressors. At the same time, however, no evidence suggests that a level of intensity similar to that often provided to children with autism will have additional short- or long-term benefits compared to more conventional, less intensiveprograms. In this case, intensity should be guided by the magnitude of stressors facing individual children and families.

INCLUSION

Within the past few years, efforts have continued to provide supports and services in natural environments and to maximize the participation of children with disabilities with typically developing children in virtually all service and community activities. Inclusion as a value system, philosophy, service model, and legal right is gradually becoming an accepted principle and practice (Guralnick, in press-b). Indeed the development and evaluation of inclusive practices has received considerable attention by researchers and program developers. As described below, evidence continues to mount suggesting that inclusive practices are best practices.

Evaluations of inclusive programs for young children with disabilities have revealed that they can be accomplished in a 'feasible' manner (Guralnick, in press-b). That is, the integrity of early childhood programs is maintained even when children with disabilities participate. Accommodations to children's developmental skills and abilities readily occur, and patterns of interactions with materials, peers, and adults are similar for all children given their developmental status, as is their level of engagement in activities (Kontos, Moore, and Giorgetti, 1998; McCormick, Noonan, and Heck, 1998; Stoiber, Gettinger, and Goetz, 1998). Inclusive programs can also achieve reasonable levels of developmental appropriateness (Bredekamp and Copple, 1997) for preschool children (La Paro, Sexton, and Snyder, 1998) and for toddlers (Bruker and Staff, 1998). Moreover, with adequate training and resources, needed curriculum adaptations can be accomplished (Wolery and Fleming, 1993). Similarly, integrated therapy models are highly compatible with inclusive practices and can be an effective approach (McWilliam, 1996a). Even children who pose unique challenges, such as those with autism or hearing impairments, can be accommodated successfully in inclusive programs (Antia and Levine, in press). Although inclusive practices appear to be feasible, success is highly dependent on proper staff training, availability of adequate related services and resources, and a willingness of all individuals to adopt new approaches and collaborative models.

When the progress of children in feasible inclusive programs (that is, well-established community programs or research models) is compared to that of children in specialized programs, children with and without disabilities do well in both settings. A comprehensive analysis of 22 studies by Buysse and Bailey (1993) and others (Bruder and Staff, 1998; Guralnick, Connor, Hammond, Gottman, and Kinnish, 1996a; Guralnick, Connor, Hammond, Gottman, and Kinnish, 1996b; Hundert, Mahoney, Mundy, and Vernon, 1998) have revealed that progress of children in all developmental domains, including social, is essentially unaffected by participation in inclusive programs. No negative effects have been found in any of the studies. When differences have emerged, benefits in terms of increased social interactions with peers for children with disabilities have been associated with inclusive settings (Guralnick et al., 1996a).

Taken together, it is clear that inclusive programs can be feasibly carried out and that expected developmental progress for all children participating is the result. Given the philosophical, ethical, and legal bases for inclusion and the absence of any obvious benefits associated with specialized programs, inclusive programs should be considered best practice. As with all intervention programs, appropriate attention must be given to issues of program design, training, resources, collaborative models, and other aspects of the program to ensure its feasibility.

SOCIAL COMPETENCE

Extensive research has established the unusual social competence difficulties, particularly with regard to peers, affecting a disproportionately large number of young children with developmental problems (Craig and Washington, 1993; Gertner, Rice, and Hadley, 1994; Guralnick, 1990; Guralnick, in press-d; Ross, Lipper, and Auld, 1990; Wilson, 1999). The quality of social exchanges with peers is affected, as are children's friendships (Buysse, 1993; Guralnick, Gottman, and Hammond, 1996). Unless this developmental trajectory is altered, future adjustment problems and accompanying social isolation are likely to result (Parker and Asher, 1987; Williams and Asher, 1992). Importantly, social separation does exist between children with and without disabilities in inclusive settings, a circumstance that can be primarily attributed to difficulties in peer-related social competence (Guralnick, 1999b; Guralnick, in press-d).

Despite numerous efforts to influence children's peer-related competence within the early intervention framework, sustained and generalizable effects have been difficult to achieve (McEvoy, Orom, and McConnell, 1992). Gains that occur in related developmental domains, such as cognition and language, are associated with only small changes in social competence. Nevertheless, developing meaningful, productive relationships with peers continues to be a high priority among parents and practitioners (Guralnick, 1999b; Guralnick, Connor, and Hammond, 1995). Consequently, best practice in early intervention should include a special focus on promoting children's social competence with peers.

Recent developmental research has had success in identifying the social strategies and underlying social processes that govern children's peer-related social competence. By combining this knowledge with a comprehensive and long-term intervention program involving families and peer group settings (day care, preschool, playgroups), more positive outcomes in the future may well be achieved (Guralnick, in press-d; Guralnick and Neville, 1997).

EARLY IDENTIFICATION

It is generally accepted that the earlier problems are identified, the greater the likelihood that interventions will produce meaningful effects. In some circumstances the benefits are more obvious, such as the early identification of hearing impairments (Yoshinaga-Itano, Sedey, Coulter, and Mehl, 1998). However, other circumstances can be compelling as well. As noted in previous sections of this chapter, for many children at risk and those with established disabilities the duration of the intervention matters, thereby requiring as early a start as reasonable. Moreover, some early developmental patterns such as the formation of secure attachments between parents and children are more difficult to accomplish for children with disabilities (Atkinson et al., 1999). Even resolution in the context of the early identification and diagnostic process itself can affect attachment formation (Marvin and Pianta, 1996). Since early attachment patterns are associated with later developmental outcomes, including peer relations (Guralnick and Neville, 1997), early identification provides an opportunity to minimize future difficulties. Perhaps most importantly, early identification allows families and the early intervention system time to gather the resources to address promptly and efficiently the stressors that can compromise family interaction patterns. As a result, early identification is clearly a best practice.

EVALUATION

Processes and procedures for evaluating goals and objectives at every level of a system, including the early intervention system, constitute a generally accepted best practice. Both ongoing and long-term outcome assessments consistent with specific objectives and the broader conceptual framework of what is important are essential. Evaluation systems not only yield feedback as to process and product outcomes, but also serve to refine assessments as well as guide modifications of goals and objectives themselves. In a meaningful way evaluation systems help focus programs and contribute to their design and structure. Perhaps as much as any other factor, program structure, which depends on a strong evaluation domain, is essential for early intervention effectiveness (Shonkoff and Hauser-Cram, 1987).

Summary: Best Practice Domains

Examination of related issues in early intervention has clearly indicated that best practice requires attention to the following domains:

- Long-term effectiveness—with special reference to intensity and specificity
- Inclusion—operating as a guiding principle for program design and community involvement
- Social competence—requiring a programmatic focus on promoting social competence, particularly peer competence
- Early identification—preventing unnecessary problems from developing and maximizing long-term benefits
- Evaluation—a process necessary for success at all levels of the system

A Developmental-Systems Approach

This chapter has provided a conceptual framework and corresponding research support for a set of best practices in the field of early intervention for vulnerable children. Three categories were described:

(1) best practices based on a conceptual model;

(2) best practices associated with specific program components; and

(3) best practices associated with a number of important related domains.

The vital question that follows from this analysis is how can early intervention systems translate these best practices into a reality that can be observed in daily interactions with children and families? Across North America, one can find excellent examples of clusters of these best practices, but no systematic, comprehensive program has yet emerged in a major community. An approach is needed that can incorporate these best practices into a set of decision rules and criteria to ensure their application. One such model is presented in Figure 3.4. Diamonds indicate decision points whereas rectangles indicate systems activities. Where appropriate, the types of processes or activities are indicated below each rectangle.

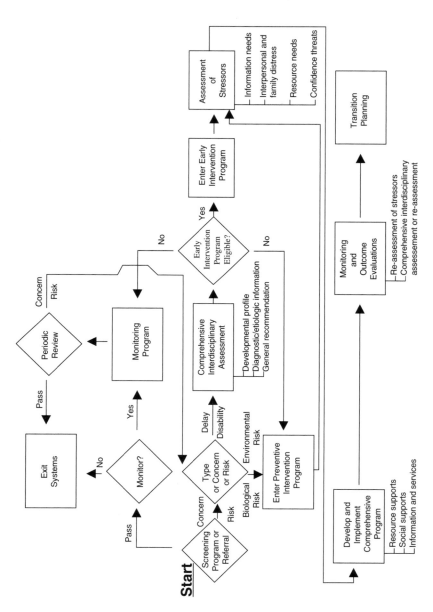

Figure 3.4   A developmental systems model incorporating best practices

Significantly, this Developmental-Systems Model is consistent with, and based upon, the major themes described in this chapter. With support from family-friendly, reliable, and valid assessment tools and procedures, an adequate supply of well-trained professionals, the availability of information, materials, and related resources that can assist practitioners and families to acquire and apply knowledge of interventions that hold most promise for individual children and families, the existence of an infrastructure to encourage systems integration, and an administrative and evaluation framework to ensure its continued development and refinement, a maximally effective early intervention system for vulnerable children and their families will emerge. Although this will certainly require considerable time and resources, an optimally effective service and support system using resources in the most effective way is well worth the investment.

REFERENCES

Achenbach, T.M., Howell, C.T., Aoki, M.F., and Rauh, V.A. (1993). Nine-year outcome of the Vermont intervention program for low birth weight infants. *Pediatrics*, 91(1), 45-55.

Als, H., Lawhon, G., Duffy, F.H., McAnulty, G.B., Gibes-Grossman, R., and Blickman, J.G. (1994). Individualized developmental care for the very low-birth-weight preterm infant: Medical and neurofunctional effects. *Journal of the American Medical Association*, 272, 853-858.

Antia, S.D., and Levine, L.M. (in press). Educating deaf and hearing children together: Confronting the challenges of inclusion. In M.J. Guralnick (Ed.), *Early childhood inclusion: Focus on change*. Baltimore, MD: Brookes.

Atkinson, L., Chisholm, V.C., Scott, B., Goldberg, S., Vaughn, B.E., Blackwell, J., Dickens, S., and Tam, F. (1999). Maternal sensitivity, child functional level, and attachment in Down syndrome. *Monographs of the Society for Research in Child Development*, 64(3), Serial No. 258.

Bailey, D.B., Jr. (1987). Collaborative goal-setting with families: Resolving differences in values and priorities for services. *Topics in Early Childhood Special Education*, 7(2), 59-71.

Bailey, D.B., Jr. (1997). Evaluating the effectiveness of curriculum alternatives for infants and preschoolers at high risk. In M.J. Guralnick (Ed.), *The effectiveness of early intervention* (pp. 227-247). Baltimore, MD: Brookes.

Bailey, D.B., Jr., and Winton, P.J. (1989). Friendship and acquaintance among families in a mainstreamed day care center. *Education and Training in Mental Retardation*, 24, 107-113.

Barnett, W.S. (1995). Long-term effects of early childhood programs on cognitive and school outcomes. In R.E. Behrman (Ed.), *The future of children: Vol. 5 - Long-term outcomes of early childhood Programs* (pp. 25-50). Los Altos, CA: The Center for the Future of Children, The David and Lucile Packard Foundation.

Baumrind, D. (1993). The average expectable environment is not good enough: A response to Scarr. *Child Development*, 64(5), 1299-1317.

Beckman, P.J., and Pokorni, J.L. (1988). A longitudinal study of families of preterm infants: Changes in stress and support over the first two years. *Journal of Special Education*, 22(1), 55-65.

Behrman, R.E. (Ed.) (1993). *The future of children: Vol. 3 - Home visiting.* Los Altos, CA: The Center for the Future of Children, The David and Lucile Packard Foundation.

Belsky, J. (1984). The determinants of parenting: A process model. *Child Development*, 55, 83-96.

Berry, P., Gunn, V.P., and Andrews, R.J. (1984). Development of Down's syndrome children from birth to five years. In J.M. Berg (Ed.), *Perspectives and progress in mental retardation: Vol. 1 - Social, psychological, and educational aspects* (pp. 167-177). Baltimore, MD: University Park Press.

Birenbaum, A., Guyot, D., and Cohen, H.J. (1990). Health care financing for severe developmental disabilities. *Monographs of the American Association on Mental Retardation*, 14.

Black, M.M., Dubowitz, H., Hutcheson, J., Berenson-Howard, J., and Starr, R.H., Jr. (1995). A randomized clinical trial of home intervention for children with failure to thrive. *Pediatrics*, 95(6), 807-814.

Blair, C., and Ramey, C.T. (1997). Early intervention for low-birth-weight infants and the path to second generation research. In M.J. Guralnick (Ed.), *The effectiveness of early intervention* (pp. 77-97). Baltimore, MD: Brookes.

Blair, C.B., Ramey, C.T., and Hardin, J.M. (1995). Early intervention for low birth weight, premature infants: Participation and intellectual development. *American Journal on Mental Retardation*, 99, 542-554.

Booth, C.L., and Kelly, J.F. (1999). Child-care and employment in relation to infants' disabilities and risk factors. *American Journal on Mental Retardation*, 104(2), 117-130.

Bradley, R.H., Rock, S.L., Whiteside, L., Caldwell, B.M., and Brisby, J. (1991). Dimensions of parenting in families having children with disabilities. *Exceptionality*, 2, 41-61.

Bradley, R.H., Whiteside, L., Mundfrom, D.J., Casey, P.H., Kelleher, K.J., and Pope, S.K. (1994). Early indications of resilience and their relation to experiences in the home environments of low birthweight, premature children living in poverty. *Child Development*, 65(2), 346-360.

Bredekamp, S., and Copple, C. (1997). *Developmentally appropriate practice in early childhood programs* (Rev. ed.). Washington, DC: National Association for the Education of Young Children.

Bristol, M.M. (1987). The home care of children with developmental disabilities: Empirical support for a model of successful family coping with stress. In S. Landesman and P.M. Vietze (Eds.), *Living environments and mental retardation* (pp. 401-422). Washington, DC: American Association on Mental Retardation.

Bronfenbrenner, U. (1979). *The ecology of human development. Experiments by nature and design.* Cambridge, MA: Harvard University Press.

Brooks-Gunn, J., Gross, R.T., Kraemer, H.C., Spiker, D., and Shapiro, S. (1992). Enhancing the cognitive outcomes of low birth weight, premature infants: For whom is the intervention most effective? *Pediatrics*, 89, 1209-1215.

Brooks-Gunn, J., McCarton, C.M., Casey, P.H., McCormick, M.C., Bauer, C.R., Bernbaum, J.C., Tyson, J., Swanson, M., Bennett, F.C., Scott, D.T., Tonascia, J., and Meinert, C.L. (1994). Early intervention in low-birth-weight premature infants: Results through age 5 years from the Infant Health and Development Program. *Journal of the American Medical Association*, 272(16), 1257-1262.

Bruder, M.B. (1996). Interdisciplinary collaboration in service delivery. In R.A. McWilliam (Ed.), *Rethinking pull-out services in early intervention* (pp. 27-48). Baltimore, MD: Brookes.

Bruder, M.B. (1997). The effectiveness of specific educational/developmental curricula for children with established disabilities. In M.J. Guralnick (Ed.), *The effectiveness of early intervention* (pp. 523-548). Baltimore, MD: Brookes.

Bruder, M.B., and Bologna, T. (1993). Collaboration and service coordination for effective early intervention. In W. Brown, S.K. Thurman, and L.F. Pearl (Eds.), *Family-centered early intervention with infants and toddlers: Innovative cross-disciplinary approaches* (pp. 103-127). Baltimore, MD: Brookes.

Bruder, M.B., and Staff, I. (1998). A comparison of the effects of type of classroom and service characteristics on toddlers with disabilities. *Topics in Early Childhood Special Education*, 18(1), 26-37.

Bryant, D., and Maxwell, K. (1997). The effectiveness of early intervention for disadvantaged children. In M.J. Guralnick (Ed.), *The effectiveness of early intervention* (pp. 23-46). Baltimore, MD: Brookes.

Burchinal, M.R., Campbell, F.A., Bryant, D.M., Wasik, B.H., and Ramey, C.T. (1997). Early intervention and mediating processes in cognitive performance of children of low-income African American families. *Child Development*, 68, 935-954.

Buysse, V. (1993). Friendships of preschoolers with disabilities in community-based child care settings. *Journal of Early Intervention*, 17(4), 380-395.

Buysse, V., and Bailey, D.B., Jr. (1993). Behavioral and developmental outcomes in young children with disabilities in integrated and segregated settings: A review of comparative studies. *Journal of Special Education*, 26, 434-461.

Campbell, F.A., and Ramey, C.T. (1994). Effects of early intervention on intellectual and academic achievement: A follow-up study of children from low-income families. *Child Development*, 65, 684-698.

Cicchetti, D., and Beeghly, M. (1990). An organizational approach to the study of Down syndrome: Contributions to an integrative theory of development. In D. Cicchetti and M. Beeghly (Eds.), *Children with Down syndrome: A developmental perspective* (pp. 29-62). Cambridge: Cambridge University Press.

Cicchetti, D., and Toth, S.L. (1995). Developmental psychopathology and disorders of affect. In D. Cicchetti and D.J. Cohen (Eds.), *Developmental psychopathology: Vol. 2 - Risk, disorder, and adaptation* (pp. 369-420). New York: Wiley.

Clarke-Stewart, K.A. (1988). Parents' effects on children's development: A decade of progress? *Journal of Applied Developmental Psychology*, 9, 41-84.

Cooley, W.C. (1994). The ecology of support for caregiving families. Commentary. *Journal of Developmental and Behavioral Pediatrics*, 15, 117-119.

Craig, H.K., and Washington, J.A. (1993). Access behaviors of children with specific language impairment. *Journal of Speech and Hearing Research*, 36, 322-337.

Duncan, G.J., Brooks-Gunn, J., and Klebanov, P.K. (1994). Economic deprivation and early childhood development. *Child Development*, 65, 296-318.

Dunst, C.J. (1985). Rethinking early intervention. *Analysis and Intervention in Developmental Disabilities*, 5, 165-201.

Dunst, C.J., Trivette, C.M., Cross, A.H. (1986). Mediating influences of social support: Personal, family, and child outcomes. *American Journal of Mental Deficiency*, 90, 403-417.

Duwa, S.M., Wells, C., and Lalinde, P. (1993). Creating family-centered programs and policies. In D.M. Bryant and M.A. Graham (Eds.), *Implementing early intervention* (pp. 92-123). New York: Guilford.

Dyson, L.L. (1993). Response to the presence of a child with disabilities: Parental stress and family functioning over time. *American Journal on Mental Retardation*, 98, 207-218.

Elardo, R., Bradley, R.H., and Caldwell, B.M. (1977). A longitudinal study of the relations of infants' home environments to language development at age three. *Child Development*, 48, 595-603.

Emery, R.E., and Kitzmann, K.M. (1995). The child in the family: Disruptions in family functions. In D. Cicchetti and D.J. Cohen (Eds.), *Manual of developmental psychopathology: Risk, disorder, and adaptation - Vol. 2.* (pp. 3-31). New York: Wiley.

Feldman, M.A. (1997). The effectiveness of early intervention for children of parents with mental retardation. In M.J. Guralnick (Ed.), *The effectiveness of early intervention* (pp. 171-191). Baltimore, MD: Brookes.

Gallimore, R., Coots, J., Weisner, T., Garnier, H., and Guthrie, D. (1996). Family responses to children with early developmental delays II: Accommodation intensity and activity in early and middle childhood. *American Journal on Mental Retardation*, 101, 215-232.

Gallimore, R., Keogh, B.K., and Bernheimer, L.P. (1999). The nature and long-term implications of early developmental delays: A summary of evidence from two longitudinal studies. In L.M. Glidden (Vol. Ed.), *International Review of Research in Mental Retardation* (Vol. 22, pp. 105-135). San Diego: Academic Press.

Gertner, B.L., Rice, M.L., and Hadley, P.A. (1994). Influence of communicative competence on peer preferences in preschool classroom. *Journal of Speech and Hearing Research*, 37, 913-923.

Gibson, D., and Harris, A. (1988). Aggregated early intervention effects for Down's syndrome persons: Patterning and longevity of benefits. *Journal of Mental Deficiency Research*, 32, 1-17.

Goffman, E. (1963). *Stigma: Notes on the management of spoiled identity.* Englewood Cliffs, NJ: Prentice-Hall.

Gorman, K.S. (1995). Malnutrition and cognitive development in children: Evidence from experimental/quasi-experimental studies among the mild-to-moderately malnourished. *Journal of Nutrition*, 125, 2239S-2244S.

Guralnick, M.J. (1988). Efficacy research in early childhood intervention programs. In S.L. Odom and M.B. Karnes (Eds.), *Early intervention for infants and children with handicaps: An empirical base* (pp. 75-88). Baltimore, MD: Brookes.

Guralnick, M.J. (1990). Peer interactions and the development of handicapped children's social and communicative competence. In H. Foot, M. Morgan, and R. Shute (Eds.), *Children helping children* (pp. 275-305). Sussex, England: John Wiley & Sons.

Guralnick, M.J. (1993). Second generation research on the effectiveness of early intervention. *Early Education and Development*, 4, 366-378.

Guralnick, M.J. (1996). Future directions in early intervention for children with Down syndrome. In J.A. Rondal, J. Perera, L. Nadel, and A. Comblain (Eds.), *Down syndrome: Psychological, psychobiological and socio-educational perspectives* (pp. 147-162). London: C. Whurr.

Guralnick, M.J. (Ed.). (1997a). *The effectiveness of early intervention.* Baltimore, MD: Brookes.

Guralnick, M.J. (1997b). Second generation research in the field of early intervention. In M.J. Guralnick (Ed.), *The effectiveness of early intervention* (pp. 3-22). Baltimore, MD: Brookes.

Guralnick, M.J. (1998). The effectiveness of early intervention for vulnerable children: A developmental perspective. *American Journal on Mental Retardation*, 102, 319-345.

Guralnick, M.J. (1999a). Developmental and systems linkages in early intervention for children with Down syndrome. In J.A. Rondal, J. Perera, and L. Nadel (Eds.), *Down syndrome: A review of current knowledge* (pp. 51-63). London: Colin Whurr.

Guralnick, M.J. (1999b). The nature and meaning of social integration for young children with mild developmental delays in inclusive settings. *Journal of Early Intervention*, 22, 70-86.

Guralnick, M.J. (2000). Early childhood intervention: Evolution of a system. In M. Wehmeyer and J.R. Patton (Eds.), *Mental retardation in the 21st century* (Figure reprinted from p. 40). Austin, TX: PRO-ED.

Guralnick, M.J. (in press-a). The early intervention system and out-of-home child care. In D. Cryer and T. Harms (Eds.), *Infants and toddlers in out-of-home care*. Baltimore, MD: Brookes.

Guralnick, M.J. (in press-b). A framework for change in early childhood inclusion. In M.J. Guralnick (Ed.), *Early childhood inclusion: Focus on change*. Baltimore, MD: Brookes.

Guralnick, M.J. (in press-c). Interdisciplinary team assessment for young children: Purposes and processes. In M.J. Guralnick (Ed.), *Interdisciplinary clinical assessment for young children with developmental disabilities*. Baltimore, MD: Brookes.

Guralnick, M.J. (in press-d). Social competence with peers and early childhood inclusion: Need for alternative approaches. In M.J. Guralnick (Ed.), *Early childhood inclusion: Focus on change*. Baltimore, MD: Brookes.

Guralnick, M.J., and Bricker, D. (1987). The effectiveness of early intervention for children with cognitive and general developmental delays. In M.J. Guralnick and F.C. Bennett (Eds.), *The effectiveness of early intervention for at-risk and handicapped children* (pp. 115-173). New York: Academic Press.

Guralnick, M.J., Connor, R., and Hammond, M. (1995). Parent perspectives of peer relationships and friendships in integrated and specialized programs. *American Journal on Mental Retardation*, 99, 457-476.

Guralnick, M.J., Connor, R., Hammond, M., Gottman, J.M., and Kinnish, K. (1996a). Immediate effects of mainstreamed settings on the social interactions and social integration of preschool children. *American Journal on Mental Retardation*, 100, 359-377.

Guralnick, M.J., Connor, R., Hammond, M., Gottman, J.M., and Kinnish, K. (1996b). The peer relations of preschool children with communication disorders. *Child Development*, 67, 471-489.

Guralnick, M.J., Gottman, J.M., and Hammond, M.A. (1996). Effects of social setting on the friendship formation of young children differing in developmental status. *Journal of Applied Developmental Psychology*, 17(4), 625-651.

Guralnick, M.J., and Neville, B. (1997). Designing early intervention programs to promote children's social competence. In M.J. Guralnick (Ed.), *The effectiveness of early intervention* (pp. 579-610). Baltimore, MD: Brookes.

Hart, B., and Risley, T.R. (1995). *Meaningful differences in the everyday experience of young American children*. Baltimore, MD: Brookes.

Hauser-Cram, P., Warfield, M.E., Shonkoff, J.P., Krauss, M.W., Upshur, C.C., and Sayer, A. (1999). Family influences on adaptive development in young children with Down syndrome. *Child Development*, 70(4), 979-989.

Heneghan, A.M., Silver, E.J., Bauman, L.J., Westbrook, L.E., and Stein, R.E.K. (1998). Depressive symptoms in inner-city mother of young children: Who is at risk? *Pediatrics*, 102, 1394-1400.

Hodapp, R.M., Dykens, E.M., Evans, D.W., and Merighi, J.R. (1992). Maternal emotional reactions to young children with different types of handicaps. *Journal of Developmental and Behavioral Pediatrics*, 13, 118-123.

Holm, V.A., and Dinno, N.D. (in press). Neurodevelopmental pediatrics in the interdisciplinary team assessment process: Emphasis on etiology. In M.J. Guralnick (Ed.), *Interdisciplinary clinical assessment of young children with developmental disabilities*. Baltimore, MD: Brookes.

Hundert, J., Mahoney, B., Mundy, F., and Vernon, M.L. (1998). A descriptive analysis of developmental and social gains of children with severe disabilities in segregated and inclusive preschools in Southern Ontario. *Early Childhood Research Quarterly*, 13(1), 49-65.

Infant Health and Development Program (IHDP) (1990). Enhancing the outcomes of low-birth-weight, premature infants: A multisite, randomized trial. *Journal of the American Medical Association*, 263, 3035-3042.

Keating, D.P., and Hertzman, C. (Eds.) (1999). *The developmental health and wealth of nations: Social, biological and educational dynamics.* New York: Guilford.

Kennell, J.H. (1999). Authoritative knowledge, evidence-based medicine, and behavioral pediatrics. *Journal of Developmental and Behavioral Pediatrics,* 20, 439- 445.

Kontos, S., Moore, D., and Giorgetti, K. (1998). The ecology of inclusion. *Topics in Early Childhood Special Education,* 18, 38-48.

Ladd, G.W., Profilet, S.M., and Hart, C.H. (1992). Parents' management of children's peer relations: Facilitating and supervising children's activities in the peer culture. In R.D. Parke and G.W. Ladd (Eds.), *Family-peer relationships: Modes of linkage* (pp. 215-253). Hillsdale, NJ: Erlbaum.

La Paro, K.M., Sexton, D., and Snyder, P. (1998). Program quality characteristics in segregated and inclusive childhood settings. *Early Childhood Research Quarterly,* 13, 151-167.

Liaw, F-R., and Brooks-Gunn, J. (1993). Patterns of low-birth-weight children's cognitive development. *Developmental Psychology,* 29, 1024-1035.

Lovaas, O.I. (1987). Behavioral treatment and normal educational and intellectual functioning in young autistic children. *Journal of Consulting and Clinical Psychology,* 55, 3-9.

Mahoney, G., and Filer, J. (1996). How responsive is early intervention to the priorities and needs of families. *Topics in Early Childhood Special Education,* 16, 437- 457.

Mahoney, G., Kaiser, A., Girolametto, L., MacDonald, J., Robinson, C., Safford, P., and Spiker, D. (1999). Parent education in early intervention: A call for a renewed focus. *Topics in Early Childhood Special Education,* 19, 131-140.

Marvin, R.S., and Pianta, R.C. (1996). Mothers' reactions to their child's diagnosis: Relations with security of attachment. *Journal of Clinical Child Psychology,* 25, 436-445.

McBride, S.L., and Peterson, C. (1997). Home-based early intervention with families of children with disabilities: Who is doing what? *Topics in Early Childhood Special Education,* 17, 209-233.

McCarton, C.M., Brooks-Gunn, J., Wallace, I.F., Bauer, C.R., Bennett, F.C., Bernbaum, J.C., Broyles, S., Casey, P.H., McCormick, M.C., Scott, D.T., Tyson, J., Tonascia, J., and Meinert, C.L. (1997). Results at age 8 years of early intervention for low-birth-weight premature infants. The Infant Health and Development Program. *Journal of the American Medical Association,* 277, 126-132.

McCormick, L., Noonan, M.J., and Heck, R. (1998). Variables affecting engagement in inclusive preschool classrooms. *Journal of Early Intervention,* 21, 160-176.

McEachin, J.J., Smith, T., and Lovaas, O.I. (1993). Long-term outcome for children with autism who received early intensive behavioral treatment. *American Journal on Mental Retardation,* 97, 359-372.

McEvoy, M.A., Odom, S.L., and McConnell, S.R. (1992). Peer social competence intervention for young children with disabilities. In S.L. Odom, S.R. McConnell, and M.A. McEvoy (Eds.), *Social competence of young children with disabilities: Issues and strategies for intervention* (pp. 113-133). Baltimore, MD: Brookes.

McWilliam, R.A. (1996a). A program of research on integrated versus isolated treatment in early intervention. In R.A. McWilliam (Ed.), *Rethinking pull-out services in early intervention* (pp. 71-102). Baltimore: Brookes.

McWilliam, R.A. (1996b). *Rethinking pull-out services in early intervention.* Baltimore, MD: Brookes.

Melson, G.F., Ladd, G.W., and Hsu, H-C. (1993). Maternal support networks, maternal cognitions, and young children's social cognitive development. *Child Development,* 64, 1401-1417.

Meyer, E.C., Garcia Coll, C.T., Seifer, R., Ramos, A., Kilis, E., and Oh, W. (1995). Psychological distress in mothers of preterm infants. *Journal of Developmental and Behavioral Pediatrics*, 16, 412-417.

Murphey, D.A. (1992). Constructing the child: Relations between parents' beliefs and child outcomes. *Developmental Review*, 12, 199-232.

New York State Department of Health (undated). *Autism/pervasive developmental disorders: Assessment and intervention for young children (ages 0-3 years)*. (Clinical Practice Guideline Report of the Recommendations). New York: NYS DOH Early Intervention Program.

NICHD Early Child Care Research Network (1999). Child outcomes when child care center classes meet recommended standards for quality. *American Journal of Public Health*, 89, 1702-1707.

Olsen, H.C., and Burgess, D.M. (1997). Early intervention for children prenatally exposed to alcohol and other drugs. In M.J. Guralnick (Ed.), *The effectiveness of early intervention* (pp. 109-145). Baltimore, MD: Brookes.

Osofsky, J.D. (1995). The effects of violence exposure on young children. *American Psychologist*, 50(9), 782-788.

Parker, J.G., and Asher, S.R. (1987). Peer relations and later personal adjustment: Are low-accepted children at risk? *Psychological Bulletin*, 102(3), 357-389.

Ramey, C.T., Bryant, D.M., Wasik, B.H., Sparling, J.J., Fendt, K.H., and LaVange, L.M. (1992). Infant health and development program for low birth weight, premature infants: Program elements, family participation, and child intelligence. *Pediatrics*, 89(3), 454-465.

Ramey, C.T., and Campbell, F.A. (1984). Preventive education for high-risk children: Cognitive consequences of the Carolina Abecedarian Project. *American Journal of Mental Deficiency*, 88, 515-523.

Rauh, V.A., Achenbach, T.M., Nurcombe, B., Howell, C.T., and Teti, D.M. (1988). Minimizing adverse effects of low birthweight: Four-year results of an early intervention program. *Child Development*, 59, 544-553.

Roach, M.A., Orsmond, G.I., and Barratt, M.S. (1999). Mothers and fathers of children with Down syndrome: Parental stress and involvement in childcare. *American Journal on Mental Retardation*, 104, 422-436.

Ross, G., Lipper, E.G., and Auld, P.A.M. (1990). Social competence and behavior problems in premature children at school age. *Pediatrics*, 86, 391-397.

Rubin, S., and Quinn-Curran, N. (1985). Lost, then found: Parents' journey through the community service maze. In M. Seligman (Ed.), *The family with a handicapped child: Understanding and treatment* (pp. 63-94). New York: Grune & Stratton.

Sameroff, A.J. (1993). Models of development and developmental risk. In C.H. Zeanah, Jr. (Ed.), *Handbook of infant mental health* (pp. 3-13). New York: Guilford.

Sameroff, A.J., Seifer, R., Barocas, R., Zax, M., and Greenspan, S. (1987). Intelligence quotient scores of 4-year-old children: Social-environmental risk factors. *Pediatrics*, 79, 343-350.

Santelli, B., Turnbull, A.P., Marquis, J.G., and Lerner, E.P. (1995). Parent to parent programs: A unique form of mutual support. *Infants and Young Children*, 8(2), 48-57.

Scarr, S., and McCartney, K. (1988). Far from home: An experimental evaluation of the mother-child home program in Bermuda. *Child Development*, 59, 531-543.

Shonkoff, J.P., and Hauser-Cram, P. (1987). Early intervention for disabled infants and their families: A quantitative analysis. *Pediatrics*, 80, 650-658.

Shonkoff, J.P., Hauser-Cram, P., Krauss, M.W., and Upshur, C.C. (1992). Development of infants with disabilities and their families. *Monographs of the Society for Research in Child Development*, 57(6), Serial No. 230.

Sontag, J.C., and Schacht, R. (1994). An ethnic comparison of parent participation and information needs in early intervention. *Exceptional Children*, 60(5), 422-433.

Sparling, J., Lewis, I., Ramey, C.T., Wasik, B.H., Bryant, D.M., and LaVange, L.M. (1991).
Partners: A curriculum to help premature, low birthweight infants get off to a good
start. *Topics in Early Childhood Special Education*, 11, 36-55.

Spiker, D., and Hopmann, M.R. (1997). The effectiveness of early intervention for children
with Down syndrome. In M.J. Guralnick (Ed.), *The effectiveness of early intervention* (pp.
271-305). Baltimore, MD: Brookes.

Stoiber, K.C., Gettinger, M., and Goetz, D. (1998). Exploring factors influencing parents' and
early childhood practitioners' beliefs about inclusion. *Early Childhood Research Quarterly*, 13, 107-124.

Stoneman, Z. (1993). The effects of attitude on preschool integration. In C.A. Peck, S.L.
Odam, and D.D. Bricker (Eds.), *Integrating young children with disabilities into community
programs* (pp. 223-248). Baltimore, MD: Brookes.

Strain, P., McGee, G., and Kohler, F.W. (in press). Inclusion of children with autism in early
intervention settings: An examination of rationale, myths, and procedures. In M.J. Guralnick (Ed.), *Early childhood inclusion: Focus on change*. Baltimore, MD: Brookes.

Taylor, L., Zuckerman, B., Harik, V., and Groves, B.M. (1994). Witnessing violence by young
children and their mothers. *Journal of Developmental and Behavioral Pediatrics*, 15, 120-
123.

Thyen, T., Kuhlthau, K., and Perrin, J.M. (1999). Employment, child care, and mental health
of mothers caring for children assisted by technology. *Pediatrics*, 103, 1235-1242.

Wachs, T.D. (1992). *The nature of nurture*. Newbury Park, CA: Sage Publications.

Wasik, B.H., Ramey C.T., Bryant, D.G., and Sparling, J.J. (1990). A longitudinal study of two
early intervention strategies: Project CARE. *Child Development*, 61, 1682-1696.

Wehmeyer, M., and Patton, J.R. (Eds.) (2000). *Mental retardation in the 21st century*. Austin,
Texas: Pro-Ed.

Wikler, L.M. (1986). Family stress theory and research on families of children with mental
retardation. In J.J. Gallagher and P.M. Vietze (Eds.), *Families of handicapped persons* (pp.
167-195). Baltimore, MD: Brookes.

Williams, G.A., and Asher, S.R. (1992). Assessment of loneliness at school among children
with mild mental retardation. *American Journal on Mental Retardation*, 96(4), 373-385.

Wilson, B. (1999). Entry behavior and emotion regulation abilities of developmentally delayed boys. *Developmental Psychology*, 35(1), 214-222.

Wolery, M., and Fleming, L.A. (1993). Implementing individualized curricula in integrated
settings. In C.A. Peck, S.L. Odam, and Diane D. Bricker (Eds.), *Integrating young children with disabilities into community programs* (pp. 109-132). Baltimore, MD: Brookes.

Yoshinaga-Itano, C., Sedey, A.L., Coulter, D.K., and Mehl, A.L. (1998). Language of early-
and later-identified children with hearing loss. *Pediatrics*, 102, 1161-1171.

Sudden Infant Death Syndrome: A Literature Review and a Summary of BC Trends

4

L.T. Foster*, W.J. Kierans**, J. Macdonald**

*BC Ministry for Children and Families, **BC Vital Statistics Agency*

with up-date to original work of Fisk, Macdonald, and Vander Kuyl, 1998

INTRODUCTION

The death of a child is doubtless the most tragic and shocking event a parent may face. The sudden, unanticipated death of an apparently healthy infant must be the most devastating of all. Compounding the grief is the subsequent revelation that the cause of death is unknown.

Sudden Infant Death Syndrome is widely understood to be the sudden and unexpected death of a baby and it is the leading cause of death for both Canadian babies between the ages of 28 days and 1 year old (Health Canada, 1999a) and also in BC in 1999 in that age group. Consideration of the age of the baby and precisely what constitutes "sudden" and "unexpected" is reduced to insignificance by the event itself. Currently most widely known by its acronym SIDS, it has been referred to as cot death (Hiley and Morley, 1994; Scragg, Mitchell, Tonkin, and Hassall, 1993), SUDI (sudden and unexpected death in infancy) (Alessandri et al., 1995; de Jonge, Burgmeijer, Engleberts, Hoogenboezem, Kostense, and Sprij, 1993), and crib death (Committee on Child Abuse and Neglect, 1994). Each name partially describes the circumstances, but there is no indication or mention of an underlying pathology or etiology. To compound the diagnostic difficulties, child abuse and SIDS share some common risk factors and, at times, a lack of physical evidence (Committee on Child Abuse and Neglect, 1994; Botash, Fuller, Blatt, Church, and Weinberger, 1995; Willinger, 1995). In 1994, a committee of the American Academy of Pediatrics cited evidence that child abuse accounted for a small proportion of sudden and unexpected infant deaths (3% to 5%) and SIDS accounted for a large proportion (59.4%). In situations needing further investigation (temporarily classified as 'unknown cause'), a diagnosis of 'probable SIDS' would be "...correct about 95% to 98% of the time" (Committee on Child Abuse and Neglect, 1994). Definitions of SIDS vary slightly in terms of age of infant and nature of investigation (Committee on Child Abuse and Neglect, 1994; Willinger, Hoffman, and

Hartford, 1994; Millar and Hill, 1993; Ambershi, 1994) and has been aptly summarized by the Canadian Foundation for the Study of Infant Deaths (1993) as follows:

> *the sudden and unexpected death of an apparently healthy infant less than one year of age, which remains unexplained even after a full investigation* (Health Canada, 1993).

Sudden Infant Death Syndrome (SIDS) has drawn the attention of researchers and health professionals since it was recognized that some sudden unanticipated deaths shared non-causal, identifiable characteristics. The common characteristics were subsequently identified as a "syndrome." Since that time, there have been an increasing number of studies published in medical/health journals examining epidemiology, risk factors/characteristics, prevention/intervention and incidence. The literature review summary provided in the introductory and background section of this chapter is intended primarily to familiarize readers with the central topics concerning SIDS but cannot fully represent the broad spectrum of SIDS research.

Even a cursory review of national and international studies points to two trends: SIDS has been decreasing in most countries and the decrease has been attributed to widening public awareness of risk factors, particularly prone sleeping. Considering that the certification of a SIDS death is still determined by the exclusion of other potential causes, the question arises as to whether the decline in SIDS world wide and in BC is valid or merely a function of changes in reporting practices of coroners or improved investigative and pathology techniques. This issue is examined later in this chapter in an up-dated evaluation of the decline in SIDS (Fisk, Macdonald, and Vander Kuyl, 1998) (relative to other causes of infant death—specific and undefined) as experienced in BC from 1985 to1998.

EPIDEMIOLOGY

Average SIDS incidence rates in Japan, the Netherlands, and Canada for 1988 to 1990 have been reported as less than one per 1,000 live births. Rates in Sweden (1.01 per 1,000), US (1.37), UK (1.79), and New Zealand (3.24) were all above the Canadian average rate (Mitchell, Brunt, and Everard, 1994).

The National Institute of Child Health and Human Development (NICHD) in the US reported SIDS incidence rates from 1985 to 1992 for Australia, Britain, New Zealand, the Netherlands, Norway, and the US. It was determined that each country, except Sweden and the US, had reduced their initial rate by at least 50% during the period. The decline in New Zealand was dramatic given a comparatively high initial rate of 3.7 SIDS deaths per 1,000 live births. The rate in the US decreased little and, in Sweden, it progressively increased during the same period.

In the 18 year period 1981 to 1997, Canada (Willinger, 1995) and BC (Fisk et al., 1998) reported declining mortality due to SIDS. Since 1981 BC has been higher than the national rate (Figure 4.1). While there has been a decrease in the Canadian rate (from 1.17 in 1983 to 0.44 in 1997), the decline in BC has been more dramatic (2.18 to 0.56). The Canada rate for 1998 was not available at the time of this review, but at 0.35 per 1,000 live births, BC's rate may be below the Canadian rate for the first time, at least in historical memory. As recently as 1995, SIDS was still reported as the leading cause of death for infants between 1 month and 1 year in each province and territory (Miller and Hill, 1993) and in other jurisdictions around the world (Committee on Child Abuse and Neglect, 1994; Willinger, 1995; Rhoades, Brenneman, Lyle, and Handler, 1992).

Rate per 1000 live births

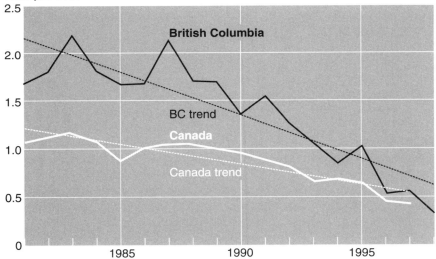

1998 Data for Canada not available.
Source: BC Vital Statistics Agency and Statistics Canada.
Prepared by: Non-Communicable Disease Epidemiology.

Figure 4.1   SIDS* rates, BC and Canada, 1981 to 1998

An epidemiological study from Western Australia (Alessandri et al., 1995) evaluated the validity of cultural differences among inhabitants of the same geographic region. In 1980, the Western Australia SIDS rate was 1.6 deaths per 1,000 live births for non-Aboriginal infants, and 3.9 for Aboriginals. By 1989, the non-Aboriginal rate was 1.3 while the Aboriginal rate had increased to 7.0 (Alessandri et al., 1995). During the same period, overall infant mortality ranged from 6.7 to 8.8 per 1,000 live births for non-Aboriginals and from 19.6 to 31.1 for Aboriginal infants (Alessandri, Read, Stanley, Burton, and Dawes, 1994).

The investigators noted there had been a decrease in Aboriginal deaths due to birth defects and low birth weight. Also, a higher proportion of Aboriginal SIDS had occurred in the first month of life (Alessandri et al., 1995). The results suggested that the apparent increase in Aboriginal SIDS might have been an artifact of the diagnostic process. The diagnostic reliability of SIDS as the appropriate cause of death was tested by an independent review of pathologists resulting in excellent agreement with the original diagnostic findings. The investigators confirmed the reliability of the increase in the SIDS death rate among Aboriginals and its relative stability among non-Aboriginals from 1980 to1989. Diagnostic consistency has been reported by others (Willinger, 1995).

As was found in Australia and New Zealand, a disparate proportion of SIDS has been noted among Status Aboriginal infants in BC (Figure 4.2). Of the 627 SIDS cases occurring in BC during 1987 to 1998, 171 were Status Aboriginal infants. BC Status Aboriginal live births have made up 6% to 7% of the provincial total while, from 1987 to 1998, this group accounted for an average of 28.2% of all SIDS. In that time period there was a steady decline in SIDS among non-Aboriginal infants particularly notable after 1995. Until 1998, however, Aboriginal infants did not experience the same decreasing pattern, but rather remained disproportionately high and actually appeared to increase proportionally from 1995 to 1997 (Figure 4.3). Due to certain data quality issues, this may be an artifact of under-ascertainment of Status Indian identity.

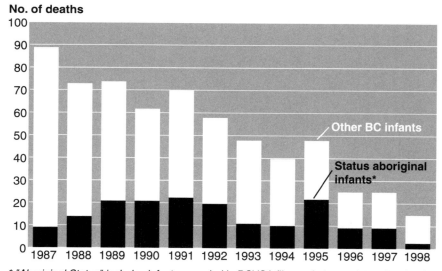

* "Aboriginal Status" includes infants recorded in BCVSA files as being registered under the Indian Act, while "Other BC infants" includes all other infants resident in the Province.
        Source: BC Vital Statistics Agency.
    Prepared by: Non-Communicable Disease Epidemiology.

Figure 4.2   SIDS counts, Status Aboriginal and other BC infants, 1987 to 1998

Percent

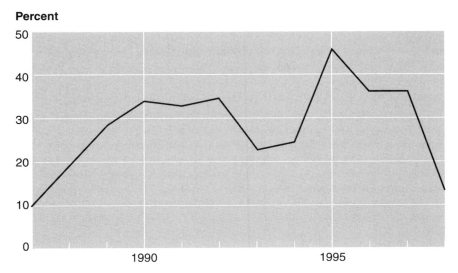

* *"Aboriginal Status" includes infants recorded in*
BCVSA files as being registered under the Indian Act.
       Source: BC Vital Statistics Agency.
Prepared by: Non-Communicable Disease Epidemiology.

Figure 4.3   SIDS in Status Aboriginal infants** as a proportion of provincial total SIDS, 1987 to 1998

This rate disparity between indigenous peoples and local non-indigenous infants has been reported for BC Status Aboriginal (Ambershi, 1994; Fisk et al., 1998; Foster, Macdonald, Tuk, Uh, and Talbot, 1995), New Zealand Maori (Hiley and Morley, 1994; Mitchell et al., 1994), US American Indians and Alaska Natives (Rhoades et al., 1992), and Western Australia Aboriginals (Alessandri, Read, et al., 1995; Alessandri et al., 1994). The higher rates among so-called "fourth world" (Alessandri et al., 1994) populations have been particularly apparent during the post-neonatal period (28- 365 days after birth). In BC, Status Aboriginal SIDS in the post-neonatal period was almost four times that of non-Aboriginals, and most of the excess was associated with mothers over age 35 (Foster et al., 1995).

There have been other reports of similar rate disparities concerning SIDS among Aboriginal Peoples in North America (Rhoades et al., 1992). On the other hand, certain cultural groups consistently exhibit a low SIDS incidence rate of less than 1 in 1,000 live births. Infants born to ethnic Chinese mothers rarely succumb to SIDS whether they be in Hong Kong (Bradshaw, 1996; Lee, Chan, Davies, Lau, and Yip, 1989), BC (Mitchell, Fitzpatrick, and Waters, 1998), or the US (Rhoades et al., 1992; Kraus and Borhani, 1972). South Asian cultures also exhibit low rates (Kierans and Hu, 1996).

RISK FACTORS

For the purposes of this review, a distinction has been made between epide-miological reports and risk factor studies, although this distinction is largely arbitrary. Analyses of demographic factors and prevalence have led to the identification of common SIDS characteristics that overlap assessments of risk. It should be noted that the comparative designs and statistical methods that have been used for SIDS research permit conclusions between an association between SIDS and certain risk factors but not a causal relationship.

An early case control study (Steele and Langworth, 1996) of SUDI done in Ontario in 1960 and 1961 was important as it included pre- and postnatal inter-views with mothers that, for the first time, allowed for examination of behav-ioural and socio-demographic variables. Several benchmark variables showed statistically significant differences between mothers of cases and controls—high risk for smokers, young mothers, young fathers, delayed prenatal visits, low birth weight babies, bottle feeding, and preterm deliveries.

Maternal smoking during pregnancy has been amply demonstrated to be associated with increased risk for SIDS as it has for other unfavourable birth outcomes. Consistent evidence of the positive relationship between mothers' prenatal smoking and SIDS persisted in those studies (Anderson and Cook, 1997) that reported statistical adjustment for confounding variables such as birth weight or mother's age. Father's tobacco use and maternal postnatal smoking was identified as a risk factor, but in the case of the former the strength and reliability of the effect varied, and the latter was not well differentiated between pre- and postnatal maternal smoking.

A more recent Canadian retrospective case control study (Millar and Hill, 1993) used 1986 to 1988 vital statistics records. The results indicated that male infants, unmarried mothers, and infants born small for their gestational age were at greater risk. Most SIDS infants died at about 3 months of age. There was also an initial quick reduction in risk up to maternal age 24 then a levelling off and an apparent increase after age 35. In addition to male gender, analyses of Canadian vital statistics birth and death records identified higher risk for infants between 2 and 4 months of age (Millar and Hill, 1993; Ambershi, 1994). First order births were found to be the least risky (Millar and Hill, 1993), but risk increased with each subsequent birth.

Variations in SIDS mortality have been reported based on north/south geography (Rhoades et al., 1992), on east/west geography (Foster, 1993), on environmental temperature, and on altitude (Kohlendorfer, Kiechl, and Sperl, 1999). In New Zealand, the higher rates found on the southern island with a cooler more temperate climate suggested "...a relationship between SIDS and environmental temperature" (Mitchell et al., 1994). In the US, SIDS was noted to be twice as common in the Pacific and Mountain regions and an extensive statistical analysis showed that SIDS was less prevalent in industrial states, but occurred most often in states with elevated soil levels of selenium, calcium, strontium, and sodium. Further analysis suggested that high SIDS rates may be related to a maternal iodine deficiency accompanied by an excess or deficiency of selenium, resulting in a thyroid hormone imbalance (Foster, 1993). In Austria, in the Tyrol and Salzburg regions, both of which share common geographical and climatic conditions, a marked seasonality (winter preponderance) in late SIDS has been noted (Kohlendorfer et al., 1999). It has been proposed that cooler temperatures may encourage room heating and thermal insulation that could lead to hyperthermia in some infants (Ponsonby, Dwyer, Gibbons, Cochrane, and Wang, 1993). Hyperthermia has often been associated with SIDS. Face down positioning of the infant exacerbates the risk because the face is an important site to dissipate body heat (Bradshaw, 1996). Swaddling, heating the infant's room, over wrapping, heavy blanketing, and soft bedding are said to contribute. The contribution of some of these factors and their interaction with prone sleeping was demonstrated using Tasmanian birth and death data (Ponsonby et al., 1993). Swaddling potentiated the adverse effects of prone sleeping fourfold, natural fibre (very soft) mattresses twentyfold, and room heating tenfold. Altitude of residence has also been recently identified as an independent risk factor, and may be related to not only lower outdoor temperatures but also to oxygen desaturation (Kohlendorfer et al., 1999).

Prone sleeping has been repeatedly associated with SIDS. A study done in New Zealand (Hassall and Vandenberg, 1985) contributed to a greater understanding of infant sleep dynamics, especially with respect to sleep positioning. Surveys conducted in the US in 1992 and 1993 found that 80% of infants that had been placed prone were in the same position when "checked during the night," whereas 50% of infants that had been placed on their side rolled onto their back (Willinger et al., 1994). Only 10% of infants placed on their side had moved onto their stomach. Virtually all of the studies that analysed the risks associated with SIDS concurred that infants who sleep on their stomachs were at increased risk of SIDS (Willinger, 1995; Willinger et al., 1994; Ponsonby, Dwyer, Kasl, Cochrane, and Newman, 1994; Schlaud et al., 1999). The consensus has prompted some authorities, including those in BC, to implement public health programs to eradicate prone crib placement (Scragg, Mitchell, Tonkin, and Hassall, 1993), whereas other authorities debate the widespread application of the research findings (Botash et al., 1995; Bradshaw, 1996; Long and Barron, 1992). Many infants sleep quite safely on their stomachs. Yet, a higher proportion of prone sleepers die of SIDS compared to supine (back) or lateral (side) sleepers. There have been attempts to explain the dangers inherent in placing a newborn front-down in its cot. Possibly modern crib mattresses contain a toxic inhalable substance (Reid and Tervit, 1995). Perhaps bedding that is too soft restricts the infants breathing (Botash et al., 1995; Willinger, 1995), or suffocation occurs when some infants are unable to turn their head sideways to breathe properly (Bradshaw, 1996). After a comprehensive review (Willinger, 1995; Willinger et al., 1994) of research reports on the relationship between

sleeping position and SIDS, the American Academy of Pediatrics (AAP) recommended that healthy babies be placed in the supine or lateral position, but
also noted exceptions (certain medical conditions and illness) where prone
should be the position of choice. More recently, US researchers have noted that
SIDS is nearly three times as likely to occur in day care settings, primarily home
day care rather than organized, licensed child care centres, than in the baby's
home setting. Authorities believe that caregivers may not be heeding advice to
have babies sleep on their backs (Gottlieb, 2000).

In 1998, the New York Times reported that researchers in Wichita, Kansas,
using autopsy results, had found persistent high levels of hemoglobin-F (HgF)
in victims of SIDS in the weeks or months after birth—well after those levels
should have declined. The newspaper reported that British studies with a different focus had shown similar persistent levels. Hemoglobin is the blood component that attaches itself to oxygen for distribution throughout the body. It
normally switches from the HgF type predominant in newborns to hemoglobin
A, which is normally dominant in adults, within the first few months of life.
HgF does not release oxygen to the tissues as readily as hemoglobin A. The
researchers found that the elevated HgF correlated with the presence of some
of the risk factors associated with SIDS, including maternal urinary tract infection, placental complications, a pregnancy weight gain of 20 pounds or less,
and restricted infant growth. Medical professionals have commented that in
several HgF and SIDS studies over the past 10 years, some have shown significant elevations and some have not (Hunt, 1999). The method used for
measurement has been a source of some debate, and the availability of suitable
controls has also been an issue.

> The HgF elevation in SIDS victims appears to be of potential im-
> portance only to the extent that it sheds additional light on a mecha-
> nism for SIDS. Based on the data reported in the medical literature,
> there is no likelihood that HgF screening in young infants would be
> of any value in identifying infants at risk for SIDS—there is too
> much individual overlap between SIDS values and control values
> (Hunt, 1999).

PREVENTIVE PROGRAMS

A long list of factors has been statistically associated with a higher risk for SIDS.
Some were directly related to the mother's or the infant's behaviour and condition, some were related to the intrauterine environment, and some were purely
environmental or geographic in nature. Obviously, prone sleeping, maternal
tobacco use, and sleeping with adults can be prevented. A youthful pregnancy
can be avoided, but being between 1 and 4 months old cannot. Thus, risk
factors that are preventable and amenable to widespread intervention have
been targeted.

Currently in Canada, SIDS prevention material is disseminated to prospective mothers through prenatal classes and to new mothers before hospital discharge. In BC, information on SIDS is included in *Baby's Best Chance* (BC Ministry of Children and Families, 1998), distributed through prenatal classes, physicians, birthing hospitals, and pharmacies.

The most widely reported prevention program was carried out in New Zealand in response to a very high SIDS mortality rate. The National Cot Death Prevention Program (Mitchell, Aley, and Eastwood, 1992) was initiated late in 1989 to reduce the prevalence of prone sleeping position, maternal tobacco use, and non-breast feeding. Programs to reduce prone sleeping have been similarly initiated (Willinger, 1995) in the Netherlands in 1987, in Norway in 1990, in Australia and Britain in 1991, and in parts of Austria in 1992 (Einspieler, Löscher, Kurz, Schober, Rosanelli, Rosegger, Roll, Kenner, and Haidmayer, 1993; Einspieler, Kerbl, and Kenner, 1997; Kenner, Einspieler, Haidmayer, and Kurz, 1998; Botash et al., 1995; Menzies Foundation, 1991).

National and community-based preventive activities have been shown to precede large reductions in SIDS incidence. In addition, home monitoring of infants' respiratory function has been recommended (Willinger, 1995; Millar and Hill, 1993; Canadian Paediatric Society, 1992) for some high risk infants. There have been anecdotal reports that confirmed the benefits of monitoring, but there have been no formal evaluations regarding SIDS prevention (Canadian Paediatric Society, 1992).

THE DECLINE OF SIDS—A BRITISH COLUMBIA EVALUATION

The prevention of SIDS has centred substantially on the reduction of prone sleeping and few other risk factors. Promotion has relied almost completely on public information programs. Based on national mortality data, declines in SIDS occurred in those countries where prone sleeping reduction programs had been initiated. In New Zealand, SIDS mortality was relatively stable from 1986 to 1989, but in 1990 there was a substantial decrease followed by lesser decreases in 1991 and 1992. However, the successes were largely among non-Maori, leading evaluators to believe that the written message may not reach all segments of the population at risk. The same explanation may be responsible for a disparate decline of SIDS among North American Aboriginal peoples.

The program in the Netherlands (1987) was the first national program initiated to combat prone sleeping and the Netherlands was the first western country to report a reduction in their SIDS rate (de Jonge et al., 1993; Bradshaw, 1996). Willinger summarized longitudinal parent survey data in six industrialized world regions and reported that prone sleeping had diminished in each of five areas to less than 5% by 1992 (Willinger, 1995). The SIDS rate also was shown to decrease in the countries that had shown the reduction.

As shown in Figure 4.1, there has been a substantial decline in SIDS mortality rates in Canada, and notably in BC. Since a diagnosis of SIDS is determined through ruling out all other explanations, the question has been raised (Fisk et al., 1998) as to whether there is a real decrease in SIDS or whether the decrease can be explained by changing diagnostic, investigative, or reporting practices. In BC, for cases awaiting autopsy and/or a coroner's investigation, infant deaths are temporarily placed in the "unknown cause" category by the Vital Statistics Agency in BC. A later re-assignment from "unknown cause" to SIDS may occur, the cause may be left as "undetermined," or the cause may be assigned to some other condition, as determined by further investigation.

In BC, the number and rate of infant deaths that remained unassigned as to cause or were deemed undeterminable was generally stable until the more recent years of 1997 and 1998 (Table 4.1). Investigation for final cause of death can be a lengthy and protracted process that is not yet complete for more recent years of data. A relatively high rate in 1992 may be reflective of reporting and updating practices anomalous in that year. However, it is evident that even if all infant deaths of unknown/undetermined cause were actually SIDS, the SIDS decline would still be seen to persist (Figure 4.4).

In terms of rates per 1,000 live births, if the SIDS and unknown/undetermined cause are combined, on the presumption that the unknown cases should have been diagnosed as SIDS, this would only have had a minor effect on the declining SIDS trend (Figure 4.5).

While the SIDS rate has declined in BC in recent years, so has total infant mortality and infant mortality for causes other than SIDS (Figure 4.6). Thus, the decline in SIDS, while not accounted for by an increase in deaths from unknown/undetermined cause, has occurred within an overall pattern of declining infant mortality.

It is evident from BC vital statistics data that the decline in SIDS is not just a question of corresponding increases in unresolved or undeterminable cases. Evaluation of the validity of the SIDS decrease must also consider the possibility of assignment of cause of death to some other category or pathology. Figure 4.7 shows the major causes of infant mortality in BC for the period 1985 to 1991 compared to 1992 to 1998. In both time periods, SIDS was the third most common major cause of death after Certain Perinatal Conditions and Congenital Anomalies. From the perspective of preventing post-neonatal mortality from 28 days to 12 months of age, SIDS takes on greater significance as mortality due to Certain Perinatal Conditions has largely already occurred within the first month of life and mortality due to Congenital Anomalies is less readily preventable at this stage because of the severity of medical problems associated with these conditions. With the exception of death from Unknown Cause (previously discussed), rates for all other major causes were less in the more recent, "SIDS-declined" time period. Further, comparative shifts in the proportions that each major cause contributed to overall infant deaths was most markedly reduced for SIDS.

Table 4.1   Infant deaths in BC due to SIDS and
                  unknown/undetermined causes

| Year | SIDS* | | Unknown cause** | |
	Number	Rate***	Number	Rate***
1985	72	1.68	0	0.00
1986	70	1.67	2	0.05
1987	89	2.14	0	0.00
1988	73	1.70	2	0.05
1989	74	1.70	4	0.09
1990	62	1.37	2	0.04
1991	70	1.54	3	0.07
1992	58	1.26	9	0.20
1993	48	1.05	4	0.09
1994	40	0.85	2	0.04
1995	48	1.03	2	0.04
1996	25	0.54	3	0.07
1997	25	0.56	8	0.18
1998	15	0.35	12	0.28

*   ICD 798.0

**   ICD 798.1, 798.2, 798.9, 799

***   Rate per 1,000 live births

Further examination of the mortality patterns for these other major causes of infant deaths are shown in Figures 4.8 to 4.11. The causes of Certain Perinatal Conditions originate within the period of time just before, during, and after delivery. The great majority of these deaths occur during the first 6 days of life (85%), with most of the remainder (13%) occurring within the next 7 to 27 days of life (BC Vital Statistics Agency, 1998; BC Vital Statistics Agency, 1999). Thus, if the condition(s) noted on the record of death are clearly perinatal in origin, they are coded as such even if the infant's age exceeds the generally defined perinatal period of less than 28 days. Examination by age of infant of deaths due to perinatal conditions over the entire period indicated consistent coding practices over time. As evident in Figure 4.8, mortality due to Certain Perinatal Conditions declined slightly over the 14 year period. Infant deaths due to

No. of deaths

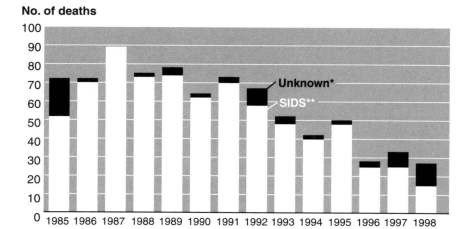

* *Selected Other Ill-Defined and Unknown Causes of*
Morbidity and Mortality (ICD 798.1-798.9, and 799).
** *Sudden Infant Death Syndrome (ICD 798.0).*
Source: BC Vital Statistics Agency. Prepared by: Non-Communicable Disease Epidemiology.

Figure 4.4   Infant deaths due to SIDS** and unknown/undetermined
                  causes*, BC 1985 to 1998

Rate per 1000 live births

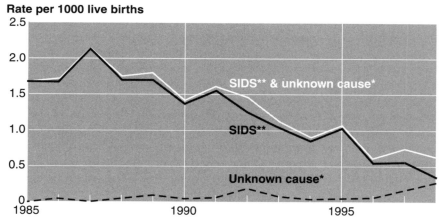

* *Selected Other Ill-Defined and Unknown Causes of Morbidity and Mortality*
(ICD 798.1-798.9, and 799)
** *Sudden Infant Death Syndrome (ICD 798.0).*
Source: BC Vital Statistics Agency.
Prepared by: Non-Communicable Disease Epidemiology.

Figure 4.5   Infant mortality rates due to SIDS** and unknown/
                  undetermined causes*, BC 1985 to 1998

Rate per 1000 live births

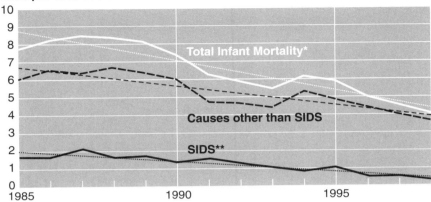

* All deaths in children aged < 1 year.
** Sudden Infant Death Syndrome (ICD 798.0).
Source: BC Vital Statistics Agency.
Prepared by: Non-Communicable Disease Epidemiology.

Figure 4.6   Comparison of total infant mortality* and SIDS** rates,
BC 1985 to 1998

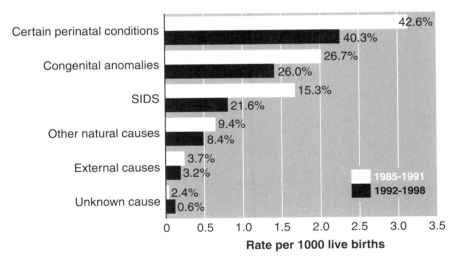

% is proportion of total infant deaths
Source: BC Vital Statistics Agency
Prepared by: Non-Communicable Disease Epidemiology.

Figure 4.7   Comparison of total infant mortality* and SIDS** rates,
BC 1985 to 1998

Rate per 1000 live births

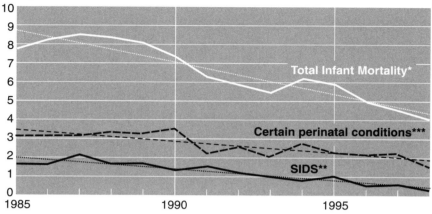

* All deaths in infants aged < 1 year. ** Sudden Infant Death Syndrome (ICD 798.0).
*** Certain Conditions Originating in the Perinatal Period (ICD 760-779).
Source: BC Vital Statistics Agency.
Prepared by: Non-Communicable Disease Epidemiology.

Figure 4.8　　Infant mortality due to SIDS and certain perinatal conditions, BC 1985 to 1998

Rate per 1000 live births

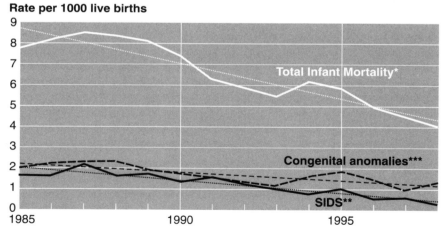

* All deaths in infants aged < 1 year. ** Sudden Infant Death Syndrome (ICD 798.0).
*** Developmental and genetic abnormalities (ICD 740-759).
Source: BC Vital Statistics Agency.
Prepared by: Non-Communicable Disease Epidemiology.

Figure 4.9　　Infant mortality due to SIDS and congenital anomalies, BC 1985 to 1998

Rate per 1000 live births

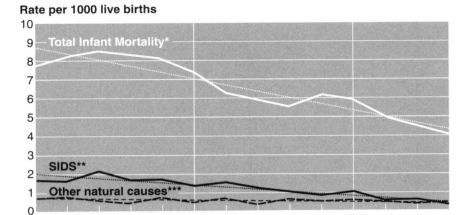

* All deaths in infants aged < 1 year.   ** Sudden Infant Death Syndrome (ICD 798.0).
*** All other natural causes except SIDS, Certain Perinatal Conditions, Congenital
Anomalies, and Unknown Cause.
Source: BC Vital Statistics Agency. Prepared by: Non-Communicable Disease Epidemiology.

Figure 4.10   Infant mortality due to SIDS and other natural causes,
BC 1985 to 1998

Rate per 1000 live births

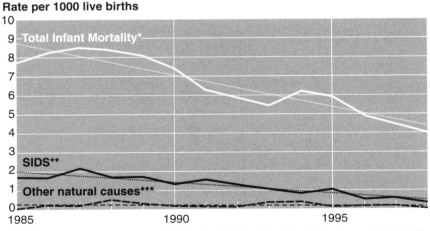

*   All deaths in infants aged < 1 year.   **   Sudden Infant Death Syndrome (ICD 798.0).
*** All External Causes (ICD E800-E999).
Source: BC Vital Statistics Agency.
Prepared by: Non-Communicable Disease Epidemiology.

Figure 4.11   Infant mortality due to SIDS and external causes,
BC 1985 to 1998

Congenital Anomalies also declined (Figure 4.9). Mortality due to Other Natural Causes (e.g., neurological disorders, pneumonia, infections) showed a fairly flat trend with a slight decline in the 1990s. This grouping encompasses a wide range of different diseases which individually are such rare causes of infant mortality that separate analysis is unlikely to be informative in terms of suggesting a diagnostic preference sufficient to offset the decline in SIDS. Infant mortality due to External Causes (a category that includes unintentional injury, poisoning, violence, etc.) is examined in Figure 4.11. These are very rare causes of infant death and the trend was fairly flat, with minor variation over the 14 year period.

In the course of examining BC infant mortality for diagnostic and reporting consistency relative to SIDS of "unknown/undetermined" and other major causes of infant mortality, similar trend patterns were exhibited for Status Aboriginal infants as for the province as a whole. However, it was noted that Status Aboriginal infants, in addition to having approximately 5 times the risk for SIDS, also had an increased risk of mortality due to Unknown Causes which was about 9 times the risk for other BC infants (Table 4.2).

Table 4.2   Cumulative relative risk of infant mortality due to SIDS and unknown causes, BC 1989 to 1998

	Aboriginal infants*		Other BC infants	
Cause of death	Mortality rate	Relative risk	Mortality rate**	Relative risk
SIDS	4.96	6.62	0.75	1.00
Unknown cause	0.27	2.76	0.10	1.00
Total infant mortality	12.02	2.21	5.44	1.00

*   "Aboriginal Status" includes children in BCVSA files and those identified through record linkage with MSP and INAC as being registered under the Indian Act while "Other BC Infants" includes all other children resident in the Province.

**   Rate per 1,000 live births

This disproportionate assignment of Unknown Cause probably means that there has been undercounting of SIDS (and possibly, to a lesser extent, of External Causes) among Status Aboriginal infants. For general comparison, the relative risk for total infant mortality in Status Aboriginal infants was 2.1 times higher than for other BC infants. The higher SIDS mortality in Aboriginal infants was positively associated with a high mortality due to Unknown Causes and the lower SIDS in other BC infants was positively associated with a lower mortality due to Unknown Causes (Figure 4.12).

Rate per 1000 live births

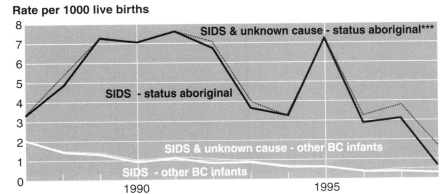

* *Sudden Infant Death Syndrome (ICD 798.0).* ** *Selected Other Ill-Defined and Unknown Causes of Morbidity and Mortality (ICD 798.1-798.9, and 799).*
*** *"Status Aboriginal" includes infants recorded in BCVSA files as being registered under the Indian Act, while "Other BC Infants" includes all other (non-Status Aboriginal) infants in the Province. Source: BC Vital Statistics Agency.*
Prepared by: Non-Communicable Disease Epidemiology.

Figure 4.12   Infant mortality due to SIDS* and unknown/undetermined causes**, combined Status Aboriginal*** and other BC infants, BC 1985 to 1998

SUMMARY, CONCLUSIONS AND RECENT DEVELOPMENTS

Despite a lack of substantive advancement in determining etiological cause(s) of SIDS, there has been considerable progress in the identification of the risk factors associated with it. The introduction of public health programs to reduce particular risks has resulted in subsequent reductions in SIDS incidence which are continuing. The literature review has portrayed prone sleeping placement as an important risk associated with SIDS which is the most amenable to prevention. Although the mechanisms by which prone sleeping position can result in death are not actually understood, there is no doubt that if prone sleeping is reduced, so is SIDS.

Such decline has been noted in many jurisdictions throughout the world, including BC which has seen rates drop from 2.14 per 1,000 births in 1987 to 0.35 in 1998. This decline was not an artifact of changing diagnostic or coroner reporting practices. Over the last 14 years, the decline in SIDS has been accompanied by a decline or stability in other major causes of infant mortality. Special attention was paid to the impact on potential SIDS mortality by deaths for which a cause was not provided or determined. In BC, deaths still under investigation are submitted to the Vital Statistics Agency as "interims." These deaths are coded as being due to "Unknown Cause" and manner of death is marked "pending." As investigations are completed, these deaths are updated appropriately. What remain as "Unknown Cause" deaths are those considered to be natural but the exact cause was never definitively determined, and those still "pending" at the time the data are extracted (September 1999 for 1997 and 1998 data used in this report). Some inconsistency was noted in the numbers of infant deaths due to "Unknown Cause" as well as an understandable increase of these in the more recent years under review. However, even if one were to consider all "Unknown Cause" infant deaths as being due to SIDS, which is highly unlikely, the Unknown Cause/SIDS combined rates still demonstrated a marked decline—from 2.14 per 1,000 births in 1987 to 0.63 in 1998. The decline of SIDS in BC is a very real phenomenon.

As was previously noted, for whatever reasons the tendency to "Unknown Cause" is considerably higher for BC Status Aboriginal Infants than for other infants in the province (Table 4.3a and b). However, this had no effect on the relative differences in SIDS and/or Unknown Cause rates between Status Aboriginal and non-Aboriginal infants. In the previous study to 1996 by Fisk et al., which has formed the basis of the second half of this chapter, it was noted that, not only was the rate of SIDS considerably higher for Status Aboriginal infants, but an apparent slight decline did not occur as early or as markedly as was found among non-Aboriginal infants. Further, the proportion of total SIDS that were Status Aboriginal remained disparately high to 1996 (29.2%). These findings suggest that information related to risk factors for SIDS may not have been reaching this at risk segment of the BC population and that a specific campaign for the Status Aboriginal subgroup is required as suggested for subgroups elsewhere (Schlaud et al., 1999). The addition of two more years of data to Fisk's study provides evidence for cautious optimism (based on small numbers) as the slightly reduced mortality rate of Status Aboriginal SIDS/Unknown Cause which was noted in 1996 (3.23 per 1,000 live births) persisted in 1997 and dropped dramatically to a rate of 1.69 in 1998, although the 1998 figures are still awaiting some confirmation, and may be confounded by the quality of the data related to Status Indian designation. The proportion of total SIDS/Unknown Cause that are Aboriginal has also declined to 18.5%.

The reasons for this more recent reduction cannot yet be determined, but the Ministry for Children and Families developed an inter-ministry working group in February 1998 to develop improved public information material, especially geared to low literacy populations (Byrne, 1999). This group includes representatives from both the Ministry for Children and Families and the Ministry of Health and their respective Aboriginal policy and health branches to ensure Aboriginal perspectives are recognized. Since its inception the group has revised information about SIDS contained in *Baby's Best Chance*, which was released in the Spring of 1998 and provided at no cost to all pregnant women in BC (BC Ministry for Children and Families, 1998). In addition, a fact sheet on SIDS has been developed (White, 1999). Posters titled *Smoke Free Zone—Baby in House* have been produced, in consultation with Aboriginal

Table 4.3a Causes of infant mortality, BC total, 1985 to 1998

Year	Total live births	Other natural causes	Other natural causes rate	Congenital anomalies	Congenital anomalies rate	Certain perinatal causes	Certain perinatal causes rate	SIDS	SIDS rate	External causes	External causes rate	Unknown	Unknown rate	Infant deaths	Infant mortality	SIDS and unknown rate	Infant mortality less SIDS and certain perinatal causes	Infant mortality less SIDS
1985	42,965	32	0.74	87	2.02	137	3.19	72	1.68	4	0.09	0	0.00	332	7.73	1.68	2.86	6.05
1986	41,825	33	0.79	93	2.22	135	3.23	70	1.67	10	0.24	2	0.05	343	8.20	1.72	3.30	6.53
1987	41,652	26	0.62	96	2.30	133	3.19	89	2.14	10	0.24	0	0.00	354	8.50	2.14	3.17	6.36
1988	42,886	20	0.47	100	2.33	143	3.33	73	1.70	21	0.49	2	0.05	359	8.37	1.75	3.33	6.67
1989	43,599	34	0.78	86	1.97	142	3.26	74	1.70	13	0.30	4	0.09	353	8.10	1.79	3.14	6.40
1990	45,390	22	0.48	80	1.76	160	3.53	62	1.37	9	0.20	2	0.04	335	7.38	1.41	2.49	6.01
1991	45,328	31	0.68	71	1.57	102	2.25	70	1.54	8	0.18	3	0.07	285	6.29	1.61	2.49	4.74
1992	45,983	16	0.35	61	1.33	119	2.59	58	1.26	7	0.15	9	0.20	270	5.87	1.46	2.02	4.61
1993	45,932	30	0.65	56	1.22	96	2.09	48	1.05	16	0.35	4	0.09	250	5.44	1.13	2.31	4.40
1994	46,820	25	0.53	76	1.62	130	2.78	40	0.85	17	0.36	2	0.04	290	6.19	0.90	2.56	5.34
1995	46,646	26	0.56	86	1.84	107	2.29	48	1.03	6	0.13	2	0.04	275	5.90	1.07	2.57	4.87
1996	45,923	23	0.50	70	1.52	101	2.20	25	0.54	7	0.15	3	0.07	229	4.99	0.61	2.24	4.44
1997	44,383	17	0.38	44	0.99	100	2.25	25	0.56	7	0.16	8	0.18	201	4.53	0.74	1.71	3.97
1998	42,987	21	0.49	58	1.35	66	1.54	15	0.35	2	0.05	12	0.28	174	4.05	0.63	2.16	3.70
Total	622,319	356	0.57	1,064	1.71	1,671	2.69	769	1.24	137	0.22	53	0.09	4,050	6.51	1.32	2.59	5.27

Table 4.3b Causes of infant mortality for Status Indians*, BC 1985 to 1998

Year	Total live births	Other natural causes	Other natural causes rate	Congenital anomalies	Congenital anomalies rate	Certain perinatal causes	Certain perinatal causes rate	SIDS	SIDS rate	External causes	External causes rate	Unknown	Unknown rate	Infant deaths	Infant mortality	SIDS and unknown rate	Infant mortality less SIDS and certain perinatal causes	Infant mortality less SIDS
1987	2,707	6	2.22	10	3.69	10	3.69	9	3.32	2	0.74	0	0.00	37	13.67	3.32	6.65	10.34
1988	2,849	6	2.11	1	0.35	5	1.76	14	4.91	5	1.76	1	0.35	32	11.23	5.27	4.56	6.32
1989	2,885	2	0.69	7	2.43	15	5.20	21	7.28	2	0.69	0	0.00	47	16.29	7.28	3.81	9.01
1990	2,965	5	1.69	5	1.69	7	2.36	21	7.08	0	0.00	0	0.00	38	12.82	7.08	3.37	5.73
1991	3,022	10	3.31	3	0.99	8	2.65	23	7.61	2	0.66	0	0.00	46	15.22	7.61	4.96	7.61
1992	2,970	8	2.69	6	2.02	10	3.37	20	6.73	1	0.34	1	0.34	46	15.49	7.07	5.39	8.75
1993	2,981	8	2.68	5	1.68	6	2.01	11	3.69	4	1.34	1	0.34	35	11.74	4.03	6.04	8.05
1994	3,056	1	0.33	5	1.64	11	3.60	10	3.27	4	1.31	0	0.00	31	10.14	3.27	3.27	6.87
1995	3,043	11	3.61	2	0.66	9	2.96	22	7.23	1	0.33	0	0.00	45	14.79	7.23	4.60	7.56
1996	3,095	5	1.62	6	1.94	11	3.55	9	2.91	0	0.00	1	0.32	32	10.34	3.23	3.88	7.43
1997	2,885	5	1.73	1	0.35	10	3.47	9	3.12	0	0.00	2	0.69	27	9.36	3.81	2.77	6.24
1998	2,961	3	1.01	2	0.68	2	0.68	2	0.68	0	0.00	3	1.01	12	4.05	1.69	2.70	3.38
Total	35,419	70	1.98	53	1.50	104	2.94	171	4.83	21	0.59	9	0.25	428	12.08	5.08	4.32	7.26

* Status Indians refers to individuals noted in BCVSA files as registered under the Indian Act.

Source: BC Vital Statistics Agency, rates per 1,000 live births. Prepared by: Non-Communicable Disease Epidemiology.

health representatives for education purposes (BC Ministry for Children and Families, 1999). Also, a video featuring Aboriginal, Asian, and low income families has been produced to help educate to minimize SIDS (BC Ministry for Children and Families, 2000). It is being distributed widely within the province, along with a joint statement from several Canadian groups (Health Canada, 1999b) and a supporting brochure (*Back to Sleep*) on reducing the risk of SIDS.

While much progress has clearly been made and SIDS rates are now very low, nearly 160 deaths still occur in Canada every year, although BC has the lowest rate, next of PEI, Newfoundland, and the Yukon (Health Canada, 1999a). In BC, Aboriginal communities are still disproportionately represented whether in the care of natural parents or in the care of the state (Fisk, 1999). It remains to be seen whether the work of the inter-ministry working group will reach those at risk and result in further successful outcomes until such time as medical research may determine the actual cause(s) of SIDS and an effective means of prevention.

REFERENCES

Alessandri, L.M., Read, A.W., Stanley, F.J., Burton, P.R., and Dawes, V.P. (1994). Sudden infant death syndrome and infant mortality in Aboriginal and non-Aboriginal infants. *Journal of Paediatrics and Child Health*, 30, 242-247.

Alessandri, L.M., Read, A.W., et al. (1995). Pathology review of sudden and unexpected death in Aboriginal and non-Aboriginal infants. *Paediatric and Perinatal Epidemiology*, 9, 406-419.

Ambershi, H. (1994). Sudden infant death syndrome in British Columbia: 1981 to 1993. *Vital Statistics' Quarterly Digest*, 3(4), 19-35.

Anderson, H.R., and Cook, D.G. (1997). Passive smoking and sudden infant death syndrome: Review of epidemiological evidence. *Thorax*, 52, 1003-1009.

Botash, A.S., Fuller, P.G., Blatt, S.D., Church, C.C., and Weinberger, H.L. (1995). Child abuse, sudden infant death syndrome, and attention-deficit hyperactivity disorder. *Current Opinion in Pediatrics, 7,* 235-9.

Bradshaw, C.M. (1996). Sleeping position and sudden infant death syndrome. *Indiana Medicine*, January-February, 64-73.

BC Ministry for Children and Families (1998). *Baby's best chance: Parent's handbook of pregnancy and baby care* (5th Ed.). Victoria, BC: Ministry for Children and Families.

BC Ministry for Children and Families (1999). *No smoking—Baby in house.* Victoria, BC: Ministry for Children and Families.

BC Ministry for Children and Families (2000). *SIDS: Reducing the risks* (video). Victoria, BC: Ministry for Children and Families.

BC Vital Statistics Agency (1998). *Selected vital statistics and health status indicators: Annual report, 1997.* Victoria, BC: Ministry of Health and Ministry Responsible for Seniors.

BC Vital Statistics Agency (1999). *Selected vital statistics and health status indicators: Annual report, 1998.* Victoria, BC: Ministry of Health and Ministry Responsible for Seniors.

Byrne, R.M. (1999). Reducing the risk of SIDS in BC. Working Group Status. Victoria, BC: Ministry for Children and Families, Personal Communication, October 1999.

Committee on Child Abuse and Neglect (1994). Distinguishing sudden infant death syndrome from child abuse fatalities. *Pediatrics*, 94, 124-26.

de Jonge, G.A., Burgmeijer, R.J.F., Engelberts, A.C., Hoogenboezem, J., Kostense, P.J., and Sprij, A.J. (1993). Sleeping position for infants and cot death in the Netherlands, 1985-91. *Archives of Disease in Childhood*, 69, 660-663.

Einspieler, C., Kerbl, R., and Kenner, T. (1997). Temporaral disparity between reduction of prone sleeping prevalence. *Early Human Development*, 43, 123-133.

Einspieler, C., Löscher, W.N., Kurz, R., Schober, P., Rosanelli, K., Rosegger, H., Roll, P., Kenner, T., and Haidmayer, R. (1993). Prospective application of the Graz scoring system (SRFB-Graz) for identifying infants at risk for SIDS on 6000 infants. In A.M. Walker, C. McMillen, National SIDS Council of Australia (Eds.), *Second SIDS International Conference and First SIDS Global Strategy Meeting*, Sydney, Australia, February 1992 (pp. 129-136). Ithaca, NY: Perinatology Press.

Fetus and Newborn Committee, Canadian Pediatric Society (1992). The infant home monitoring dilemma. *Canadian Medical Association Journal*, 147(11), 1661-1664.

Fisk, R. (1999). Personal Communication. Consultant Epidemiologist, BC Ministry of Health, May 1999.

Fisk, R., Macdonald, J., and Vander Kuyl, W. (1998). The declining trend of Sudden Infant Death Syndrome: Comparison with other major causes of infant mortality and infant deaths due to unknown causes, BC, 1985 to 1996. *Vital Statistics' Quarterly Digest*, 7(4) 1998, 19-25.

Foster, H.D. (1993). Sudden infant death syndrome: The Bradford Hill criteria and the evaluation of the thyroxine deficiency hypothesis. *Journal of Orthomolecular Medicine*, 8(4), 201-225.

Foster, L.T., Macdonald, J., Tuk, T.A., Uh, S.H., and Talbot, D. (1995). Native health in British Columbia: A vital statistics perspective. In P.H. Stephenson, S.J. Elliott, L.T. Foster, and J. Harris (Eds.), *A persistent spirit: Aboriginal health in British Columbia* (pp. 43-94). Victoria, BC: University of Victoria, Department of Geography, Western Geographical Series, Vol. 31.

Globe and Mail (1998). "Clues found to sudden infant death syndrome" per *New York Times* Service, Dec. 1, 1998, A23.

Gottlieb, S. (2000). More "cot deaths" occur in day care than at home. *British Medical Journal*, 321, 529.

Hassall I.B., and Vandenberg, M. (1985). Infant sleep position: A New Zealand survey. *New Zealand Medical Journal*, 98, 97-99.

Health Canada (1993). *Joint Statement: Reducing the Risk of SIDS in Canada*, Canadian Foundation for the Study of Infant Deaths, Canadian Institute of Child Health and Canadian Paediatric Society, August, 1993.

Health Canada (1999a). Sudden infant death syndrome. Canadian Perinatal Surveillance System, September, Ottawa.

Health Canada (1999b). *Reducing the risk of sudden infant death syndrome in Canada*. Joint statement: Canadian Foundation for the Study of Infant Deaths, Canadian Institute of Child Health, Canadian Paediatric Society, and Health Canada. Ottawa: Health Canada.

Hiley, C.M.H., and Morley, C.J. (1994). Evaluation of government's campaign to reduce the risk of cot death. *British Medical Journal*, 309, 703-4.

Hunt, C. Comments from Medical Professionals [Re. HgF], chunt@mco.edu.

Kenner, T., Einspieler, C., Haidmayer, R., and Kurz, R. (1998). Sudden infant death syndrome: Risk factor profiles for distinct subgroups. Letter to the Editor. *American Journal of Epidemiology*, 149, 785-786. In response to Kohlendorfer, U., Kiechl, S., and Sperl,

W. (1998). Sudden infant death syndrome: Risk factor profiles for distinct subgroups. *American Journal of Epidemiology*, 147, 960-968.

Kierans, W.J., and Hu, W. (1996). *A community health mosaic: Immigrants of Chinese origin.* BC Vital Statistics Agency, Victoria, BC.

Kohlendorfer, U., Kiechl, S., and Sperl, W. (1998). Living at high altitude and risk of sudden infant death syndrome. *Archives of Disease in Childhood*, 79, 506-509.

Kohlendorfer, U., Kiechl, S., and Sperl, W. (1999). The Author's Reply. *American Journal of Epidemiology*, 149, 780.

Kraus, J.F., and Borhani, N.O. (1972). Post-neonatal sudden unexpected death in California: A cohort study. *American Journal of Epidemiology*, 95, 497.

Lee, N.N., Chan, Y.F., Davies, D.P., Lau, E., and Yip, D.C. (1989). Sudden infant death in Hong Kong: Confirmation of low incidence. *British Medical Journal*, 298, 721-722.

Long, C.A., and Barron, D. (1992). SIDS and infant positioning: Implications for critical care. *Pediatric Nursing*, 18(5), 524-529.

Menzies Foundation (1991). A scientific review of the association between prone sleeping position and Sudden Infant Death Syndrome. *Journal of Paediatrics and Child Health*, 27, 323-324.

Millar, W.J., and Hill, G.B. (1993). Prevalence of and risk factors for sudden infant death syndrome in Canada. *Canadian Medical Association Journal*, 149(5), 630-635.

Mitchell, E.A., Aley, P., and Eastwood, J. (1992). The national cot death prevention program in New Zealand. *Australian Journal of Public Health*, 16, 158-161. See also: Nelson, T. (1996). Sudden infant death syndrome and child care practices. M.D. thesis. University of Otago.

Mitchell, E.A., Brunt, J.M., and Everard, C. (1994). Reduction in mortality from sudden infant death syndrome in New Zealand: 1986-92. *Archives of Disease in Childhood*, 70, 291-294.

Mitchell, E.A., Fitzpatrick, M.G., and Waters, J. (1998). SIDS and the toxic gas theory revisited. *New Zealand Medical Journal*, 111, 219-221.

Ponsonby, A.L., Dwyer, T., Gibbons, L.E., Cochrane, J.A., and Wang, Y-G. (1993). Factors potentiating the risk of sudden infant death syndrome associated with prone position. *New England Journal of Medicine*, 329, 377-82.

Ponsonby A.L., Dwyer, T., Kasl, S.V., Cochrane, J.A., and Newman, N.M. (1994). An assessment of the impact of public health activities to reduce the prevalence of prone sleeping position during infancy: The Tasmanian cohort study. *Preventive Medicine*, 23, 402-408.

Reid, G.M., and Tervit, H. (1995). Sudden infant death syndrome and superoxide/nitric oxide. *Medical Hypotheses*, 45, 395-397.

Rhoades, E.R., Brenneman, G., Lyle, J., and Handler, A. (1992). Mortality of American indian and Alaska native infants. *Annual Review of Public Health*, 13, 269-85.

Schlaud, M., Eberhard, C., Trumann, B., Kleemann, W.J., Poets, C.F., Tietze, K.W., and Schwartz, F.W. (1999). Prevalence and determinants of prone sleeping position in infants: Results from two cross sectional studies on risk factors for SIDS in Germany. *American Journal of Epidemiology*, 5(1), 51-57.

Scragg, L.K., Mitchell, E.A., Tonkin, S.L., and Hassall, I.B. (1993). Evaluation of the cot death prevention programme in South Auckland. *New Zealand Medical Journal*, 106(948), 8-10.

Steele, R., and Langworth, J. (1966). The relationship of antenatal and postnatal factors to sudden unexpected death in infancy. *Canadian Medical Association Journal*, 94, 1165-1171.

White, A. (1999). Public Health Nurse Consultant. November 1999. Personal communication.

Willinger, M. (1995). SIDS prevention. *Pediatric Annals*, 24(7), 358-364.

Willinger, M., Hoffman, H.J., and Hartford, R.B. (1994). Infant sleep position and risk for sudden infant death syndrome: Report of meeting held January 13 and 14, 1994, National Institutes of Health, Bethesda, MD. *Pediatrics*, 93(5), 814-819.

World Health Organization (1975). *International Classification of Diseases, 1975 Revision*. Geneva: World Health Organization.

Quality Child Care and Community Development: What is the Connection?

5

Jessica Ball, Alan Pence, Allison Benner
University of Victoria

INTRODUCTION

The challenge of reforming services to children and families in order to approximate more closely the goals of protecting and promoting children's well-being has been taken up by numerous provinces and states across North America (Dombro, O'Donnell, Galinsky, Melcher, and Farber, 1996), including British Columbia (Morton, 1996). There are widespread efforts to coordinate and integrate services for children and families and to bring them closer to the community. There is also a broad recognition of the importance of the early years in shaping children's later lives, including their capacity to be productive, independent citizens in the future (Carnegie Corporation, 1994; Keating and Hertzman, 1999; Shonkoff and Phillips, 2000). Increasingly, the importance of quality child care in promoting the healthy development of children is recognized as a central component of policies, programs, and implementation practices intended to protect and promote the well-being of children and families (McCain and Mustard, 1999; To, Cadarette, and Liu, 2000). There is striking similarity in the language used across North America in calls to reform service delivery systems and to give families a greater voice in service provision (Schorr, 1988; Cornell Empowerment Project, 1989; Cochran, 1991a and 1991b; Adams and Nelson, 1995; Bouchard, 1996; Dombro et al., 1996; Healthy Child Development Project, 1996; Morton, 1996).

This overarching similarity in rhetoric, however, conceals very different understandings about: who is to be included in the definition of community; the extent to which communities should be involved in service planning, delivery and evaluation; practical strategies for bringing community goals and viewpoints into focus; and the overall purpose of community involvement.

Accordingly, there is considerable variability among North American program approaches with regard to: the degree to which they planfully and actively seek and support community involvement; the extent to which decision-making authority is devolved to communities; and the breadth of involvement of the whole community rather than only community leaders and service providers. Often, what is described as 'community involvement' means only an invitation to attend a public meeting or to provide feedback on a strategic plan (Dombro et al., 1996). This is a limited, tokenistic vision of community participation which may ultimately alienate community members from involvement in program development (Fullan and Miles, 1992).

The basic premise of this chapter is that quality child care and community development can be reciprocally enhancing processes that can co-evolve as both means and ends. We argue that this potential is worth serious exploration in reconceptualizing child care policy and capacity building in Canada. In this chapter, we describe several child care initiatives that have actively sought to bring elements of the community into focus and to enlist the active participation of community members in the interest of ensuring quality child care and other family services. These examples are discussed with a view to how they can stimulate and guide a reconceptualization of the child care systems and the relationship of child care systems to other elements in the broader ecology of Canadian families and communities.

We begin with a rationale for challenging prevailing approaches to child care policies, program design, and service delivery strategies. We then review illustrative approaches to mobilizing and involving community in the design and/or implementation of child care programs. Finally, we describe a child care capacity building initiative involving the first two authors and eight First Nations communities in western Canada from 1989 to the present. This training initiative explicitly links the development of child care services and the development of the participating communities as both means and ends. A recently completed evaluation of these 'First Nations Partnership Programs' (Ball, 2001) provides evidence of the effectiveness of this approach, and yields guidelines for changing approaches to child care policy and programs in order to ensure their relevance and utility in achieving developmental goals of children, families, and communities.

Problematizing Conceptions of 'Quality'

To answer the question posed in this chapter, "Is there a connection between quality child care and community development?", the ways in which quality has been conceptualized needs to be problematized. The examples of approaches to community development in the context of child care and other family services discussed in this chapter are intended to suggest that quality child care can play a positive role in the development of "high quality" communities. However, the connection between optimum community development and quality child care may not be transparent. This is in part because of the limited way that quality child care has been conceptualized in North America.

A major undertaking of child care researchers over the past two decades has been to identify key features of quality child care (Phillips, 1987; Melhuish, 2001). Canadian research has confirmed that a number of features, including licensing/regulation, child care training/professional development, and low child/staff ratios, are associated with enhanced physical, emotional, social, and cognitive development for children (Goelman and Pence, 1987; Doherty and Stuart, 1996; Doherty, Lero, Goelman, Tougas, and LaGrange, in press; To et al., 2000). Child care programs that include these regulatable features generally receive higher scores on global aspects of quality, as measured by instruments such as the Early Childhood Environment Rating Scale – Revised (Harms, Clifford, and Cryer, 1998) and Quality of Day Care Environment Scale (Bradley, Caldwell, Fitzgerald, Morgan, and Rock, 1996), than programs that do not. Because these features are specific and measurable, they lend themselves to the development of policies and programs that support quality child care, as this concept has been operationally defined in North American child care research findings.

Katz (1993) identifies five perspectives on quality in early childhood programs:

- top-down: quality as seen by the adults in charge of the program;
- bottom-up: quality as experienced by the children participating in the program;
- inside-outside: quality as experienced by the families served by the program;
- inside: quality from the perspective of the staff working in the program; and
- outside or ultimate: quality as seen by the community and the larger society served by the program.

North American conceptions of quality child care tend to be dominated by the "top-down" perspective, which typically takes into account such program features as: staff/child ratios, staff qualifications and working conditions, characteristics of adult-child relationships, quality and quantity of equipment, materials and physical space, and health and safety provisions (Katz, 1993). These features, often included in licensing standards, are associated with positive developmental outcomes for children (Goelman and Pence, 1988; Harms and Clifford, 1980; Howes, 1988; Howes and Smith, 1995), but they only constitute one aspect of quality, within the framework offered by Katz. These features do not take into consideration the perspectives of children, parents, caregivers, or the community at large—or the complex inter-relationships among these perspectives.

The features associated with the "top-down" approach, as described above, have come to dominate the "discourse of quality" (Moss, 1997; Dahlberg, Moss, and Pence, 1999). As Moss notes, while these features are useful, it is important to recognize that their esteem derives primarily from a business model of

quality assurance, where the primary objectives are "standardisation, reliability and objectivity of measurement, the aim being to reduce the complexity of
the service to basic measurable parameters; and reduction in the variation of
products, since variation is equated with defects" (Moss, 1997, p. 9). The trend
towards promoting universal 'standards' of quality can be found not only in
North America but also in Europe (Dahlberg and Asen, 1994; Jensen, 1994).
This trend has led a Danish child care expert to reflect:

> In the past, 'quality' was generally used to provide a brief reference
> point in describing an experience and as a way of expressing in
> shorthand a complexity which was hard to define otherwise with-
> out using thousands of words—and even if thousands of words were
> used, the feeling remaining would often be that the description had
> only scratched the surface of what had actually been experienced.
> The concept of quality is used differently today, especially in Dan-
> ish business life where the subject has been addressed for some time.
> The results achieved do not look promising, at least for child care
> services. The key words seem to be 'quality management' and 'qual-
> ity control,' and **there is no mention of the kind of quality
> which might lead to indefinable change**. These days, quality
> has to be defined and measured precisely. **Perhaps true quality is
> no longer really required.** Perhaps the main aim is simply to
> achieve tighter management and tighter control (Jensen, 1994, p.
> 156, our emphasis).

These reflections, although they may be dismissed by some as nostalgia or
disenchantment, serve nonetheless to place "top-down" conceptions of the
discourse of quality into question.

Indeed, an expert-driven conception of quality is by no means universal,
or without historical context. Recently, some child care researchers have begun to question the foundation on which these conceptions rest. Research in
'minority' community settings in North America (Bernhard, Corson, Gonzalez-
Mena, Stairs, and Langford, 1996) and elsewhere (Nsamenang, 1992; Kagitcibasi,
1996; Woodhead, 1996) has highlighted the relative, context-dependent meaning and measurement of 'quality' (Moss and Pence, 1994; Dahlberg, Moss, and
Pence, 1999) and of child development (Katz, 1996; Lubeck, 1996; Masten,
1999; Stott and Bowman, 1996). The emerging impetus among early childhood educators to re-think foundational aspects of the field is oriented towards
deconstructing the knowledge base that has informed child care research and
practice for the past few decades in order to recognize, make explicit, and
problematize the culturally constructed, values-based nature of the field. For
example, conceptions of child development and quality child care that are rooted
in a dominant North American cultural context tend to privilege cognitive over
social competence, individual over group development, measurable over in-
tangible goals, and professional over lay perspectives (New, 1997; Rosenthal,
1999). These values conflict with, diminish, or even extinguish the potential

contributions of 'lay' communities to the development of a quality child care system, even as child care researchers and practitioners increasingly recognize the importance of community involvement in developing and delivering child care services (Moss and Pence, 1994; Dombro et al., 1996; Kagan et al., 1996; Woodhead, 1996). As stated by Moss:

> ... 'quality' in early childhood services is a relative concept, not an objective reality. Definitions of quality reflect the values and beliefs, needs and agendas, influence and empowerment of various 'stakeholder' groups having an interest in these services. 'Quality' is also a dynamic concept; definitions evolve over time. The process of defining quality involves stakeholder groups, and is not only a means to an end but is important in its own right (Moss, 1994, p. 1).

Within this context, professionally-driven conceptions of quality child care may be seen to compromise the development of community-oriented conceptions of quality care. More significantly, the dialogue that could support negotiation on these differing conceptions has, with a few exceptions, not yet begun. North American social systems do not provide, on a broad scale, meaningful opportunities to engage in this kind of dialogue.

This discussion highlights the need for a "counter-discourse" which:

> ... needs to be able to accommodate features of advanced modernity which the 'discourse of quality' is not well equipped to handle: increasing diversity and multiple perspectives; increasing change; uncertainty; reflexivity; contradictions and ambivalence; and subjectivity. It should be based on the concept of citizenship, defining a place for all its members, children and adults, and on values that are not easily accommodated in the 'discourse on quality: solidarity and reciprocity; democracy and inclusion; tolerance and trust; mutual respect; dialogue and confrontation. Finally, the counter-discourse needs to include a concept of services for young children as societal institutions, with cultural and social significance, where varied cultural and social projects take place... (Moss, 1997, p. 11).

Clearly this kind of discourse, which is simultaneously a counter-discourse to the established discourse of quality and an integral component of a broader conception of quality, can only take place with the full participation of the community. Within this framework, quality child care—its definition and implementation—is inseparable from community development. How can such participation be encouraged? Where can it take place? Are communities interested in participating in this kind of dialogue?

In the next section of this chapter we present a number of examples of participatory processes that draw upon and stimulate community development processes in relation to child and family services. We have drawn these examples from international literature and our own work in partnerships with First Nations in Canada. Our aim is not to provide a comprehensive, exhaustive account of community development strategies from around the world. Rather, the examples have been chosen as a means of promoting the dialogue on child care and community which is necessary to support a quality child care system that embodies and furthers the child care goals, knowledge, and experiences within communities.

THE CONTINUUM OF COMMUNITY AND COMMUNITY INVOLVEMENT

Before moving on to examples of various approaches to community involvement, it is useful to reflect on what is implied in the terms "community" and "community involvement." A community may be defined as "a group of people brought together by geography, culture, or common interests" (Dombro et al., 1996, p. 7). Within that community, a variety of groups exist. Schaeffer (1995) identifies a range of "internal" and "external" actors. "Internal actors" may include: nuclear and extended families; voluntary, community, and non-governmental organizations; religious organizations; agencies of local government; and local private enterprise and media. "External actors" include: national and international non-government organizations; agencies of national and provincial governments; and national media. Community development involves mobilizing all these community members.

Similarly, community participation exists along a continuum. At one end lies the simple use of a service. Moving along the continuum to greater degrees of participation are: passive involvement through attendance at meetings; participation in consultation on particular issues; involvement in the actual delivery of a service; and decision-making power with respect to services (Schaeffer, 1995). It is our position that only the greatest degrees of community involvement are likely to result in widely endorsed, sustainable, quality services that are seen as having 'quality' and that yield lasting benefits to children, families, and communities. Our position is echoed by a growing number of child care advocates, community service providers, and governments (Bouchard, 1996; Dombro et al., 1996; Kretzmann and McKnight, 1993; McKnight, 1995). The challenge lies in putting that principle into practice and learning to distinguish community from its counterfeits (McKnight, 1995).

There are a variety of factors that make community mobilization a challenge. As Schaeffer points out, "despite the way 'the community' is often conceptualised, as a seemingly homogeneous force capable of organising itself for the common good, the fact is that communities are usually extremely heterogeneous entities" (Dalais, Landers, and Fuertes, 1996, p. 19). Also, community members, from the most powerful to the most marginalized, may lack the attitudes, skills, experiences, and resources to participate in collaborative discussion and decision-making that benefits the entire community. In order for community involvement to be effective, the culture in which it is grounded must genuinely value the input of all of its citizens, and must promote the development of problem-solving skills and the ability to respect and respond creatively to differing points of view (Dombro et al., 1996). In reviewing the examples presented below from North America, Europe/Australasia, and Majority World (or "developing") countries, it is useful to consider whether the full range of community members is involved in the development of services; to what degree they are involved; and to what extent the culture in question promotes the values and skills that allow community involvement to be most effective.

North America

Across North America, within the past decade, the trend in child and family services has been to improve coordination and integration of a continuum of services at the local level. Related to this trend is a call for greater community involvement in the planning, delivery, and evaluation of services. Several sometimes conflicting factors provide the impetus for such change, including the rising incidence of family stress and child poverty, producing an ever larger "at risk" population (Canadian Council on Social Development, 1996), as well as the need to manage public funds more efficiently. The following description of current activity in the United States reflects the current situation across North America:

> It has become increasingly evident that to improve the well-being of young children, the service delivery systems that support them must be significantly changed. This requires identifying and leveraging areas where flexibility currently exists and encouraging state and local policymakers, program supervisors, and frontline staff to determine where additional flexibility would enable them to better meet the needs of children and families. It requires recognizing the diversity in states, communities, and individual families as well as their concerns, priorities, and resources. It entails exploring the constraints of the current system and experimenting with promising strategies to simplify and rationalize that system (Dombro et al., p. 313).

One approach to empowering communities in the management and delivery of child and family services is to move decision-making to the local level. However, the degree to which communities have control over the decision-making process can impact the usefulness of this approach. The contrasting experiences of North Carolina's Smart Start initiative and Indiana's Step Ahead initiative illustrate differences in commitment to community empowerment and the consequences for community development.

North Carolina's Smart Start initiative, introduced in 1993, was intended to guarantee every child access to comprehensive, integrated, high quality services, including early childhood education, child care, and health care. Through the initiative, partnerships of families, child care providers, health and human service agencies, businesses, schools, churches, and local governments were established in 32 counties to develop and implement innovative local plans to meet children's needs. To support and guide the county partnerships, and to enforce state-wide standards, a central, non-profit, public/private corporation was established (Dombro et al., 1996). A preliminary evaluation of the Smart Start initiative indicated that the initial emphasis on local decision-making power was limited by plan approval mechanisms, budgetary deadlines, and state-wide standards required by the central government. Local participants indicated that while, in theory, Smart Start operated on a "bottom-up" model of governance, genuine decision-making authority was maintained centrally (North Carolina Department of Human Resources, 1994).

In contrast, Indiana's Step Ahead initiative, which is similar in intent to Smart Start, genuinely delegates decision-making power to the local level. Through the initiative, each of the state's 92 counties formed local councils with representation from parents, local and state agencies, schools, churches, businesses, and community services, to develop comprehensive service delivery systems for children and families. Early child development, including child care and preschool service, is a particular focus of the initiative (Kagan et al., 1995). The experience with Step Ahead suggests that when communities have genuine authority over decision-making, community ownership and enhanced civic participation are possible. One local council member, following a survey of licensed child care providers, describes the impact of Step Ahead in strengthening her community:

> Our data reflected that families' needs were being met in town but not in rural areas. This was important information but even more valuable was how the process brought us together and gave us a new way of looking at how best to support families. Now that we've gained experience and gotten a large cross-section of the community involved in the Council, we are reframing our work. Rather than think about how we can spend the money we get... we are looking at how we can get the whole community involved and use our resources to meet our needs (Dombro et al., 1996, p. 57).

A common theme in the North American literature on child and family services is the need to support community-based prevention and early intervention initiatives, rather than focus resources on problems once they have already occurred (Dombro et al., 1996; Morton, 1996). Early intervention and prevention initiatives, often directed at disadvantaged families, vary widely in the degree to which they focus on family strengths rather than weaknesses, and in the extent to which they promote family and community involvement in defining issues, developing solutions, and providing services.

One highly regarded program in the United States is Healthy Start, a home-based intervention program which originated in Hawaii and has been adapted in 20 other states. Healthy Start provides postpartum screening assessment, paraprofessional home visitation, child care, parent support groups, and community education to disadvantaged families. Services are voluntary and continue until children reach the age of five. The program has been successful in substantially reducing the incidence of child abuse and neglect among families considered at risk, from 18 to 20% in the disadvantaged population generally, compared to less than 1% among program participants (Dombro et al., 1996).

Healthy Start is a good example of a flexible, coordinated, family-centred program delivered at the community level which generates positive outcomes for its intended beneficiaries. By North American standards, it might be called a "high quality" program. Yet it is also an example of a program which defines families by their deficiencies rather than by their strengths, and which provides participating families with few opportunities to be involved in the actual management and delivery of the services that touch their lives. With this program, as with many other similar programs across North America (e.g., New Brunswick's Early Childhood Initiatives), families are at the "receiving end" of a program which may assist them to "fit into," but not necessarily to shape, their communities; a program which protects them against risk factors in their lives, but may not help them to thrive.

It is only by way of contrast with other approaches to early intervention and prevention that the limited potential of programs like Healthy Start to strengthen families and communities is made visible. The American Head Start program, for instance, is also a comprehensive, multi-service, family-centred program targeted to disadvantaged families. In contrast, however, it explicitly aims to build on the strengths of low-income families in their own neighbourhoods. The direct involvement of parents in the management and delivery of the services (often including employment in the services) is one of the tangible ways this commitment is demonstrated (Schorr, 1988). One central feature of strength-oriented as opposed to deficit-oriented approaches is that the former provides families and communities with opportunities to transform the social and economic conditions which make them disadvantaged in the first place, while the latter tend to leave these 'macrosystem' conditions intact (Kretzmann and McKnight, 1993; McKnight, 1995).

The innovative 1,2,3, Go! project in Greater Montreal is an example of a strength-oriented initiative aimed at empowering children and families within a holistic conception of community:

> *1,2,3 Go! is an experimental project whereby some communities of the Greater Montreal area were selected and invited to mobilize whatever resources they needed, be they material, intellectual, social or political, in order to develop and sustain a culture concerned with the well-being and development of their 0 to 3 year olds.... Although there is a specific concern with offering the project to communities in which risks are higher for children for developing problems,...*

> *the overall objective is more in line with a health or well-being pro-*
> *motion approach than with a prevention or remedial approach. As*
> *such it relies on three main strategies: enhancement of individual*
> *competencies, institutional and organizational changes and mass*
> *influence.... 1,2,3 Go! results in the postulate that communities can*
> *and ought to empower themselves around the issue of children's*
> *development and well-being* (Bouchard, 1996, p. 3).

Results to date indicate that the program has been effective in mobilizing communities (including parents) to collaborate in identifying problems, setting
priorities, and developing solutions (Bouchard, 1996). Another Canadian initiative with a similarly holistic focus is Ontario's Better Beginnings, Better
Futures initiative (Peters and Russell, 1996).

While direct, intensive mobilization of communities presents challenges,
experience suggests that the greater the autonomy in local decision-making on
the part of those directly affected by services, the greater the impact in strengthening the community as a whole (Adams and Nelson, 1995; McKnight, 1995).
"Clients" are afforded their rightful recognition as citizens.

An example from New Mexico's Family Development Program shows how
the development of early childhood services by and for families can become
the vehicle for community development in a broader sense. In 1985, a group of
families in low-income, predominantly minority families were provided with
the opportunity to design an early childhood program to meet their own needs.
These families created a comprehensive preschool program, including parent
involvement and education, family support, infant and toddler services, and
an after-school program for older children. Evaluations of the program showed
benefits for children and parents in these families, including improved school
performance among the children, economic independence for many of the
families, and a greater degree of civic involvement (Dombro et al., 1996, p. 330).
Although the program was originally designed to address parents' child care
needs, it became the vehicle for broader involvement in community development. As noted by the program coordinator:

> *Community action is becoming a reality: program parents have pe-*
> *titioned the city school board to obtain better transportation for their*
> *older children, the police department for more effective patrolling,*
> *the city waste management division for neighbourhood clean-up*
> *services, and the neighbourhood public schools to establish parent-*
> *teacher associations* (van der Eyken, 1991, p. 8).

The foregoing examples of community development approaches by no
means capture the extent of activity underway in the reform of child and family services across North America. Fortunately, we are seeing a small but growing number of programs in Canada and the United States which genuinely
give communities authority over program planning and delivery, and which
value citizen involvement in child and family services as a means of enriching

the community as a whole. If these approaches are implemented more broadly, they have the potential to support community dialogue and action towards creating a comprehensive system of services for children and families, including quality child care.

Europe/Australasia

Child care in Europe and Australasia is distinct from child care in North America in a number of ways, primarily in the extent of publicly funded services available, and in the presence of strong national policies for children and families— minimally in countries in the United Kingdom and maximally in the Nordic countries, with most other countries falling somewhere in the middle of this continuum (Cochran, 1993; European Commission Network on Child Care, 1996). Generally, the presence of national systems of early childhood education and comprehensive family policies make for a more stable, well resourced child care system, and a stronger basis for community development and public dialogue on issues pertaining to child and family services. Examples of efforts to enhance community involvement in child care are described below.

In the late 1980s, New Zealand undertook a major reform of its child care system with the introduction of a system of chartering:

> *Chartering is a process where various stakeholders (parents, staff and the community) are given the opportunity to define quality at the individual centre level in negotiation with a government agency. The intent of the process is to strike a balance between centrally determined criteria of quality and the philosophy and local needs of centres.... Charter documents contain an outline of centre policies, philosophies and characteristics.... The charter is a quality assurance mechanism for government. The funding of individual centres ... is linked to the development and approval of charters with the Ministry according to the level of quality the government is prepared to support* (Smith and Farquhar, 1994, pp. 123, 125).

In theory, chartering provides a mechanism for the greater involvement of parents and the community to shape individual child care centres, while maintaining a minimum standard of quality nationwide, allowing for a conception of quality which is relative but not arbitrary. Yet the experience of chartering in New Zealand highlights the need for processes which promote ongoing, meaningful involvement in the definition and implementation of quality child care.

Smith and Farquhar (1994) studied the effects of the charter in four kindergartens, three child care centres and two play centres. Generally, the charter was considered a useful statement of a centre's goals, objectives, and policies, but was consulted more frequently by staff than parents, and proved not to be a particularly useful way of meaningfully involving child care providers, parents, or the community in discussions of quality child care. As noted by Smith

and Farquhar, many child care providers perceived the charter as a bureaucratic exercise. As for parent participation:

> *Many centres did not find it easy to get parents interested or involved
> in writing the charter. All centres experienced some difficulty in
> getting parents to participate and many lowered their expectations
> after an initial failed attempt.... The process of charter development
> was perceived as making large physical and emotional demands on
> staff and parent time* (Smith and Farquhar, 1994, p. 131).

Given that the charter was a requirement in order to access public funds, and
that its form and content were, to some extent, predetermined by the central
government, it is not surprising that it may have been experienced by many as
an elaborate grant application. Also, the nature and variability of parent and
community participation may not have been conducive to producing a meaningful, "living document":

> *There were many variations in the methods of consultation and the
> number of people who participated in consultation and discussion
> in different centres. These methods included written procedures
> such as displaying the charter on notice boards, notices or news-
> letters sent home with children; more systematic data gathering pro-
> cedures such as the use of questionnaires or telephone interviews;
> and more interactive procedures varying in formality from small
> subcommittees intensively working together and public meetings
> to informal conversations and social events* (Smith and Farquhar,
> 1994, p. 131).

The consultation methods described above cannot, in isolation from provisions
for ongoing dialogue and involvement of parents and community members
on child care, support true community involvement in the development of a
quality child care centre, let alone a quality child care system.

By contrast, Denmark has employed a different mechanism to provide a
balance between centralized standards and development of quality at the
centre level:

> *... the [Danish] system is... characterized by a high level of autonomy
> for individual centres.... The state and communities lay down only
> a few general guidelines and targets, leaving the rest up to the child
> care centre concerned... decentralization has led to great activity in
> and around individual child care centres, and children, staff and
> parents all feel that they can contribute to an active democratic
> process in which changes are allowed and even approved of. This
> means that children, parents and staff at child care centres can be
> given the chance to be the leading figures in their own centre...
> They have great influence on daily routines, the way groups are
> made up, the activities and rules in the centre, and so on. This has*

*led to a more flexible and open understanding of what is required
and an ability to put good ideas quickly into practice* (Jensen, 1994,
p. 154).

The contrasting experiences of New Zealand and Denmark, both of which enjoy comprehensive public funding and provision of child care, suggest that
national policies can support or detract from communities' ability to meet local child care needs. Furthermore, this contrast illustrates that the nature of the
processes intended to support community decision-making is critical. If the
involvement takes place at a few distinct points in time, rather than on an ongoing basis, and if the involvement is indirect as opposed to direct, the impact
of the processes on quality care will differ significantly.

However, it is important to recognize that the decentralized structure and
processes described by Jensen do not exist in isolation; they exist within a culture that supports children's rights, parental involvement in the daily routines
and overall management of child care centres, highly trained and committed
child care staff, and "a strong underlying coherence in the system due to generally shared cultural values which manifest themselves in widespread support for certain priority objectives: fellowship, the importance of children's
own play, self-determination" (Jensen, 1994, p. 156). Without this supportive
cultural context, it is possible that a decentralized system would produce little
public involvement in child care, and perhaps even poor quality environments
for children.

In discussing the European (and particularly the Nordic) conceptions of
community involvement in quality child care, it is useful to highlight the extent to which children are increasingly perceived as active citizens with useful
contributions to make—a view that receives scant consideration in the North
American literature on "community stakeholders." In North America, childhood is usually conceived as a preparatory phase; children are citizens of the
future, but not of the present (Mayall, 1996). In contrast, a number of European
initiatives, including the European Childhood as Social Phenomenon Project
(Qvortrup, Bardy, Sgritta, and Wintersberger, 1994), the *BASUN* (Childhood,
Society and Development in the Nordic Countries) Project, and the Danish Children as Citizens Project (Langsted, 1994) seek to understand childhood from
children's perspectives and to promote children's greater involvement in civic
life, including decision-making. These projects extend the concept of children's
rights and agency even to very young children. For example, one component
of the Danish Children as Citizens Project involved a nursery for children from
six months to three years:

*Here the staff [had] been preoccupied with rules, frequently regulat-
ing the behaviour of children by prohibitions. On the assumption
that even very young children have the right to control themselves
in their everyday life, and that they are able to do so, the staff have
reviewed the rules and try to listen more to the children. This means,*

> *among other things, that children have got the right to say 'no'....*
> *One of the consequences is that there are fewer conflicts between*
> *adults and children. On the other hand there are more conflicts*
> *between the children. But this is seen as another right that children*
> *have—the right to try to solve their own conflicts. And on many*
> *occasions they are able to do so* (Langsted, 1994, p. 32).

Within this framework, child care settings may be seen not only as part of the community, or as a means for community development, but as communities in development. They provide children, parents, caregivers, and community members with opportunities to interact in new ways that break down barriers between adults and children, between caregivers and parents, between different socio-economic and ethnic groups within the community, and between families and the larger community (Woodhead, 1996; New, 1997). The *creches parentales* in France provide an interesting example of how parent involvement in the provision of child care can effect such changes.

The *creches parentales*, or parent-run day care centres, comprise a minority of the child care provided for preschool children in France, which has one of the highest levels of publicly funded child care in Europe (Cochran, 1993). Parent-run day care centres are now recognized as a valuable alternative to centre- and family-based child care. Participating parents spend approximately one half day per week working with their own and other people's children; all *creches* employ some professional caregivers to ensure continuity and support for children and parents. Over the past 20 years, use of the *creches* has mostly been confined to professional, middle class parents, but recently the *creche parentale* model has been extended to multicultural and disadvantaged families, with approximately 40 multicultural *creches* in operation (Woodhead, 1996). The description of one *creche* presents a contrast to that typically observed in "traditional" child care settings:

> *The families using the* creche *live mainly in the apartments above,*
> *or within walking distance of the* creche. *As parents arrive to take*
> *their children home, there are lots of hugs and talks. The atmos-*
> *phere is very informal. Parents wander into the playroom, the*
> *kitchen, and the bedroom in search of their little ones. One even*
> *lingers for a coffee. This is the moment when the contrast with a*
> *conventional nursery is most clear—these parents are chatting with*
> *the 'staff' as if they are old friends, but then they are old friends, or*
> *if not, at least there are no status or professional barriers that might*
> *distance them. There are two more* creche parentale *within a few*
> *miles of this one. They are all different, but all using premises that*
> *have been adapted and all locally managed by parents themselves.*
> *The one thing they have in common is the enthusiasm to provide a*
> *child care system, by parents and for parents* (Woodhead, 1996,
> p. 34).

This description would not be so striking were it not for the very different situation revealed by much current research into the relationships between parents and caregivers in North America:

> *Although the idea of 'parent-professional partnerships' is widely touted, few professionals have been trained or feel prepared to manage relationships with parents. Training is needed to prepare professionals to relate to parents as equals, not only as experts, and to help them understand the implications of cultural diversity for programme practices and relationships with families. Even with training, however, it will be difficult for professionals to invite parents to join them as full and equal partners in discussions of child care and its quality, since that necessarily involves sharing control and relinquishing status* (Larner and Phillips, 1994, p. 58).

A study of the multicultural *creches parentales* suggested that parental involvement of this scope not only produced a greater sense of community cohesion, but resulted in improved outcomes for both children and parents:

> *The study of* creches parentales *illustrates the possibilities for bridging the gulf between the micro-systems of* creche *and home, institutional and familial care, and professional and parental care giving.... Parental participation mediates the relation between social or ethnic membership and the level of cognitive interaction.... when parents... are present and involved in the daily educational activities of the parent-run day care centre, they participate, and get the children to participate, in more complex cognitive interactions .... The parents acquire a sense of pedagogical responsibility in the day care centre: they see themselves as 'teachers,' they think about pedagogical issues and thus develop their pedagogical capacity* (Woodhead, 1996, pp. 35, 36, and 79).

Parental and community involvement in child care supports the reflectiveness necessary for communities to engage in meaningful dialogue about quality child care and the role of child care in the lives of children, families, communities, and society. Without meaningful involvement, parental and community input to such processes as public meetings, charters, or strategic plans has a shaky foundation, and is easily co-opted by more powerful stakeholders, or by the particular dictates of the chosen process (e.g., the limited time of a public meeting; the accepted format of a strategic plan). If communities are not meaningfully involved in child care (or in any issue that affects their lives), the agenda is more or less set in advance. As Dahlberg and Asen point out in discussing Swedish efforts to renew the public sector:

> *The goals of economy and efficiency are presented as value-free, to be shared by everyone, while political and values-based questions, such as whose welfare the reforms improve, are avoided (Olsen, 1991).*

> *We are convinced that the question of how to restore legitimacy under existing conditions can only be tackled if the economic aspects are more closely connected with the pedagogical and values-based aspects of early childhood education. A prerequisite for this is that pedagogical practice and its functions must be made visible outside the world of schools and child care centres and become a part of public discourse... this requires the participation of a variety of concerned groups and a pedagogical practice based on empowerment, participation and reflective discourse between parents, staff, administrators and politicians* (Dahlberg and Asen, 1994, p. 166).

Dahlberg and Asen propose an "associative model" of child care governance to complement the existing political and professional models and to counter the increasingly powerful "market-oriented goal-governing model." To support the associative model, it is necessary "to create forums or arenas for discussion and reflection where people can engage as citizens with devotion and vision— not only as stakeholders positioned in an administrative perspective" (Dahlberg and Asen, 1994, p. 166). Within recent years, a number of "arenas" or "plazas" have developed in Sweden. Dahlberg and Asen believe these forums may provide a basis for the broader dialogue on child care quality which is called for in the associative model:

> *In these plazas politicians, administrators, teachers and other representatives come together to discuss different aspects of early childhood education.... The purpose is to establish a dialogue, characterized by debate, confrontation and exchange of experiences (Gothson, 1991). The plaza should not be seen primarily as the place for traders, but as the place for a dialogue between independent citizens. It is the symbol of a vibrant democracy. 'Bring forward your experience into the plaza' has been the motto for one of these plazas.... This motto refers to "the idea that exchange of experience creates respect for different approaches and conditions and counters superficial acceptance of models and general organizational solutions. ... It also refers to the idea that everyday and practical work must be the starting point for all leadership and development work"* (Gothson, 1991, p. 11, quoted in Dahlberg and Asen, 1994, p. 167).

Clearly it is impossible to uproot structures and processes that have grown up organically in other contexts and transplant them in a foreign environment. Nonetheless, it is impossible to read the description above and fail to notice the difference between the dialogue of the Swedish plaza and the exchanges that take place at most North American public meetings which are presumably designed to solicit public input, on child and family services or any other issue. In fact, it is reasonable to question whether public meetings and strategic planning processes can have any validity without structures and processes, adapted to our own contexts, that serve the purpose of the plazas: promoting the shared reflection of the entire community. Indeed, without such reflection, what is a community?

The Italian town of Reggio Emilia is an example of a community in which the child care setting itself functions as a kind of "arena" or "plaza." It is a community in which barriers to community development disappear or at least become permeable: barriers between adults and children, between care-givers and parents, between child care and the surrounding community, be-tween theory and practice, rhetoric and reality. In this environment, quality child care is not defined or discussed, then implemented; rather, it emerges in the process of definition and discussion itself, a process which engages the entire community in a constantly evolving "work in progress" (Gandini, 1992). Consider the concept of "documentation" in the Reggio Emilian con-text, particularly its contribution to quality child care and healthy child development:

> *Documentation as conceptualized in Reggio-Emilia requires that adults observe, interpret, articulate and share what it is that they have learned from young children in collaboration with one another. These additional challenges of articulation and sharing make the role of the teacher akin to that of a collaborative action researcher (New, 1994, p. 9).... Documentation's contribution to conceptions of quality and developmentally appropriate practices is especially apparent through its ability to entice adults into discussions regard-ing children's care and education.... The documentation panels that grace the halls and classroom walls of Reggio Emilian schools then serve as a starting place for prolonged deliberations among not only those who participate in the process itself but others who ultimately view its products as well. As parents and citizens of the commu-nity view and discuss the documentation, they benefit from and contribute to shared understandings of educational goals and stand-ards. In this way documentation promotes a sense of community as well as expanded knowledge of child development among all of the adults* (New, 1997, p. 10).

Like child care centres across Italy, Reggio Emilia has been required by law since 1971 to have its child care centres managed by families and representa-tives of social organizations. In addition, in Reggio Emilia there are formal meetings throughout the year for parents, teachers, and community members to discuss issues relating to the local child care programs (New, 1997). It is important to note, however, that the meetings and management structures could not, of themselves, guarantee meaningful community involvement in child care; they rest on a foundation of daily reflective practice and citizen involvement that is, in turn, rooted in a history and culture of civic involvement extending back hundreds of years (Putnam, 1993). Like the Swedish plazas, the approach to child care in Reggio Emilia cannot be replicated exactly in a different socio-political context. However, Reggio Emilia demonstrates that quality child care and community development can be both a means and an end (New, 1997). That possibility, and the means of realizing it in practice, are worth exploring in communities across North America.

Majority World

It is useful to review examples of community development in Majority World countries with respect to early childhood services because they provide important evidence that quality child care and meaningful community involvement can occur in contexts where material resources are scarce. As noted by Woodhead (1996):

> *Programmes that might be judged as "low resource" in materially affluent nations may in fact be "high resource" in a local context. Likewise, some on-the-face-of-it "high resource" programmes in affluent contexts might more appropriately be re-labelled "low resource," in terms of community endowment* (Woodhead, 1996, p. 51).

The example of Kenya serves as a particular example of a country which is economically challenged, but which has a strong national commitment to a community-based system of early childhood education (Swadener, Kabiru, and Njenga, 2000). Nearly all of Kenya's preschools, which provide care and education to approximately 30% of the 3 to 5 year-olds in the country, have developed since the country attained independence in 1963. The Kenyan early childhood system was founded on strong national values, rooted in centuries of African traditions. With independence, the Kenyan people adopted the motto "harambee," the Swahili word meaning "let us pull together." The spirit of harambee, as described in the early 1990s, continued to infuse the early childhood education system in Kenya:

> *There is much in our African heritage, especially concern and respect for others, the Harambee spirit, the dedication to integrity, and the respect for the family, which we must maintain. Indeed, we must strengthen these traditions because they, together with development, are the principal means by which we can enhance the moral and material well-being of our children. And it is through our children that we build the future of our children* (President Kenyatta, 1963, quoted in Kipkorir, 1993, p. 338).

Preschools in Kenya, frequently managed by parent/community committees, often with very few financial resources and equipment (Woodhead, 1996), have a greater claim to a community base than programs in many other countries:

> *To set up the programme in a particular location involves creating*
> *awareness in the community, formation of a committee, providing*
> *advice to the community, locating and equipping a site, and choos-*
> *ing a teacher. At the community and classroom level, running the*
> *programme can involve, in addition to classroom teaching, working*
> *with parents and community groups* (Myers, 1992, p. 6).

The Kenyan preschool curriculum draws on local stories, dances, and games, and exists in at least 13 different languages. The system is decentralised, with county, town, and municipal governments taking an active role in administering the programs in partnership with parent/community committees. While scarce resources do present challenges to the accessibility and availability of quality child care (Woodhead, 1996), the foundation of community involvement ensures that programs are responsive to diverse local needs and that community members are committed to the continued development of the child care system—key conditions for quality child care.

Colombia is another example of a country which, despite few resources, developed a community-based response to the needs of young children, while simultaneously attempting to strengthen the economic position of community members, particularly women. The Colombian programme of "Homes of Well-being" is a large-scale, neighbourhood-based system of family child care for children aged 0 to 7. The degree of community involvement in the design and delivery of the program is extensive:

> *Community members participate in an initial analysis of the com-*
> *munities [sic] needs for services, taking into account children's ages,*
> *family income and employment, and physical and environmental*
> *variables. (If services are needed that the programme cannot pro-*
> *vide, links are made to other organizations that can assist.) The*
> *community also determines the number of "Homes of Well-being"*
> *that will be necessary to meet children's needs and selects local*
> *women to become home day care mothers. Local management is the*
> *responsibility of a board consisting of parents who are responsible*
> *for purchases and payments to the community mothers.... Day care*
> *mothers receive training in the care and development of children as*
> *well as in family and community relationships, and in nutrition*
> *and health* (Myers, 1993, p. 85).

In Majority World countries, as in North America and Europe, there are many programs which focus on the child or the caregiver, using community involvement as a means to accomplish the desired goal (Myers, 1994; Dombro et al., 1996; Healthy Child Development Project, 1996). A different approach, however, is to view children as the entry point for community development, which, as noted by Myers, "is seen as the most appropriate means for fostering the improved development of children in the long run" (Myers, 1994, p. 73). One particularly striking example of this approach is the PROMESA project, which began in 1978 in the Choco region of Colombia. The PROMESA project was based on the assumption that individuals must have direct involvement in the intellectual, physical, economic, and sociocultural conditions that impact their well-being and development. As described by the project coordinators, what began as a project focused on the development of children soon evolved into a comprehensive community development process led by community members:

> *The program began by encouraging groups of mothers, under the leadership of "promotoras," to stimulate the physical and intellectual development of their preschool children by playing games with them. Gradually, during the meetings the mothers started to identify other problems related to topics such as health, nutrition, environmental sanitation, vocational training, income generation and cultural activities. Over time therefore, as individuals gained confidence and developed a greater understanding of their overall needs, PROMESA expanded into an integrated community development project, with the entire community participating in one or more aspects of the program* (International Center for Education and Human Development, quoted in Myers, 1994, p. 73).

A number of other programs are underway in Majority World countries that support children and families, while promoting community dialogue on early childhood programs and other issues affecting the community. Chile's Parents and Children Programme (PPH) is a good example. The program integrates the goals of healthy child development, personal growth for adults, and community organization, as follows:

> *To achieve these goals, weekly meetings are organized in participating rural communities.... The meetings are timed to coincide with a radio broadcast over a local radio station which uses radio dramas and other devices to pose a problem and to stimulate discussion. Discussions at the meetings centered, originally, around different aspects of the up-bringing of children.... These topics have broadened to include questions related directly to earning a livelihood. Within the project, the child development goal is also promoted through preschool exercises for children.... An evaluation of the programme has shown positive effects on the children, on their parents, and on the community at large (Richards, 1985).... The evaluation identified changes in adult attitudes and perceptions... [in] the ease with which they reached agreements, and their ability to act on conclusions. The basic change identified was from "empathy" to participation in constructive activities as a sense of self-worth was strengthened"* (Myers, 1993, pp. 92-94).

As in the discussion of community development in North America and Europe, the examples above provide a snapshot of only a fraction of the activity underway with respect to early childhood development in Majority World countries. As noted previously, many Majority World countries are successful in creating community-based early childhood services of good quality with few economic resources. In these countries, the importance of mobilizing people—often the greatest resource—is particularly evident. In some respects, Majority World countries are more successful than more affluent countries in providing coordinated, community-based services to children and families, precisely because they are constructing their systems from the ground up. By contrast, North American and European countries are faced with a different challenge: reforming highly developed service infrastructures which have grown up independently and which have become entrenched in bureaucratic structures and traditions that tend to exclude community perspectives (Pence and Benner, 1997). As such, Majority World countries provide useful examples of alternative approaches to the delivery of services to children and families; and, given their relative lack of financial wealth, provide clear evidence of the contribution of community development in promoting quality child care.

First Nations Partnership Programs

In Canada, evaluation research focusing on our own work as partners with eight First Nations community groups in British Columbia and Saskatchewan yields insights into how building capacity for quality child care can be synchronous with community development (First Nations Partnership Programs, 2001). Through these partnerships, a unique approach has evolved, which we call the 'Generative Curriculum Model', in which a socially inclusive and culturally reconstructive approach is the means to achieving both quality child care and community development (Pence, 1999).

From 1989 to the present, eight different First Nations groups, consisting of 47 communities in total, have initiated partnerships with a team based at the University of Victoria. In each case, the goal has been to strengthen the capacity of community members to meet the developmental needs of young children and families through the provision of culturally sustaining, community-appropriate child care programs and other services (Ball and Pence, 1999). This goal is consistent with priorities articulated in the Canadian Royal Commission on Aboriginal Peoples:

> *Our recommendations emphasize the importance of protecting children through culturally-appropriate services, by attending to maternal and child health, by providing appropriate early childhood education, and by making high quality child care available, all with the objective of complementing the family's role in nurturing young children* (Canadian Royal Commission on Aboriginal Peoples, Vol. 5, Ch. 1, s4.1).

All of the First Nations that initiated the partnership program had identified enhanced capacity to provide quality care for children as a top priority in
their overall community social and economic development strategies. For
example, in 1989, the first community partner to initiate a community-partici-
patory child care training program formulated their community development
strategy as follows:

> *The First Nations of the Meadow Lake Tribal Council believe that a*
> *child care program developed, administered, and operated by their*
> *own people is a vital component to their vision of sustainable growth*
> *and development. It impacts every sector of their long term plans*
> *as they prepare to enter the twenty-first century. It will be children*
> *who inherit the struggle to retain and enhance the people's culture,*
> *language, and history; who continue the quest for economic progress*
> *for a better quality of life; and who move forward with a strength-*
> *ened resolve to plan their own destiny* (Meadow Lake Tribal Coun-
> cil Vision Statement, 1989).

Systematic evaluation of the partnership programs documented positive outcomes for individuals who completed the training and subsequently have
become employed in child and family services. Across the seven partnership
programs that were evaluated, 60 to 100% of students completed the 2 year,
diploma level training. Most program graduates have 'given back' to their
community by remaining and starting new programs: 87% are currently employed, primarily in programs for children 0 to 6 years of age. Children's
programs initiated or staffed by program graduates have included: centre-
based daycares in licensed care facilities; in-home family daycares; Aboriginal
Head Start; infant development programs; home-school liaison programs;
parent support programs; individualized supported child care for special needs;
language enhancement programs; and after-school care programs. Immediate
and extended family members of students have reported enhanced commitment to effective parenting and family cohesion. Program evaluation research
also yielded abundant evidence of positive outcomes for the partner communities as a whole, including: cultural revitalization; community-wide advocacy for child well-being initiatives; community empowerment; development
of a cohort of skilled community leaders; social cohesion; cultural healing/
recovery of cultural pride. As described by a representative of the Meadow
Lake Tribal Council:

> *There's much more talk in the communities these days about im-*
> *proving the environment for children. There's definitely a ripple*
> *effect. And it took a program like this to get things rolling.*

Evaluation of the First Nations Partnership Programs provided evidence
that the key to success in these capacity building initiatives was the socially
inclusive nature of the approach. As the employment and training director at

Mount Currie First Nation who initiated the training program in her community described:

> *There was extensive community involvement all the way through, from planning and delivering the training program to creating and delivering the new services for children and families here in our community. The program wasn't just for the students who took it. It involved the elders, other parents, children, and other community members who participated in various ways. Everyone benefited and everyone will continue to benefit because our cultural traditions are integrated right into the programs we are developing through our social services department.*

First Nations Partnership Programs continue to be delivered through partnerships between First Nations communities and a team at the University of Victoria. In each case, the program is operated by First Nations administrators, who recruit and contract with instructors, intergenerational facilitators, and students. The training program is delivered in the community, enabling many community members in addition to those who register as students to participate in various ways in the program delivery. In most of the partnership programs, this has led to the consolidation of an inclusive, enduring, mutually supportive 'community of learners.'

The two year diploma program in Early Childhood Education is designed with an 'open architecture' requiring community input into course content and community involvement throughout the teaching and learning process. In each partner community, instructors and Elders who have taught the program facilitate dialogue among community members about their own contemporary and historical child care practices and about Euro-western research and practices for promoting optimal child development.

This open-ended, co-constructed curriculum model encourages and accommodates variations from one community partner to another with regard to socio-cultural characteristics and local circumstances that shape child care. Elders' involvement in co-constructing the training curriculum has resulted in a good 'fit' between the attitudes and skills reinforced through the training program and the specific goals, needs, and circumstances of the children and families in their particular cultural community. Louise Underwood, an Elder in that partnership with Cowichan Tribes, described:

> *In order to ensure that our culture would be reflected in the structure of children's services, we had to bring the training program to the community and bring the community into the training program. It was like a big circle.*

Because the community is actively involved in co-creating and delivering the program, the community members who complete the training program experience high levels of community support and participation in programs for children and families that they initiate following program completion.

The core message in the findings of evaluation is that capacity building initiatives must be anchored deeply in the community's context, existing strengths, potential for cultural reconstruction, and ability to push forward their own agendas towards self-identified goals. Research evaluating the programs identified several interacting factors that account for the synchronous progress towards provision of quality child care and community development goals in the partnering communities:

(1) Community initiated and driven agenda.

(2) Partnership, involving reciprocal guided participation of willing community and institutional partners.

(3) Community-based delivery that enabled access and community inclusion in all phases of program planning, delivery, and follow-up.

(4) Student cohort involvement in capacity building that was always accountable to—and supported by—the community.

(5) Open architecture curriculum that depended upon cultural input by community members.

(6) Intergenerational facilitation of cultural teaching and learning involving Elders.

The evaluation showed that the *combined effects* of these program elements, embedded in a community-driven agenda, were causally related to positive program outcomes consistent with each partner community's child care and social development objectives. At present dollars are being sought to continue the evaluation process, following up on children and families who have participated in the services that have been developed in the communities since the partnership training and those that are staffed by graduates of the program.

CONCLUSION

This chapter has reviewed findings of program evaluations, anecdotal commentaries, and interpretive analyses of program models that link community development, cultural congruence, and quality child care. The range of examples chosen illustrate some of the approaches taken within and beyond a North American context to foster an environment that would support public engagement in issues relating to the needs of children and families. The examples chosen do not necessarily represent the most evolved state of community development within a global context. They do, nonetheless, highlight some of the movements underway that, at the very least, provide a starting point for outlining the foundations upon which a genuine public commitment to children and families might be constructed.

Insights derived from understanding these examples are only as useful as there are willing "users" who are positioned to make a difference in how we think about quality child care and how to achieve it within the widely varying community and cultural contexts in which children and families live. Training and development assistance institutions, policy-making bodies, and agencies which are involved in establishing and enforcing criteria for funding and delivering training and services for children all have a role. The examples underscore the need for institutions to: open up the foundations of how programs to develop and refine services for children are conceived and delivered; how optimal child care and development is defined; and how communities can play leading roles in ensuring quality child care while strengthening social cohesion and furthering community development goals.

REFERENCES

Adams, P., and Nelson, K. (1995). *Reinventing human services: Community- and family-centred practice.* New York, NY: Aldine de Gruyter.

Ball, J. (2001). *First nations partnership programs generative curriculum model: Program evaluation report.* Victoria, BC: FNPP.

Ball, J., and Pence, A. (1999). Beyond developmentally appropriate practice: Developing community and culturally appropriate practice. *Young Children,* March, 46-50.

Bernhard, J.K., Corson, P., Gonzalez-Mena, J., Stairs, N., and Langford, R. (1996, June). *Culturally situated explorations of child development. A home visit project in an early childhood education preparation program.* Paper presented at the annual meeting of the Canadian Association for Researchers in Early Childhood Education, St. Catherine's, Ontario.

Bouchard, C. (1996). *The community as participative learning environment: The case of Centraide of Greater Montreal 1,2,3 Go! project.* Paper presented to the Canadian Institute for Advanced Research, 14th conference of the International Society for the Study of Behavioural Development, Quebec, August 1996.

Bradley, R.H., Caldwell, B.M., Fitzgerald, J.A., Morgan, A.G., and Rock, S.L. (1996). Experiences in day care and social competence among maltreated children. *Child Abuse and Neglect,* 10, 181-189.

Carnegie Corporation of New York (1994). *Starting points: Meeting the needs of our youngest children.* Waldorf, MD: Carnegie Corporation of New York.

Cochran, M. (1991a). Child care and the empowerment process. *Networking Bulletin— Empowerment and Family Support,* 2(1), 1-3.

Cochran, M. (1991b). The Minnesota early childhood family education program: An interview with Lois Engstrom, Program Supervisor. *Networking Bulletin—Empowerment and Family Support,* 2(1), 4-9.

Cochran, M. (1993). *International handbook of child care policies and programs.* Westport, CT and London: Greenwood Press.

Cornell Empowerment Project (October 1989). Evaluation consistent with the empowerment process. *Networking Bulletin—Empowerment and Family Support,* 9(2), 10-12.

Dahlberg, G., and Asen, G. (1994). Evaluation and regulation: A question of empowerment. In P. Moss and A. Pence (Eds.), *Valuing quality in early childhood services* (pp. 157-171). London: Paul Chapman Publishing Ltd.

Dahlberg, G., Moss, P., and Pence, A. (1999). *Beyond quality in early childhood education and care: Postmodern perspectives.* London: Falmer Press.

Dalais, C., Landers, C., and Fuertes, P. (1996). *Early childhood development revisited: From policy formulation to programme implementation.* Florence, Italy: Unicef.

Doherty, G., and Stuart, B. (1996). *A profile of quality in Canadian child care centres.* Guelph, ON: Department of Family Studies, University of Guelph.

Doherty, G., Lero, D.S., Goelman, H., Tougas, J., and LaGrange, A. (in press). *Caring and learning environments: Quality in regulated family child care across Canada.* Guelph, ON: Centre for families, work and well-being, Department of Family Relations and Applied Nutrition, University of Guelph.

Dombro, A., O'Donnell, N., Galinsky, E., Melcher, S., and Farber, A. (1996). *Community mobilization: Strategies to support young children and their families.* New York, NY: Families and Work Institute.

European Commission Network on Childcare (January 1996). *A review of services for young children in the European Union.* London: Author.

Fullan, M., and Miles, M. (June 1992). Getting reform right: What works and what doesn't. *Phi Delta Kappan*, x(x), 745-752.

Gandini, L. (1992). *A message from Loris Malaguzzi. An interview by Lella Gandini, April, 1992, La Villetta School, Reggio Emilia.* Amherst, Massachusetts: Performanetics.

Goelman, H., and Pence, A.R. (1988). Children in three types of child care experiences: Quality of care and developmental outcomes. *Early Childhood Development and Care*, 33, 67-76.

Harms, T., and Clifford, R.M. (1980). *Early Childhood Environment Rating Scale.* New York: Teachers College Press.

Harms, T., Clifford, R.M., and Cryer, D. (1998). *Early childhood environmental rating scale— Revised.* New York: Teachers College Press.

Healthy Child Development Project (1996). *Healthy children, healthy communities. A compendium of approaches from across Canada.* Ottawa, ON: Author.

Howes, C. (1990). Can the age of entry into child care and the quality of child care predict adjustment in kindergarten? *Developmental Psychology*, 26, 292-303.

Howes, C., and Smith, E.W. (1995). Relations among child care quality, teacher behaviour, children's play activities, emotional security, and cognitive activity in child care. *Early Childhood Research Quarterly*, 10, 381-404.

Jensen, C. (1994). Fragments for a discussion about quality. In P. Moss and A. Pence (Eds.), *Valuing quality in early childhood services* (pp. 142-156). London, Paul Chapman Publishing Ltd.

Kagitcibasi, C. (1996). *Family and human development across cultures: A view from the other side.* London: Erlbaum.

Katz, L. (1996). Child development knowledge and teacher preparation: Confronting assumptions. *Early Childhood Research Quarterly*, 11, 135-146.

Keating, D., and Hertzman, C. (Eds.) (1999). *Developmental health as the wealth of nations.* New York: Guilford Press.

Kipkorir, L. (1993). Kenya. In M. Cochran (Ed.), *International handbook of child care policies and programs* (pp. 333-352). Westport, Connecticut and London: Greenwood Press.

Kretzmann, J., and McKnight, J. (1993). *Building communities from the inside out: A path toward finding and mobilizing a community's assets.* Chicago, IL: ACTA Publications.

Langsted, O. (1994). Looking at quality from the child's perspective. In P. Moss and A. Pence (Eds.), *Valuing quality in early childhood services* (pp. 28-42). London: Paul Chapman Publishing Ltd.

Larner, M., and Phillips, D. (1994). Defining and valuing quality as a parent. In P. Moss and A. Pence (Eds.), *Valuing quality in early childhood services* (pp. 43-60). London: Paul Chapman Publishing Ltd.

Lubeck, S. (1996). Deconstructing "child development knowledge" and "teacher preparation." *Early Childhood Research Quarterly*, 11, 147-167.

Masten, A. (Ed.) (1999). *Cultural processes in child development: The Minnesota Symposia on Child Psychology*. Vol. 29. Mahwah, NJ: Lawrence Erlbaum.

Mayall, B. (1996). *Children, health and the social order*. Buckingham and Philadelphia: Open University Press.

McCain, M.N., and Mustard, J.F. (1999). *Early years study final report: Reversing the real brain drain*. Toronto, ON: Publications Ontario.

McKnight, J. (1995). *The careless society: Community and its counterfeits*. New York: Basic Books, HarperCollins Publishers Inc.

Melhuish, E.C. (2001). The quest for quality in early day care and preschool experience continues. *International Journal of Behavioural Development*, 25(1), 1-6.

Morton, C. (1966). *British Columbia's child, youth and family serving system. Recommendations for change*. Victoria, BC: Queen's Printer for British Columbia.

Moss,P. (1997). Early childhood services in Europe. *Policy Options*, 18(1), 27-30.

Moss, P. (1994). Defining quality: Values, stakeholders and processes. In P. Moss and A. Pence (Eds.), *Valuing quality in early childhood services* (pp. 1-9). London: Paul Chapman Publishing Ltd.

Moss, P., and Pence, A. (Eds.) (1994). *Valuing quality in early childhood services*. London: Paul Chapman Publishing Ltd.

Myers, R. (1992, February). *Towards an analysis of the costs and effectiveness of community-based early childhood education in Kenya*. Unpublished report, the Consultative Group on Early Childhood Care and Development.

Myers, R. (1993). *Toward a fair start for children*. Programming for early childhood care and development in the developing world. Paris: UNESCO.

Myers, R. (1994, April). *Early childhood care and development: Needs and possible approaches*. Unpublished report prepared for the InterAmerican Development Bank, the Consultative Group on Early Childhood Care and Development.

New, R. (1997). Reggio Emilia's commitment to children and community: A reconceptualization of quality and DAP. *Canadian Children*, Spring, 7-12.

North Carolina Department of Human Resources (1994). *Smart Start*. Raleigh, NC: North Carolina Department of Human Resources.

Nsamenang, A.B. (1992). *Human development in cultural context*. London: Sage.

Pence, A., and Moss, P. (1994). Towards an inclusionary approach in defining quality. In P. Moss and A. Pence (Eds.), *Valuing quality in early childhood services* (pp. 172-180). London: Paul Chapman Publishing Ltd.

Pence, A., and Benner, A. (1997). *Child care in the village: Reconceptualizing child and family services*. Paper prepared for the Child Care Branch, Ministry for Children and Families.

Pence, A. (1999). "It takes a village...", and new roads to get there. In D. Keating and C. Hertzman (Eds.), *Developmental health as the wealth of nations* (pp. 322-336). New York: Guilford Press.

Peters, R. DeV., and Russell, C.C. (1996). Promoting development to prevent disorder. The Better Beginnings, Better Futures Project. In R. DeV. Peters and R.J. McMahon (Eds.), *Preventing childhood disorders, substance abuse and delinquency* (pp. 19-47). Thousand Oaks, CA: Sage Publications.

Phillips, D. (Ed.) (1987). *Predictors of quality child care*. Washington, DC: National Association for the Education of Young Children.

Putnam, R. (1993). *Making democracy work: Civic traditions in modern Italy*. Princeton, NJ: Princeton University Press.

Qvortrup, J., Bardy, J., Sgritta, G., and Wintersberger, H. (Eds.) (1994). *Childhood matters: Social theory, practice and politics.* Aldershoot, UK: Avebury Press.

Rosenthal, M.K. (1999). Out of home child care research: A cultural perspective. *International Journal of Behavioral Development, 23,* 477-518.

Schorr, L. (1988). *Within our reach: Breaking the cycle of disadvantage.* New York, London, Toronto, Sidney, and Auckland: Doubleday.

Shaeffer, S. (1995). *Community partnerships in early childhood development.* Paper presented at the Workship on Early Childhood Development Policy, International Child Development Centre, Florence, Italy, May 31 - June 6, 1995.

Shonkoff, J.P., and Phillips, D.A. (Eds.) (2000). *From neurons to neighborhoods: The science of early childhood development.* National Research Council and Institute of Medicine. Washington, DC: National Academy Press.

Smith, A., and Farquhar, S.E. (1994). The New Zealand experience of charter development in early childhood services. In P. Moss and A. Pence (Eds.), *Valuing quality in early childhood services* (pp. 123-141). London: Paul Chapman Publishing Ltd.

Stott, F., and Bowman, B. (1996). Child development knowledge: A slippery base for practice. *Early Childhood Research Quarterly, 11,* 169-183.

Swadener, B.B., Kabiru, M., and Njenga, A. (2000). *Does the village still raise the child?* Albany, NY: State University of New York Press.

To, R., Cadarette, S.M., and Liu, Y. (2000). Child care arrangement and preschool development. *Canadian Journal of Public Health, 91*(6), 418-422.

van der Eyken, W. (1991, September). Evaluating the process of empowerment. *Networking Bulletin—Empowerment and Family Support, 2*(2), 8-12.

Woodhead, M. (1996). *In search of the rainbow: Pathways to quality in large-scale programmes for young disadvantaged children.* Early Childhood Development: Practice and Reflections. Number 10. The Hague: Bernard van Leer Foundation.

Patterns and Trends in Children in the Care of the Province of British Columbia: Ecological, Policy, and Cultural Perspectives

L.T. Foster and M. Wright
Ministry for Children and Families, Victoria, BC

INTRODUCTION

Children and youth who come into the care of the state are highly vulnerable and have relatively poor health status (Millar, 1998). Children in care (c-i-c) "typically have histories of pre-natal exposure to drugs or alcohol as well as experience of neglect, abuse, and fragmented medical care" (Silver, 1999, p. 150). They also have "up to seven times more emotional adjustment problems, developmental delays and acute and chronic health problems than a comparative group of poor children" (Rosenfeld et al., 1997 as quoted by Baum, Crase, and Crase, 2001, p. 202). Sullivan and Knutson (2000) have shown that children with disabilities are 3.4 times more likely to be maltreated than non-disabled peers. Preliminary analysis of BC data suggests that over 50% of all c-i-c entering care have some form of disability (Kendall, 2001a). Furthermore, the low birth weight rate for BC c-i-c is twice the rate of the general population (102.23/1,000 compared to 51.73/1,000). These risk factors often result in substantially higher death rates (Kendall, 2001a, b; Barth and Blackwell, 1988; Ontario Child Mortality Task Force, 1997; Thompson and Newman, 1995). In addition, these factors also produce life long disadvantages and vulnerabilities. Cook-Fong (2000) has noted that adults who were in care as children had significantly higher depression scores, lower scores on marital happiness, less intimate parental relationships, and higher incidence of social isolation than adults who were never in care placements. These children have lower than average high school graduation rates and nearly 50% of those in school are in special education classes (Pallan, 2001) and often have difficulty in the transition from youth to adulthood. Many will have passed through numerous foster homes, with little permanency of care. Further, a large proportion of homeless people have passed through the child welfare system (Paliavin, 1993; Downing-Orr, 1996; Roman and Wolfe, 1997; Zlotnick, Kronstadt, and Klee, 1998) and about one third of street youth in BC communities had been in government care (McCreary Centre Society, 2001). These children are often from, and unfortunately continue in the poorest socio-economic groups in society, thus perpetuating the intergenerational effects of poverty, poor educational achievements, uncertain housing with frequent moves, earlier and longer episodes among the homeless population, and insecure parenting. A survey of youth in care in BC indicated that approximately one third did not have a regular doctor; almost 20% did not receive an explanation of their health problem and how it should be treated when they visited a doctor; and almost 40% did not feel that conversations with physicians were kept confidential. Many felt disrespected, stereotyped, judged, and patronized by health care professionals, making it difficult to discuss important issues like birth control and substance abuse because of fear of being judged (Kotovich, 1998).

This chapter provides an historical analysis of c-i-c in BC. It discusses reasons for coming into care and how these have changed over time. It links changes in patterns of c-i-c to demographic, economic, and policy influences. Within BC it examines ecological influences on the geographical patterns of c-i-c recognizing that "child maltreatment is multiply determined" (Pierson, Nelson, and Prilleltensky, 2000, p. 30). Where data allow, comparisons are made with other jurisdictions in Canada and to a lesser extent, in the US. Within BC, differing time periods for trend analysis are used based on the availability of comparative data.

CHILD PROTECTION REPORTS—REASONS FOR BEING IN CARE

Children in care are those who have been removed from their families by child protection workers because of actual or perceived high risk of abuse and neglect or an inability of parents to look after them. In addition, some parents voluntarily ask the province to care for their children because of the high health needs of a child or other factors such as parental illness or temporary parental crisis. Table 6.1 summarizes for the 12 month period ending March 31 the fundamental reasons children were taken into care by MCF over the period April 1, 1997 to March 31, 2000. As there may be up to three reasons recorded for a child needing care the total number of reasons exceeds the total number of c-i-c. Further, because a child can be in care from birth to age 18, these data reflect the total number of c-i-c at that time and not just the incidence of new cases.

By far the most common reason for a child being in care relates to protection concerns (75.4%). These include: physical, sexual, or emotional harm; neglect because a parent is unable or unwilling to care for a child; parents have abandoned a child; or death of the parent. Protection concerns have grown in both absolute and relative terms in the last 4 years (from 9,489 to 13,066 and 71.6% to 80% respectively in the period March 1997 to March 2000). Voluntary care agreements (comprising 7.6% on average in the 4 year period) cover temporary crises such as a parent receiving medical treatment or requiring time to improve parenting skills. Special needs agreements (15.6% for the same 4 year period) cover conditions related to medical fragility, behavioural, developmental, emotional, physical, or mental conditions of a child. These have diminished in terms of relative importance over the 4 year period although analysis undertaken elsewhere has shown that in the 10 year period preceding March 1996, between 10% and 15% of all c-i-c had physical disabilities (with or without intellectual or behavioural disabilities) and a further 40% had a behavioural and/or intellectual disability without a physical disability (Kendall, a, b, forthcoming).

Table 6.1   Reasons for being in care

	March 31 1997		March 31 1998		March 31 1999		March 31 2000		4 Year Average	
	#	%	#	%	#	%	#	%	#	%
Voluntary care agreement	1,247	9.4	1,364	8.7	1,238	7.4	866	5.3	1,179	7.6
Special need agreement	2,313	17.5	2,495	16.0	2,649	15.9	2,210	13.5	2,417	15.6
Protection need	9,489	71.6	11,517	73.9	12,574	75.4	13,066	80.0	11,662	75.4
Other	204	1.5	213	1.4	206	1.3	189	1.2	203	1.4
Total	13,253	100.0	15,589	100.0	16,667	100.0	16,331	100.0	15,461	100.0

Source: Based on Ministry for Children and Families Social Work Management Information System.

There are many pathways to care. Children come to the attention of government primarily through concern notification (usually by phone to a government worker) by different groups of people who come into contact with children. These include family members, school teachers and daycare workers, friends and neighbours, and state officials including police, health professionals, and government ministry workers (Table 6.2).

MCF data show that from 1993/94 (April to March) to 1999/2000 there was a 26.8% increase in the number of child protection reports received, a rate that far exceeds the rate of child population growth in this period. Schools were a main source of reports (15.3%) over the 3 year period 1997/98 to 1999/2000. Other jurisdictions have also noted that most reports come from the school system (Trocmé, McPhee, Tam, and Hay, 1994; Sedlack and Broadhurst, 1996). As has been noted elsewhere, "School personnel and teachers in particular are in a unique position to identify suspected cases of abuse because of their daily contact with children in the classroom and lunchroom, on the playground, and in after-school activities" (Health Canada, 1999a, p.1). Community professionals (13.6%) and parents themselves (11.1%) requesting help are the next most common sources of reports. Other sources include friends and neighbours (9.8%), and concerned citizens (8.8%), and relatives (7.1%), although these groups have shown a relative decline in reports over the 3 year period. By contrast, police reports (9.9%) have increased substantially over the 3 year period and are now the third most important reporting source. In recent years (likely as a conse-quence of the Gove Inquiry—see Chapter 8), police tend to bring all investi-gated cases of family violence to the attention of child protection workers as well as drug related offences. Health professionals (5.3%) account for a re-markably low percentage of concern reports, "given the high likelihood of their encountering maltreated children in a medical setting, and the expecta-tion that they are most qualified to diagnose and treat certain types of child abuse" (Health Canada, 1999b, p. 1). One reason, however, for such a low reporting percentage relates to the observation that many health care profes-sionals, despite public expectation, feel that they are not appropriately trained to identify the signs of abuse, neglect, and maltreatment (Health Canada, 1999b).

Table 6.2   Protection calls by fiscal year (April to March) by source

	1997/98 (%)	1998/99 (%)	1999/00 (%)	3 Year Average
School	14.9	15.3	15.5	15.3
Community professional	13.5	13.6	13.8	13.6
Parent	10.9	11.3	11.0	11.1
Friend/neighbour	10.2	9.9	9.2	9.8
Concerned citizen	9.9	8.3	8.1	8.8
Police	8.7	9.4	11.5	9.9
Relative	7.5	7.2	6.7	7.1
Health professional	5.6	5.1	5.1	5.3
Ministry worker	5.5	6.6	6.2	6.1
Anonymous	3.4	3.2	3.1	3.2
Subject child	3.0	2.9	2.8	2.9
Financial assistance worker	2.5	2.8	2.8	2.7
Preschool/daycare	0.9	0.9	0.9	0.9
Other	3.5	3.5	6.1	4.4
	100.0	100.0	100.0	100.0
Total Calls	31,378	33,036	34,700	33,038

Source: Based on Ministry for Children and Families Social Work Management Information System.

Boom-Bust-Echo-Bang: C-i-c Trends in the Last 50 Years

The trend in c-i-c counts in the period between the mid-1950s and early 1980s is a function of increased concern about child abuse which came to the public's attention through publicization of the "battered child syndrome" (Kempe, Silverman, Steele, Droegemueller, and Silver, 1962; Kempe and Helfer, 1972), and also a function of the demographic composition of the child population in the province (Foot and Stoffman, 1996). First, there was rapid growth throughout the 1950s and 1960s peaking in the early 1970s, followed by a two decade long reduction until late 1993. Since that time there has been a very rapid growth in the number of c-i-c (Figure 6.1) to about 10,000, or approximately 1 in 100 of all children in the province. A predictive model developed in 1983 was able to "explain," at least retroactively, most of the c-i-c figures based purely on the number of children in the province in the 0-4, 5-9, 10-14, and 15-18 year age groupings (Merner, 1983). While the model slightly underestimated the c-i-c count in the late 1970s and the early 1980s, the predictions forward were substantially overestimated (Figure 6.2), even after retroactively recalibrating the model based on actual population counts, rather than the population forecasts available in 1983. Only in the last couple of years have c-i-c figures come close to those predicted based on the number of children in the age cohorts. All of this increase has occurred since the end of 1993, when the number of c-i-c was around 6,000. Six years later, there were over 10,000 c-i-c, which is very close to the number that the recalibrated 1983 model predicted.

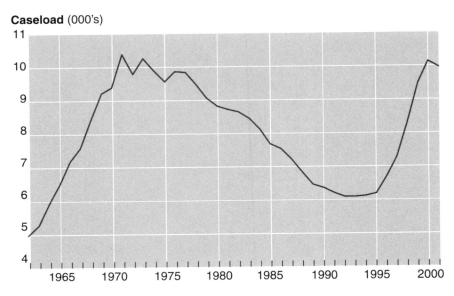

Figure 6.1 Growth in c-i-c population, 1961-2000

Caseload (000's)

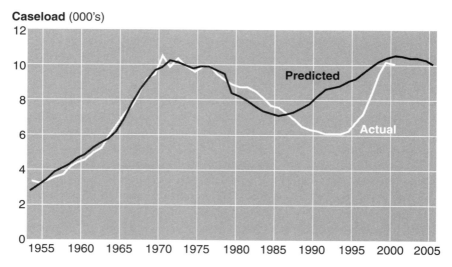

Figure 6.2   Predicted c-i-c versus actual, 1953-2005

Examining the demographic composition over time shows that the number of c-i-c, as a percentage of all children in the 0-18 age group, grew from about 0.8% in 1961, peaked at just a little over 1.3% in 1970 and then fell to just less than 0.7% in early 1994 (Figure 6.3). Since that time, growth has been slightly more rapid than in the 1960s to reach over 1% in 2000. The four main age cohorts, however, do not follow this trend equally (Figure 6.4a and Figure 6.4b).

Percent

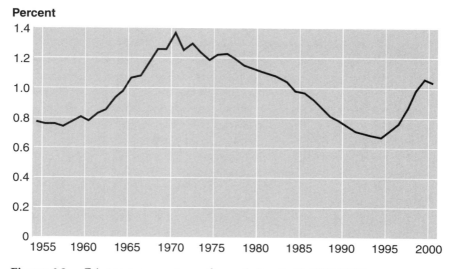

Figure 6.3   C-i-c as a percentage of population 0-18, 1954-2000

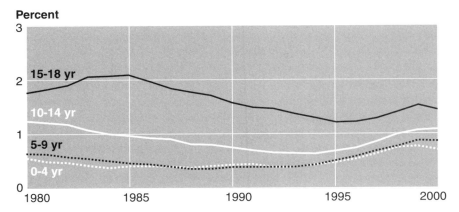

Figure 6.4a   C-i-c caseload as percentage of BC population 0-18, 1980-2000

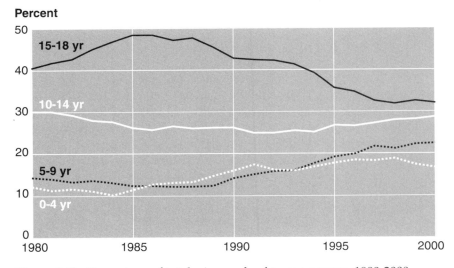

Figure 6.4b   Percentage of total c-i-c caseload to age groups, 1980-2000

15-18 Age Cohort:

This cohort has always been the largest group both relatively and absolutely, varying between 48% in 1986 and 33% in 1998 of all c-i-c over the last 2 decades (Figure 6.4b). While some of this variation can be explained by the size of the provincial cohort, there are clearly other factors at work. Approximately 2.1% of all 15 to 18 year olds were in care in 1985—an historical high. By 1995, this had fallen to 1.25% but by mid-2000 it had increased again to 1.5% (Figure 6.4a). (Part of the reason for this recent increase is related to government policy, which will be discussed later.)

10-14 Age Cohort:

Figure 6.4b shows the percentage in this cohort ranging from 30% in 1980 to a low of about 25% in 1992. The percentage of all children in the province in that age group has fallen from a high of 1.3% in 1980, to a low of 0.6% in 1994 and has climbed since to over 1%.

0-4 and 5-9 Age Cohorts:

Between March 1980 and March 2000, the pattern of c-i-c in these two age cohorts has been remarkably similar, with a slightly higher percentage of c-i-c among 5 to 9 year olds.

PROGRAMS FOR AT-RISK CHILDREN

While the demographics of the child population can explain much of the long term trend in c-i-c, particularly between 1953 and 1985, the major discrepancy between predicted and actual numbers between 1986 and 1998 requires further investigation. Other programs used for serving at-risk children are examined to evaluate their contribution to this difference.

When children cannot be adequately cared for by their parent(s), the BC government has available three alternate programs to taking or keeping a child in care. The first is supervision orders. This program was introduced with the replacement of the *1939 Protection of Children Act* by the *Family and Child Services Act* in 1981, following the work of the Berger Royal Commission on Family and Children's Law (Armitage, 1998). Supervision orders allow children to return to their families under supervision of the government. Such orders have the effect of lowering the c-i-c count.

The two other programs are part of the income security safety net (once equally cost-shared with the federal government). The Child in the Home of a Relative (CIHR) program allows children whose parents are unable to care for them to be placed with a relative who can claim a subsidy from government. The Underage Income Assistance (U19) program provides independent income assistance to older teens under the age of 19. These programs act as substitutes to taking a child into care under certain circumstances. Figure 6.5 shows the trends in children in these three programs between 1980 and 2000, along with the number of children in the c-i-c program.

The predictive model described above estimated that the c-i-c count would increase from the mid-1980s onwards, following the expected increase in the child population in the province, but it did not. The continuing fall in c-i-c between 1986 and 1994 can in part be explained by continuing growth in the CIHR and U19 programs, and (to a much lesser extent) by supervision orders. In 1980, the number of CIHR was about 2,000, and rose between 1982 and 1985, following the recession in the province. By 1986, the number of CIHR had fallen back to pre-recession figures. Between 1986 and 1995, however, the

Number of children (000's)

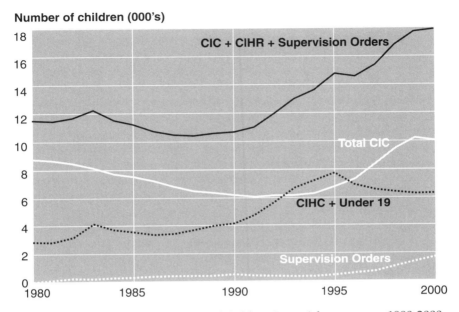

Figure 6.5 Trends in the number of children in at-risk programs, 1980-2000

number doubled to over 4,000, following the promotion of family support (rather than taking children into care) by the governments of the day during this period. First the Social Credit government invested heavily in family preservation programs in the late 1980s. Second the New Democratic government at the beginning of the 1990s also was sympathetic to keeping children with families, including relatives, and providing additional supports. Since 1995 the number has tended to level off following increased scrutiny of income assistance programs, as well as concern around the extent of government's revised liability for children in these two programs, as a result of new child protection legislation introduced in early 1996.

For the U19 program, there were approximately 1,900 youth receiving independent income assistance from about 1983 to 1990. In the first 4 years of the 1990s this number doubled to nearly 3,900 in 1994, after which time it has fallen back to levels prevalent in the 1980s. The growth in the early 1990s for U19 was part of the then New Democratic government's approach to help deal with poverty issues. In the same period, there was also a rapid growth in the number of children in income assistance families (Figure 6.6), which peaked in 1995, and has since fallen back dramatically.

Supervision orders, on the other hand, have had relatively little impact on alleviating c-i-c until the middle to late 1990s. They have grown from about 300 in 1996 to over 1,600 in 2000. A revision to legislation in June 1998 allowed some children to be covered by supervision orders, without having been in

Number of children (000's)

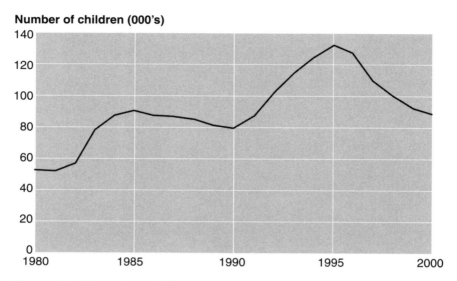

Figure 6.6   Dependent children on income assistance, 1980-2000

care, as a measure to avoid going through the court system when it was not necessary. The number in this category has grown from 15 in June 1998 to over 300 by June 2000.

Figure 6.5 shows that it is likely that fewer children were taken into care from 1986 to 1995 because of the family preservation policies that encouraged use of the CIHR program and also the support for older teens through income assistance. Had CIHR and U19 programs continued to be encouraged as they were in the mid to late 1980s and the first part of the 1990s, it is possible that the growth in c-i-c would have been less over the second half of the 1990s.

Socio-Economic Factors

The performance of the economy is also an important factor in helping to explain the number of children in these at-risk programs. Figure 6.7 shows a counter cyclical relationship (statistically significant) between the Gross Provincial Product (GPP) per capita and the number of children in at-risk programs as a percentage of all children in the province. Three year running means are used in this analysis to help account for lags in influences as well as to smooth out annual counts which can fluctuate dramatically from year to year. As GPP/capita goes down, families are affected economically, resulting in an increase in children being put at risk of neglect/abuse or parents having difficulties coping and needing to enter into voluntary agreements with the state to look after their children.

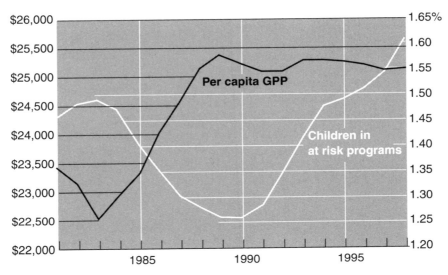

Figure 6.7   Per capita GPP and children in at-risk programs, 1981-1998

Work undertaken elsewhere has shown the importance of economic and social stress factors in child maltreatment (Trocmé, McPhee, Tam, and Hay, 1994; Wolfe and Jaffe, 1991; Cohen-Schlanger, Fitzpatrick, Hulchanski, and Raphael, 1995; Trocmé and Lindsey, 1996; Leventhal, 1996; Mayer, 1998; Wolfe, 1998; Percy, Carr-Hill, Dixon, and Jamison, 2000; Azar, 2000; Ernst, 2000; Jack, 2000; MacLeod and Nelson, 2000; Tajma, 2000). Within BC, an analysis using the regional c-i-c caseload for the average of the two fiscal years 1997/98 - 1998/99 allows us to check for the importance of certain socio-economic factors. With the creation of the MCF in September 1996, there was a 6 month period of transition work, after which the ministry was organized into the same 20 regions for administrative purposes (MCF, 1997) as those used by the Ministry of Health. Table 6.3a provides a correlation matrix which shows the relationship between average c-i-c counts as a percentage of total population 0-18 years of age in each region and specific socio-economic variables from the 1996 census known to be associated with the c-i-c count at the provincial level. These variables are:

1. **Percentage of Aboriginal children (0-18) in the regional child population averaged for the 2 year period:**

Historically, over 30% of all c-i-c are known to be of Aboriginal ancestry (Figure 6.8), an issue of major concern identified in separate provincial reports in the 1990s (Community Panel, 1992a; Petch and Scarth, 1997), and discussed later in this chapter. The poor living conditions, extreme poverty, and high mortality rates evident in some Aboriginal communities resemble those found in third world countries (BC Royal Commission on Health Care and Costs, 1991). In general terms, Aboriginal communities have "relatively low incomes, increased unemployment rates, poor housing, low duration of education and insufficient control over living and working conditions" (Millar, 1992, as quoted in Foster, Macdonald, Tuk, Uh, and Talbot, 1996).

Percent

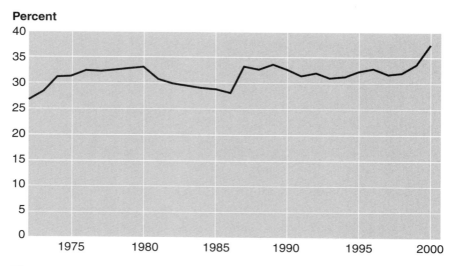

Figure 6.8   Aboriginal c-i-c as a percentage of total c-i-c, 1972-2000

2. Percentage of children in a region on Income Assistance in June 1997:

Courtney (1998) has noted the extent of overlap between c-i-c and families on income assistance. In BC, over 65% of all c-i-c are from families on income assistance at the time of admission (Figure 6.9). These combinations of factors doubly disadvantage such children. As Ross, Scott, and Kelly (1996, p. 6) note: "poor children have lower levels of educational attainment, they live in riskier environments, and they partake in riskier behaviours." In urban areas, the rate of child poverty has been shown to be four percentage points worse for children 5 and under, relative to older children (Lockhead and Shillington, 1996).

3. Percentage of lone parent families in the region in July 1996:

Over the last 15 years a large proportion of all c-i-c are from lone parent families (Figure 6.10; the reduction in percentage between 1996 and 1997 results from a change in the way data were recorded). Lone parent families, especially those headed by females (approximately 90% of lone parent families) tend to be substantially poorer than two parent families. At the same time, the cost of shelter has increased over the last decade, leaving families with less to spend on food and clothing (Sauvé, 1999). Persistent poverty characterizes almost 70% of female lone parents (Finnie, 1997) and nearly half of all poor children in

Canada lived with lone parents in 1994, (Ross, Scott, and Kelly, 1996). Some suggest that much of this is a result of the liberalization of divorce laws (Pearson and Gallaway 1998; Allen and Richards, 1999; Picot, Zyblock, and Pyper, 1999) and the resultant impacts especially on mothers. Indeed, research has shown that children are at greater risk of poor life attainments when living with a divorced single mother, than when living with a widowed, single mother or two biological parent family (Biblarz and Gottainer, 2000).

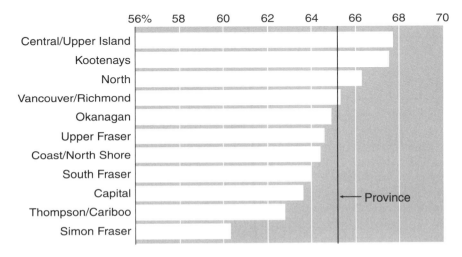

Figure 6.9 Proportion of c-i-c whose parents received Income Assistance at time of admission by region, February 28, 2001

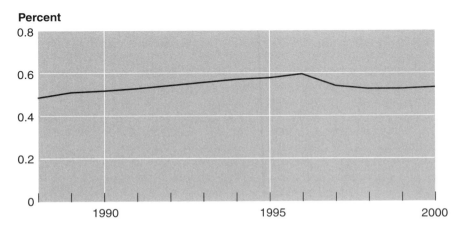

Figure 6.10 Percentage of c-i-c from single parent homes* as percentage of total c-i-c (as of March 31)

4. Unemployment rate in the region in July 1996:

Families in which the head of the household is unemployed suffer greater financial and psychological stress which increases the potential for child neglect and abuse. Part of this is related to income loss, part is related to dislocation as a result of the search for new employment and part is related to increased isolation that follows from not being able to participate meaningfully in productive daily routines. Unemployment rates, along with income inequality have been found elsewhere to be predictive of rates of child maltreatment (Trocmé and Lindsey, 1996, p. 179).

5. Percentage of population between 25 and 34 years of age in July 1996 that did not graduate from high school:

This variable is associated with young, poor families who experience difficulty adapting to a changing economy, which has been underway in the province since the recession of the early 1980s (Picot, Zyblock, and Pyper, 1999). During such periods of economic and social changes, mothers and children are most likely to feel the brunt of those changes (MCF, 1998).

   Four of the five variables chosen have statistically significant correlation coefficients. The highest is unemployment rate ($r=0.772$), followed by Aboriginal child population ($r=0.689$), the number of children in income assistance families ($r=0.639$) and finally population age 25 to 34 who did not graduate from high school ($r=0.631$). Surprisingly, lone parent families had a low and non-statistically significant correlation. One reason for this non-significant relationship may be that the lone parent variable includes all children, not just include lone parents with young children. As expected, many of the variables had significant correlations with each other. In sum this analysis, while not able to determine cause and effect, confirms the importance of ecological relationships between certain poverty related socio-economic variables and the c-i-c count across the province. It provides further statistical evidence for what practitioners know about the importance of poverty and social marginalization in influencing the c-i-c count. The Community Panel, in 1992, went as far as to say "when governments allow children to live in poverty, they are, in effect, committing systemic child neglect" (Community Panel, 1992b, p. 9).

   Many of the c-i-c in the 1997/98 to 1998/99 period would have been in care for several years—some as long as 18 years. As such, they may have been residing in a region other than the one in which they were residing in this 2 year period when they originally came into care, thus potentially calling into question the validity of the analysis just described. Accordingly, correlation coefficients are provided not only for the average c-i-c count, but also for protection reports and new admissions into care for the 1997/98 to 1998/99 period. These latter two variables are likely to be more immediately related to the socio-economic conditions of the day. This analysis is presented in Tables 6.3b and 6.3c and the results corroborate the findings of Table 6.3a, providing

Table 6.3a   Correlation matrix: c-i-c rate

	CIC	Aboriginal	Graduate	Income	Lone parent	Unemployment
CIC	1.000	0.689**	0.631**	0.639**	0.389	0.772*
Aboriginal	0.689**	1.000	0.736**	0.292	0.163	0.755**
Graduate	0.631**	0.736**	1.000	0.465*	−0.096	0.820**
Income	0.639**	0.292	0.465*	1.000	0.522*	0.643**
Lone parent	0.389	0.163	−0.096	0.522*	1.000	0.190
Unemployment	0.772**	0.755**	0.820**	0.643**	0.190	1.000

Table 6.3b   Correlation matrix: protection reports

	Report	Aboriginal	Graduate	Income	Lone parent	Unemployment
Report	1.000	0.777**	0.760**	0.462*	0.039	0.836**
Aboriginal	0.777**	1.000	0.736**	0.292	0.163	0.755**
Graduate	0.760**	0.736**	1.000	0.465*	−0.096	0.820**
Income	0.462*	0.292	0.465*	1.000	0.522*	0.643**
Lone parent	0.039	0.163	−0.096	0.522*	1.000	0.190
Unemployment	0.836**	0.755**	0.820**	0.643**	0.190	1.000

Table 6.3c   Correlation matrix: admissions

	Admission	Aboriginal	Graduate	Income	Lone parent	Unemployment
Admission	1.000	0.788**	0.718**	0.559*	0.171	0.850**
Aboriginal	0.788**	1.000	0.736**	0.292	0.163	0.755**
Graduate	0.718**	0.736**	1.000	0.465*	−0.096	0.820**
Income	0.559*	0.292	0.465*	1.000	0.522*	0.643**
Lone parent	0.171	0.163	−0.096	0.522*	1.000	0.190
Unemployment	0.850**	0.755**	0.820**	0.643**	0.190	1.000

Note: *   Statistically significant (<0.05)

　　　　**   Highly statistically significant (<0.01)

further evidence to support the conclusion of the importance of these socio-economic factors.

Throughout the province there is a tremendous variation in the relative c-i-c count among the 20 regions over the 1997-1999 period (Figure 6.11), much of it related to the variation in the socio-economic factors just discussed. Counts range from nearly 15/1000 children in the North West to as low as 4/1000 in the North Shore and Richmond regions in the South West. The highest counts are generally in the north and west of the province—regions with large Aboriginal populations and poorer economic prospects. The lowest counts are in the suburban regions around the city of Vancouver in the South West, which are relatively affluent areas with small Aboriginal populations. Vancouver itself, at over 13/1000 c-i-c, has large variations both socio-economically (Burr, Costanzo, Hayes, MacNab, and McKee, 1995) and in terms of the Aboriginal/non-Aboriginal c-i-c counts, as will be discussed later.

ECHO–BANG: 1994-2000

As indicated earlier, the number of c-i-c fell from over 10,000 (1.3% of the child population) in the early 1970s to about 6,000 (less than 0.7% of the child population) in 1993/94. Since that time there has been a dramatic growth—one that is still underway early in the new millenium.

If the long term underlying trend in the c-i-c count between 1986 (when c-i-c were forecast to start increasing along with the start of the "echo" effect of the baby boom) and late 1993 (when the c-i-c count bottomed out) had continued (Figure 6.12) there would have been substantially fewer c-i-c than the current count. As of March 2000, the province would have had about 8,300 c-i-c, rather than the approximately 10,000 recorded. The difference between actuals and predicted is remarkable, but no more remarkable than the difference between the predicted number using Merner's 1983 model (Figure 6.2) and what actually happened. It could be argued that the rapid growth since 1994 is just a "catch-up" to where the c-i-c count should have been based on historical trends. However the growth since 1994 is nothing short of phenomenal and far outstrips population growth.

Three major events hit the province of BC in fairly quick succession, which collectively "shocked" the system and resulted in a very rapid increase in the number of c-i-c. First, in January 1994, the provincial government announced that it was tightening up on its income assistance program. This followed years of BC "swimming against the current in a meaner, leaner Canada, where the link between local need and federal/provincial dollar matching was severed with the demise of the Canada Assistance Plan" (Sullivan, 1998, p. 109). Second, following intense questioning in the provincial legislature about the death of a child who was "known" to the government ministry responsible for child protection, but was not in care (Matthew Vaudreuil), government announced a

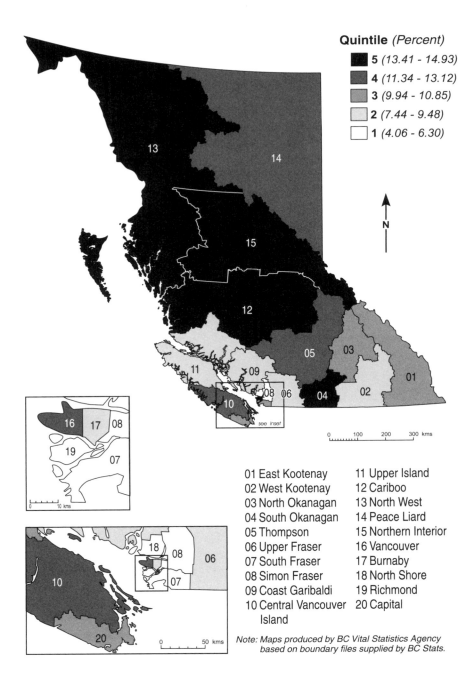

Quintile *(Percent)*

- 5 *(13.41 - 14.93)*
- 4 *(11.34 - 13.12)*
- 3 *(9.94 - 10.85)*
- 2 *(7.44 - 9.48)*
- 1 *(4.06 - 6.30)*

01 East Kootenay
02 West Kootenay
03 North Okanagan
04 South Okanagan
05 Thompson
06 Upper Fraser
07 South Fraser
08 Simon Fraser
09 Coast Garibaldi
10 Central Vancouver Island
11 Upper Island
12 Cariboo
13 North West
14 Peace Liard
15 Northern Interior
16 Vancouver
17 Burnaby
18 North Shore
19 Richmond
20 Capital

Note: Maps produced by BC Vital Statistics Agency based on boundary files supplied by BC Stats.

Figure 6.11 Average percent c-i-c in population (0-18 years) by region (BC, 1997/8-1998/9 fiscal years)

Caseload (000's)

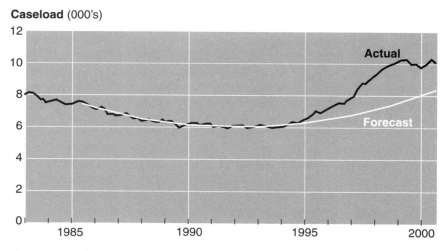

Figure 6.12   Actual c-i-c vs forecasted c-i-c based on trend

public inquiry into the death. This inquiry led to a full review of the child serving system in the province (Gove, 1995). Finally, following a review completed in late 1992 (Community Panel, 1992 a,b), the government revised its child welfare legislation which was passed in the late summer of 1994 and finally implemented in early 1996. A major provision of the new *Child, Family and Community Services Act* was a much broader definition of "risk," including emotional risk, for child protection purposes.

Income Assistance Reform

Following the announcement of the tightening of income assistance in January 1994 there was a dramatic reduction in the number of underage (U19) income assistance clients and CIHR growth was curtailed (Figure 6.4). As noted earlier, these are potential program substitutes to taking children into care. At the same time, real GPP/capita started to fall again in the province after a couple of years of respite, putting more pressure on families at the lower end of the socio-economic scale. Although BC was less ruthless than other jurisdictions in tightening its welfare net (Spigelman, 1998), further restraint measures in income assistance programs were introduced throughout 1995. In 1996, the government introduced its BC Benefits program, which saw the introduction of a new Family Bonus program for low and low/middle income families, but there was no increase for families on income assistance (Ministry of Social Services, 1996; Ministry of Social Development and Economic Security, 2000), a cause of great concern among anti-poverty groups (Mendelson, 1997). In fact no provincial increases were given for over 5 years until a 2% increase in 2000. An analysis of income assistance payments from 1990 to 1998 based on data provided by the National Council of Welfare (2000) shows that, in constant dollars, a single parent with a child and a couple with two children had increases to their welfare payments of 5.3% and 7.9% respectively between 1990 and 1994. Between 1994 and 1998, their payments fell in constant dollars by 8.6% and 6.3% respectively.

The income assistance program also changed the definition of "unemployable." Clients in this category (usually disabled people or single mothers) were not expected to go out and search for work. Prior to the reforms, a single mother on income assistance whose youngest child was under the age of 12 years was defined as "unemployable." Following the reforms, the age was lowered to 6 years, thus putting more pressure on single mothers to search for work. Further, earnings exemption allowances for those on income assistance were reduced, resulting in lower income for those who were able to earn some income to supplement their welfare cheque (Ministry of Social Services, 1996). As indicated elsewhere (see **Chapter 7**), single mothers on income assistance are at very high risk of having their children moved into government care because of neglect. The number of children in families on income assistance peaked just prior to the introduction of the BC Benefits Program and has since fallen dramatically (Figure 6.6), some argue largely as a result of the Family Bonus (Mendelson, 1997). In contrast, the number of c-i-c has continued to increase and it is highly likely that some children came into care as an unintended consequence of welfare reform.

Gove Inquiry Into Child Protection

While there were several BC studies on child welfare sponsored by the government in the 1990s, probably the one with the greatest impact was the Gove Inquiry (Gove, 1995). This public inquiry studied the death of Matthew Vaudreuil, a five year old who was suffocated by his mother. The child had, on numerous occasions, been seen and examined by a plethora of health and social service child welfare professionals. Despite numerous allegations of abuse, Matthew had not been admitted into care for protective purposes. His dramatic death, and the review of the child serving system it sparked, resulted in a major overhaul of the child welfare system in BC—an overhaul that is still underway. This has led to a great increase in the number of c-i-c since the mid-1990s (see **Chapter 8** for more information on the changes to the child welfare system). Following the establishment of the Gove Inquiry in the spring of 1994, the c-i-c count started to increase and shot up following the release of the Gove Report in late 1995. Indeed, the response was immediate; c-i-c caseloads jumped in December, a month that normally saw a seasonal decline. This upward trend continued in early and mid 1996 as an additional 325 child protection workers were hired. As indicated elsewhere, "when children known to statutory agencies die at the hands of their caregivers (an) atmosphere of blame and criticism always surrounds the public inquiries set up to investigate the deaths and becomes encapsulated in the judgemental tones of the final reports" (Reder, Duncan, and Gray, 1993, p.1). The Gove report was no exception to this, being influenced by the adversarial framework of the legal system. The report was very critical of the government (stretching back to the early 1980s), and particularly critical of staff in the Ministry of Social Services, the agency responsible for child welfare in the province. This criticism was so personal in some instances that part of the report was ordered to be removed in a judgement by Madame Justice Allan on January 12, 1998. Nevertheless, the review of Matthew's death brought intense public scrutiny to the child welfare system which resulted in an increase in calls of "reports" of potential neglect/abuse concerns. At the same time, because Matthew Vaudreuil had been a "false negative"—a child who should have been in protective care, but was not—workers became more risk averse and felt it safer to take children into care, rather than provide family support services to keep a child at home. This type of conservative, risk averse social worker practice has been described elsewhere. Not only are more children taken into care following major incidents and their reviews, but fewer children are returned home (Reder, Duncan, and Gray, 1993; Petch and Scarth, 1997; Usher, Wildfire, and Gibbs, 2000; Kinjerski and Herbert, 2000; Sengupta, 2000).

Child, Family and Community Service Act

The trend of an increasing number of c-i-c was further reinforced in early 1996 when the new *Child, Family and Community Service Act*, which was passed initially in 1994 following 2 years of public consultation (Community Panel, 1992 a,b), and modified in June 1995 following interim recommendations from Gove, was implemented. While there continues to be debate about the influence of the new legislation on child welfare practice, there is no doubt that the Act's intended approach was undermined by the acceptance of the interim recommendation from Judge Gove. The guiding principles section of the Act as drafted (Section 2) had a broad and interlocking set of principles to guide the interpretation and administration of the Act. These principles attempted to marry the dual purpose of any child welfare program—the protection of children **and** support to families so that they can safely care for their children (Armitage, 1999; Berland, 2000).

The adoption of Gove's recommendation altered this balance in a not so subtle way. A new, over-riding clause was added to the guiding principles of the Act so that the "safety and well-being of children" were listed as the "paramount considerations." This change dramatically widened the scope of the Act beyond what the original drafters had intended and opened the door for greater incursion into the lives of families. The 'well-being' rubric encouraged the Act to become the default mechanism for delivery of services to all children while the 'safety' language added to the developing risk averse culture which grew from the inquiry into the death of Matthew Vaudreuil (see **Chapter 8**).

The Act's definitions of risk in Section 13, addressed all the harms and potential harms to children identified at the time and incorporated case law decisions from across the country (see **Chapter 7** for a description of how risk is analyzed in BC). The definitions were consistent with legislation from Ontario and Nova Scotia and clarified some of the vague and general language used in the previous BC statute. The Act also provided for many avenues to step away from the traditional adversarial approach to child protection and the inevitable march through the court system that was required under the previous Act.

Provisions to enable a family conference approach (Sections 20 and 21) have not been proclaimed. Ironically, BC was one of the first North American jurisdictions to enact family conferences but has long been surpassed in implementation by US states. (In New Zealand, the home of the family conference, the c-i-c population dropped from over 7,000 to just over 2,500 after the introduction of the family conference approach.)

In September 1996 the MCF was created along with a new oversight body, the Children's Commission, adding to the two existing oversight bodies of the Ombudsman and the Child, Youth and Family Advocate. Since the creation of the ministry there has been very intense scrutiny and an accompanying growth in the number of c-i-c. This has been fuelled from time to time by critical reports from the oversight bodies (Preston, 2000; Pallan, 2000) and critical media coverage of some key cases which included publicly announced disciplinary action of workers, particularly related to "false negatives" (i.e., children determined by social workers to be low risk who in fact were high risk). One such occurrence was the Katie Lynn Baker case in the Kootenay region, where a young girl thought to have Retts Syndrome, and known to ministry workers, died from malnutrition in late 1996. Another was the Amanda Simpson case in November 1999, where a young girl from a family well known to ministry workers died in suspicious circumstances in Prince George. Following the release of the MCF report on the death of Amanda, there was a rapid growth in the c-i-c count.

Under such circumstances of perceived system failures, intense critical media scrutiny, and worker suspensions from their jobs, it is hardly surprising that the number of c-i-c has continued to climb at a rate that far outstrips population growth.

ABORIGINAL CHILDREN IN CARE

In the early 1950s less than 1% of c-i-c were of Aboriginal ancestry. During that decade, however, provincial child welfare services were extended onto reserve lands (Ministry of Social Services, 1992) and for most of the last 30 years Aboriginal c-i-c have comprised 30% or more of all c-i-c. Figure 6.8 shows growth throughout the 1970s peaking at 33% in 1980 before falling to 28% in 1986. A jump to greater than 33% was seen in 1987 following Bill C31, which redefined "Status Indian," returning Registered Indian Status to certain Aboriginal women and their children—a status recognized by the federal government and local Aboriginal Bands for benefits purposes. This increase was related to redefining the Indian status of children already in care as well as that of new children coming into care. The percentage remained between 31% and 33% until 1998. However, 1999 and 2000 have seen a very large jump to 37% of all c-i-c.

Table 6.4   Growth in Aboriginal c-i-c March 1998-March 2000

Region	Number of Aboriginal c-i-c		Percent change
	March 1998	March 2000	
Kootenays	67	65	-2.99
Okanagan	154	198	28.57
Thompson/Cariboo	229	448	95.63
Upper Fraser	183	289	57.92
South Fraser	153	182	18.95
Simon Fraser	112	142	26.79
Coast/North Shore	78	112	43.59
Central/Upper Island	428	492	14.95
North	732	772	5.46
Vancouver/Richmond	633	694	9.64
Capital	128	148	15.63
Total	**2,997**	**3,542**	**18.18**

Source: Based on Ministry for Children and Families Social Work Management Information System.

This growth (Table 6.4) has occurred in all regions of the MCF (the ministry reduced the number of administrative regions from 20 to 11 in April 1999) except the Kootenay region in the south east. This is a region that has relatively few Aboriginal people and by far the lowest number of Aboriginal c-i-c as a percentage of all Aboriginal children. The largest growth has been in the Thompson/Cariboo region in the central part of the province (95.63% increase), followed by Upper Fraser in the south west. This increase is partly driven by a delegation agreement with the Sto:lo Nation which has seen the transfer of certain Aboriginal c-i-c from the Greater Vancouver area to the Upper Fraser region. The North and Vancouver/Richmond regions which have by far the largest number of Aboriginal c-i-c have coincidentally had the lowest percentage growth over the 2 year period. Overall, there has been a growth of over 18% in the 2 year period in Aboriginal c-i-c, compared with a decline of 2.4% in non-Aboriginal c-i-c. This is a worrisome trend; analysis which is ongoing in the MCF, indicates that approximately one third of the Aboriginal increase is likely a result of more accurate recording of Aboriginal ancestry, and two thirds of the lift a real increase in Aboriginal c-i-c.

Table 6.5 and Figure 6.13 use the original 20 MCF regions to portray the geographic pattern across the province. This allows for a finer geographical pattern to be examined. Aboriginal children were 4.8 times more likely to be in care in March 1999 than non-Aboriginal children. By March 2000, this had grown to 5.65! Looked at another way, 40.7 out of every 1,000 Aboriginal children were in care in March 2000, compared to only 7.2 per 1,000 for non-Aboriginal children.

Table 6.5 C-i-c ratio, March 1999

	Percentage c-i-c of child population		Aboriginal – Non-Aboriginal Ratio
	Non-Aboriginal	Aboriginal	
E. Kootenay	0.99	1.98	2.00
W. Kootenay	0.84	0.82	0.98
N. Okanagan	1.17	2.13	1.82
S. Okanagan	1.35	3.87	2.87
Thompson	1.09	3.78	3.47
Upper Fraser	0.77	4.81	6.25
South Fraser	0.62	2.96	4.77
Simon Fraser	0.55	1.65	3.00
Coast Garibaldi	0.63	2.53	4.02
Central Vancouver Island	0.93	3.96	4.26
Upper Vancouver Island	0.81	2.68	3.31
Cariboo	0.84	4.37	5.20
North West	0.79	2.99	3.78
Peace Liard	0.69	4.09	5.93
Northern Interior	0.70	5.30	7.57
Vancouver	0.76	9.29	12.22
Burnaby	0.81	5.65	6.98
North Shore	0.40	1.92	4.80
Richmond	0.41	3.08	7.51
Capital	1.02	2.55	2.50
Total	**0.81**	**3.89**	**4.80**

Source: Based on Ministry for Children and Families Social Work Management Information System.

The differential between Aboriginal and non-Aboriginal children was noted in 1992 (Ministry of Social Services) and was the basis for major criticism by an Aboriginal panel with the publication of *Liberating Our Children – Liberating Our Nation* (Community Panel, 1992a). Since that time, conditions only seem to have worsened for Aboriginal children. The greatest difference between Aboriginal and non-Aboriginal c-i-c occurs in the lower mainland regions of Vancouver, Richmond, and Burnaby and in the Northern Interior, followed by Upper Fraser. In these regions there are high levels of Aboriginal c-i-c, in both an absolute and relative sense, when compared to non-Aboriginal children. For example, in Vancouver an astonishing 92.9 in every 1,000 Aboriginal children were in care, a number 60% higher than the next highest region, Burnaby. The regions with the lowest Aboriginal c-i-c are the two Kootenay regions in the south east, and the North Shore, Simon Fraser, and Burnaby regions to the north and east of Vancouver.

The reasons for relatively more Aboriginal children being in care are many and complex. This chapter has already noted the statistically significant correlation between socio-economic factors, particularly those related to poverty, and c-i-c numbers. The Vancouver/Richmond Health Board has estimated that, in 1997, 80% of Aboriginal children in BC lived in poverty (Save the Children Canada, 2000), while Canada-wide 24% of Aboriginal families are headed by lone parents compared with 13% for the rest of Canadians (Kinjerski and Herbert, 2000).

A very important factor in Aboriginal communities is the impact of residential schools on individuals, family life, communities, and culture (Haig-Brown, 1988). 18 residential schools operated within BC, the last only closing in 1972. Some Indian children also went to residential schools in the US. Such schools were "predicated on the basic notion that the First Nations were, 'by nature,' unclean and diseased (and) residential schooling was advocated as a means to 'save' Aboriginal children from the insalubrious influences of home life on reserve" (Kelm, 1998). What resulted was generation after generation having few parenting skills as a consequence of being removed from their family, band, and community (Sinclair, 1997). Some turned to substance misuse to escape, in later life, the memories of abuse suffered in these schools (Wade, 1996). There is a great likelihood of child neglect and abuse being high within Aboriginal communities, both on reserve and among those dislocated to urban areas like Vancouver, Nanaimo, Prince George, and Victoria. Of the approximately 200,000 Aboriginal people in BC, 50% are non-Status. Among Status Indian people, only 44% lived on reserve in 1996 (BC Stats, 1998), down from 71% a decade earlier. Many have moved to urban areas far from family and other supports because of the fragmentation of culture and family, abuse, lack of opportunities and inadequate housing. This has left some culturally and socially isolated. For those who remain on-reserve, over 15% of reserves are isolated and not accessible by road and a similar percentage are greater than 90 kilometres from the nearest physician (Elliott and Foster, 1996).

In a survey published by Statistics Canada (1993), BC Aboriginal people noted alcohol abuse (85%), drug abuse (53%), family violence (41%), and sexual abuse (31%) as being pervasive in their communities (Elliott and Foster, 1996). It is well documented that parents who experienced trauma and abuse in their childhood have a higher probability of becoming abusive parents (Ross and Roberts, 1999).

Further, high rates of alcohol and drug abuse have led to alarming rates of Aboriginal babies having Fetal Alcohol Syndrome, Fetal Narcotic Effects, and Sudden Infant Death Syndrome (Children's Commission, 2000; Save the Children Canada, 2000). All of these factors undoubtedly result in increased neglect and abuse of children. However, because of the history of the residential school system, many families who perhaps require assistance fail to seek it for fear of having their children taken by child welfare authorities. This becomes a self-fulfilling prophecy in that failure to seek and receive family support services often results in children being taken into care involuntarily and often involve longer stays in care. There is, without doubt, an inter-generational impact of being placed in care within the Aboriginal population. Given these factors, it is not unexpected that such a high proportion of Aboriginal children continue to come into care.

In a 1997 report on foster care, four main reasons for the over-representation of Aboriginal children and youth in care were noted (Petch and Scarth, 1997). First, Aboriginal cultural values and parenting practices have been evaluated from the perspective of a white, middle class dominant culture. Indeed, the risk assessment model in use in BC is not totally appropriate for Aboriginal cultures and the MCF now has plans to have a culturally appropriate tool developed. Second, some non-Aboriginal child protection workers wish to "save" Aboriginal children from traditional tribal ways of life, a perspective reminiscent of the background to the introduction of residential schools. Third, the absence of family and community support services for Aboriginal groups, especially in urban areas off-reserve, has favoured taking children away from the biological family and placing them in care. What has been traditionally and culturally acceptable amongst families on reserve may be seen as inappropriate off-reserve in a dominant white, European culture. Fourth, there has been a failure to consider the role of the extended family in Aboriginal child rearing and child development. "Children were raised, educated and protected by the adults in their community. Aunts, uncles, grand parents and natural parents provided services as part of a large pattern of mutual assistance based on reciprocal obligations within extended families and other traditional kinship relations" (Ministry of Social Services, 1992, p. 56).

Furthermore, the report noted that "the system may be putting children and youth from minority cultures at risk of harm when they are placed in the care of foster parents and social workers who are not culturally competent," thus making matters worse (Petch and Scarth, 1997). The abuse, neglect, and intergenerational problems associated with the residential school system are

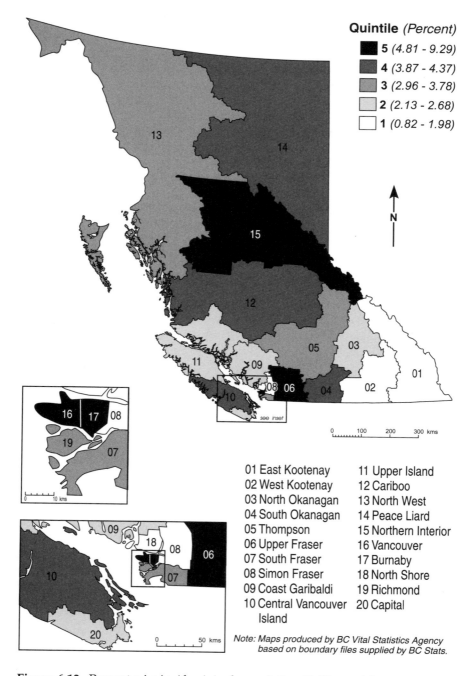

Figure 6.13 Percent c-i-c in Aboriginal population (0-18 years) by region
(BC, March 1999)

resulting in Aboriginal children accessing the child welfare system, thus potentially perpetuating those problems.

The one small glimmer of hope, if it can be called that, is that since July
1997 the number of Aboriginal c-i-c who are being looked after by Aboriginal
agencies has grown from 98 to 520 in July 2000. This represents approximately
14% of all Aboriginal c-i-c. This is consistent with the MCF Aboriginal Strategy
(MCF, 1999) which sees children and family services for Aboriginal people
being provided by Aboriginal agencies over the coming years. By the end of
2000, 18 delegation agreements had been signed with Aboriginal agencies to
provide children and family services to Aboriginal people.

OTHER CONSIDERATIONS

One of the factors plaguing the child welfare system in BC, in other provinces
(Trocmé, Fallan, Nutter, MacLaurin, and Thompson, 1999), and in other countries (Reder, Duncan, and Gray, 1993; Silver, 1999) has been the general lack
of clarity and consistency as to what the system is supposed to achieve. Certainly
the system in Canada and BC has veered between child protection and family
support (Berland, 1998; Armitage, 1998), and between child protection and child
wellbeing. Indeed, the urgency to help children has usually overshadowed
efforts to measure the effectiveness of services. Furthermore, governments have
not required accountability based on outcomes, but have rather responded to
increasing caseloads (Trocmé, MacLaurin, and Fallan 1998). Consequently,
individual workers have often used individual practice styles which undoubtedly have led to variations in the number of c-i-c, both over time and geographic region.

Assessing the practice of individual workers, however, is a very tricky
endeavour. Indeed workers "have been charged by society with an almost
impossible task—protecting children and helping to make Solomon-like
decisions about whether families should stay together" (Azar, 2000, p.644).
However, moving beyond individual cases and the other underlying factors
already described above, some of the patterns undoubtedly result from practice variations, based on experience, training, and the amount of information
available when decisions are made, as well as regional "culture." Examining
c-i-c rates among regions in BC shows tremendous variation and, as previously noted, some of this is related to socio-economic variables in addition to
the variation in child age cohorts of the regional population. The cause of the
variation is somewhat speculative at this time, but is likely to be connected to
the individual strengths and experiences of staff which go to make up the regional organizational culture. The relevant issue is culture with respect to risk
appetite, that is, making decisions about removing children from their homes
and into care. Figure 6.14 ranks regions from least (lowest standardized c-i-c
rates) to highest (highest standardized c-i-c rates). Variation is standardized

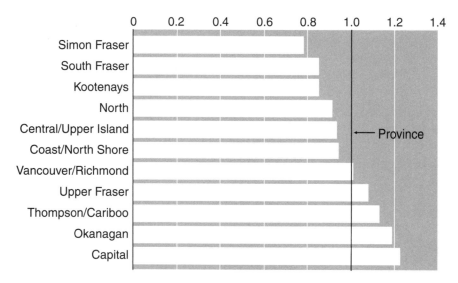

Figure 6.14 C-i-c gradient (Province = 1), December 2000

according to the provincial rate of 1.0 which takes into account a variety of socio-economic factors and the demographics of the child population. The Capital region, for example, has a "variation" 22% higher than that of the province, and 56% higher than that of the Simon Fraser Region. This may be construed as meaning that the organizational culture in the Capital region is more risk averse than that of any other region.

Elsewhere, front line workers have suggested that rapid turnover of staff has resulted in a growth in c-i-c, while managers have indicated that inexperienced staff are more likely to bring children into care and less likely to have timely discharges (Kinjerski and Herbert, 2000). Further, increased public awareness, media scrutiny, and political pressure all lead to more defensive social work practices (especially when public commentary is provided on the basis of limited information, as is often the case because of privacy policy) resulting in provincial, regional, and community variations in both child apprehension rates and the return of children to their families (Petch and Scarth, 1997; Reder, Duncan, and Gray, 1993; Kinjerski and Herbert, 2000).

Within BC, since the Gove Inquiry, it is fair to say the child welfare system has been in some turmoil, trying to find and keep its direction while dealing with rapidly increasing caseloads, increasing public and media scrutiny, and a lack of stability in leadership. Between 1996 and 2000 there have been six ministers and five deputy ministers responsible for child protection. In addition, two new oversight bodies have been created—the Children's Commission and the Child, Youth and Family Advocate—which have resulted in constant reporting on the child welfare system, with over a thousand recommended actions to which the system must respond. The rate of change was phenomenal in the last 5 years of the 1990s, and such change, which brings with it organizational uncertainty, has undoubtedly resulted in a higher caseload of c-i-c than there might have been otherwise (Kinjerski and Herbert, 2000). Also during this period, financial and human resources have been sorely stretched.

TOO SMALL – TOO BIG: THE NUMBER OF CHILDREN IN CARE

Since the 1950s, the number of c-i-c has ranged from 0.7% to 1.3% of the child population. The current rate of just over 1% is midway between these two extremes. Whether we have fewer or more c-i-c seems to have little bearing on the overall health indicators for the province's children and youth. Compared to other provinces, BC children fare very well in terms of health status (Millar, 1998; Lee, Klein, and Murray, 1999; Kendall, 2000). The growth in child welfare cases during the second half of the 1990s, however, is not restricted to BC, as shown in Figure 6.15, which plots the growth for selected provinces and for Canada (excluding Quebec, for which comparative statistics are not available). Canada and its provinces and territories do not have a consistent, comprehensive data collection system for measuring child welfare (Tromcé, MacLaurin, and Fallan, 1998; Christianson-Wood and Murray, 1999) and, as has been noted elsewhere, "Canada has placed little emphasis on documenting child welfare services" (Tromcé, McPhee, and Tam, 1995, p. 564). Since 1992, however, with the formation of the Federal/Provincial Working Group on Child and Family Services Information, this problem is in the process of being rectified. There are many difficulties in acquiring consistent data because child and family services legislation varies among the provinces with respect to basic issues such as the age definition of a child, and some provinces report only child welfare cases while others report c-i-c statistics (Federal/Provincial Working Group on Child and Family Services Information, 1994; 1996; 1999). Calls for better, consistent information on child abuse go back to the mid-1980s (Badgley, 1984), and only now is work underway to help facilitate meaningful inter-provincial comparisons (Trocmé and Wolfe, 2001). These problems are not confined to Canada, but are also systemic within the US (Goerge, Wukzyn, and Harden, 1996; Usher, Wildfire, and Gibbs, 1999). Differences in administrative data collection systems make it difficult to draw broad conclusions beyond a particular state, province, or country. Nevertheless, and with the noted cautions in mind of differing definitions and collection systems, Figure 6.15 provides a **preliminary** analysis of child welfare case trends among provinces. Between 1993/94 and 1998/99, cases across the country (excluding Quebec) have increased by over 30%, but in BC the growth at 60% has been more than twice the national rate. Other provinces, notably Alberta (75%), Nova Scotia and Ontario (nearly 30%), have also witnessed major increases. This growth is more than just the "echo" growth (Foot and Stoffman, 1996) of the child population.

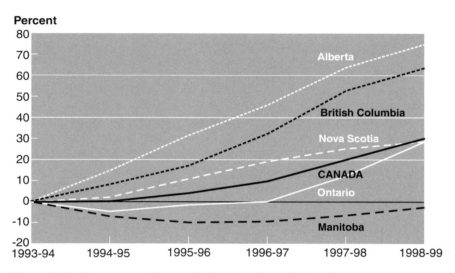

Figure 6.15   Percentage change of c-i-c for selected Canadian provinces and
               Canada (excluding Quebec), 1993/94 - 1998/99

Following years of cutbacks by the federal government in cost-shared funding for social and welfare programs and increasing provincial budget deficits,
many provinces were forced to cut back on their social and welfare programs—
some more than others. For example, Alberta went through major social and
welfare reforms in the early and mid-1990s, undertaking major cuts to its welfare system (Kinjerski and Herbert, 2000). Ontario followed in the mid-1990s.
In both cases, part of the outfall from such reforms was an increasing pressure
on families at the lower end of the socio-economic scale. Some families would
have been forced to move to even cheaper housing and would have lost any
social support system that may have been in place. These are the very families
that are most at risk of having their children taken into care due to neglect and
abuse. In both provinces, but particularly in Ontario there has also been major
scrutiny of child welfare services following intense media attention into the
deaths of c-i-c (Ontario Child Mortality Task Force, 1998). Subsequently, over
200 additional workers have been hired and new legislation was introduced in
2000 which some claim encouraged more children to be taken into care. The
combination of social and welfare program cutbacks in the US has also been
suggested as a likely cause of increases in c-i-c in some states (Courtney, 1998).
     Table 6.6 compares BC with all other provinces and territories with respect
to the child welfare population as reported to the federal government. Because
different provinces have differing age limits for child welfare, BC's c-i-c population has been truncated at different ages so that standardized comparisons
can be made. For example, Alberta stops taking children into care at age 17,
Ontario at age 15, while for BC the age is 18. To compare BC with the same

group in Alberta requires that only cases which are between the ages of 0 to 17 years be considered, thus ignoring all 18 year olds. This allows for a reasonable but (because of data quality and classification problems) far from perfect comparison between provinces and territories.

Table 6.6   Child welfare cases by province: 1995-2001

Child age definition	*Cases as percentage of child population (approx.)*			
	Province	1995	2001	1995-01 % change
	Ontario[1]	0.39	0.58	+48.7
Less than	Newfoundland	0.56	0.69	+23.3
16 years	Nova Scotia	0.75	1.10	+46.7
	Saskatchewan[2]	0.92	1.20	+30.4
	New Brunswick[3]	0.65	0.75	+15.4
	British Columbia	**0.67**	**1.01**	**+50.7**
	PEI	0.58	0.61	+5.2
Less than	Alberta	0.59	1.05	+78.0
18 years	NWT[4]	2.34	1.76	−24.8
	Manitoba	1.82	1.88	+3.3
	Yukon	2.14	2.34	+9.3
	British Columbia	**0.70**	**1.08**	**+54.3**
Less than				
19 years	**British Columbia**	**0.72**	**1.10**	**+52.8**

Notes:

[1] Unless the child is under a protection order.

[2] Extended to youth under 18 who cannot protect themselves.

[3] For disabled youth the age is under 19.

[4] Normally under 16. Voluntary services up to age 18.

Source: Based on Ministry for Children and Families Social Work Management Information Systems.

Overall, despite the large increase in cases over the last several years, BC remained firmly in the middle of the pack for both 1995 and for 2001. After Alberta, BC was the lowest in the west and north of the country in 2001. Relative to the maritime provinces, BC is at the same level as Nova Scotia but substantially higher than the other provinces, as well as Ontario, which has the lowest relative number of cases of all provinces, although its rate of growth is only marginally smaller than that of BC. Unlike other provinces, Ontario has a very extensive child and youth mental health service delivery system, which may be partly responsible for this low count.

Given this comparative analysis, it is hard to argue that BC has more or fewer c-i-c than might be expected given current policies and economic conditions. One could speculate, however, that in the mid-1990s BC may have had fewer c-i-c than might have been expected and that the rapid growth in the late 1990s was partly a "correction" that was perhaps overdue. Caseload growth may, in fact, be a positive response to societal problems (Kinjerski and Herbert, 2000). The growth in BC, however, likely occurred because of the factors noted earlier – welfare reform, child welfare system review, following the death of a child known to the system, legislative change which emphasized a child centred, rather than a family preservation approach, major media and public scrutiny and a move towards more conservative social work practice. Such a conclusion, however, is still tentative and more detailed analysis is required as many of these factors are interrelated and it is very difficult to isolate any one factor (Kinjerski and Herbert, 2000).

SUMMARY AND CONCLUSIONS

Taking children into care should be a last resort and not a "misguided notion that 'out of home care' is an end point service that 'rescues' children from their parent(s)" (Silver, 1999, p.149). Placement into a care situation is disruptive to children's lives, often removing them from their biological families, neighbourhoods, friends, and schools. In Canada, it has been concluded that "foster care does not seem to put children at additional risk of doing poorly, (but) it has not yet been proven to improve children's lives" (Tromcé, MacLaurin, and Fallan, 1998). Indeed, "there is widespread agreement that foster care is **not** the best place for children to grow" (Miller, 2000, p. 20). Clearly, we need to do a lot more research into the "causes" of c-i-c. The evidence is, however, overwhelmingly unambiguous that major risk factors for children coming into care is poverty and socio-economic stress. As one commentator has noted: "The connection between child neglect and poverty is irrefutable" (Sullivan, 1998, p. 112), while another has noted: "Poverty is the universal variable among all but a very few families receiving services from the child welfare system" (Kinjerski and Herbert, 2000, p.2). This is particularly so when combined with single mothers of Aboriginal ancestry on income assistance living off-reserve. There is a clear and pressing need to reduce the poverty gap within the province, which has been described as the worst in the country (Lee, Klein, and Murray, 1999). Reducing unemployment and its impacts through increased employment, educational opportunities, housing assistance, and child care would go a long way to supporting families to keep children at home. It would also help ensure improved development opportunities for children, thus helping to achieve the province's health goals (Ministry of Health, 1997). Further, the need to ensure better outcomes for c-i-c is an area requiring more program evaluation and research around the effectiveness of the existing services and accountability structures. It is needed if the lost public and political confidence that occurred in the child welfare system in BC and across the country throughout the 1990s is to be restored, and the broadly defined health outcomes (physical, social, emotional, educational, economic) of children served by child welfare agencies are to improve.

REFERENCES

Allen, D.W., and Richards, T. (1999). *It takes two: The family in law and finance*. C.D. Howe Institute, Policy Study No. 33. Ottawa.

Armitage, A. (1998). Lost vision: Children and the Ministry for Children and Families. *BC Studies*, 118(Summer), 93-108.

Armitage, A. (1999). Lost vision: Children and the Ministry for Children and Families. *BC Studies*, 118(Summer), 97.

Azar, S.T. (2000). Preventing burnout in professionals and paraprofessionals who work with child abuse and neglect cases: A cognitive behavioral approach to supervision. *Psychotherapy in Practice*, 56, 643-663.

Badgley, R. (1984). Report of the Committee on Sexual Offences Against Children and Youths. Minister of Supply and Services Canada, Ottawa, Ontario.

Barth, R., and Blackwell, D. (1988). Death rates among California foster care and former foster care populations. *Children and Youth Services Review*, 20(7), 577-604.

Baum, A.C., Crase, S.J., and Crase, K.L. (2001). Influences on the decision to become or not become a foster parent. *Families in Society: The Journal of Contemporary Human Services*, 82, 202-213.

BC Stats (1998). *Focus on BC Aboriginals: Living on-reserve/off-reserve*. 1996 Census Fast Facts. Victoria, BC: British Columbia Statistics, Ministry of Finance.

Berland, J. (1998). Child death reviews: What have we learned and how do we know? *Canada's Children*, 5(3), 8.

Berland, J. (2000). Executive Director, MCF. Personal Communication.

Biblarz, T.J., and Gottainer, G. (2000). Family structure and children's success: A comparison of widowed and divorced single-mother families. *Journal of Marriage and the Family*, 62, 533-548.

British Columbia Royal Commission on Health Care and Costs (1991). *Closer to home*, Volume 2. Victoria, BC: Crown Publications Inc.

British Columbia Vital Statistics Agency (2000). Analysis of Health Statistics for Status Indians in British Columbia: 1991-1998. Prepared for the Medical Services Branch, Health Canada, Vancouver, BC.

Burr, K.F., Costanzo, G.A., Hayes, M.V., MacNab, Y.C., and McKee, B. (1995). *Mortality and health status in Vancouver: An analysis by neighbourhood areas*. Victoria, BC: Ministry of Health, Division of Vital Statistics.

Child, Family and Community Service Act (1994). Victoria, BC: Ministry of Social Services.

Children's Commission (2000). Fetal alcohol syndrome – A call for action in BC. Report from the Forum hosted by the Children's Commission, November 23-24, Victoria, B.C.

Christianson-Wood, J., and Murray, J.L. (1999). Child death reviews and child mortality data collection in Canada. Ottawa: Child Maltreatment Division, Health Canada, p.4.

Cohen-Schlanger, M., Fitzpatrick, A., Hulchanski, J.D., and Raphael, D. (1995). Housing as a factor in admissions of children to temporary care: A survey. *Child Welfare*, 74, 547-562.

Community Panel, Family and Children's Services Legislation Review in British Columbia (1992a). *Liberating our children – Liberating our nations.* Report of the Aboriginal Committee. Victoria, BC: Ministry of Social Services.

Community Panel, Family and Children's Services Legislation Review in British Columbia (1992b). *Making changes: A place to start.* Victoria, BC: Ministry of Social Services.

Cook-Fong, S.K. (2000). The adult wellbeing of individuals reared in family foster care placements. *Child and Youth Care Forum*, 29(1), 7-25.

Courtney, M.E. (1998). The costs of child protection in the context of welfare reform. *Protecting Children from Abuse and Neglect*, 8(1), 88-103.

Downing-Orr, K. (1996). *Alienation and social support: A social psychological study of homeless young people in London and in Sydney.* Aldershot, England: Ashgate Publishing Ltd.

Elliott, S.J., and Foster, L.T. (1996). Mind-body-place: A geography of Aboriginal health in BC. In P.H. Stephenson, S.J. Elliott, L.T. Foster, and J. Harris (Eds). *A persistent spirit: Towards understanding Aboriginal health in British Columbia* (pp. 95-127). Victoria, BC: University of Victoria, Department of Geography, Western Geographical Series, Vol. 31.

Ernst, J.S. (2000). Mapping child maltreatment: Looking at neighborhoods in a suburban county. *Child Welfare*, 79, 555-572.

Federal/Provincial Working Group on Child and Family Services Information (1994). *Child welfare in Canada: The role of provincial and territorial authorities in cases of child abuse.* Ottawa: Health Canada.

Federal/Provincial Working Group on Child and Family Services Information (1996). *Child and family services annual statistical report.* Ottawa: Human Resources Development Canada.

Federal/Provincial Working Group on Child and Family Services Information (1999). *Foster care.* Ottawa: Human Resources Development Canada.

Foot, D.K., and Stoffman, D. (1996). *Boom, bust, echo: How to profit from the coming demographic shift.* Toronto: MacFarlan, Walter and Ross.

Foster, L.T., Macdonald, J., Tuk, T.A., Uh, S.-H., and Talbot, J. (1996). Native health in British Columbia: A vital statistics perspective. In P.H. Stephenson, S.J. Elliott, L.T. Foster, and J. Harris (Eds). *A persistent spirit: Towards understanding Aboriginal health in British Columbia* (pp. 43-93). Victoria, BC: University of Victoria, Department of Geography, Western Geographical Series, Vol. 31.

Goerge, R., Wulczyn, F., and Harden, A. (1996). New comparative insights into states and their foster children. *Public Welfare*, Summer, 12-25.

Gove, T. (1995). *Inquiry into child protection; Report of the Gove Inquiry into Child Protection*, 2 Volumes. Victoria, BC: Ministry of Attorney General.

Haig-Brown, C. (1988). *Resistance and renewal: Surviving in the Indian residential school.* Vancouver, BC: Arsenal Pulp Press.

Health Canada (1999a). *A selected, annotated bibliography of child maltreatment reporting by educational professionals.* Ottawa: Child Maltreatment Division, Health Protection Branch, Health Canada.

Health Canada (1999b). *Child abuse: Reporting and classification in health care settings.* Ottawa: Health Canada.

Jack, G. (2000). Ecological influences on parenting and child development. *British Journal of Social Work*, 30, 703-720.

Kelm, M.E. (1998). *Colonizing bodies: Aboriginal health and healing in British Columbia, 1900-50*. Vancouver: UBC Press, p. 56.

Kempe, C.H., and Helfer, R. (1972). *Helping the battered child and his family*. Philadelphia: Lippincott.

Kempe, C.H., Silverman, F.N., Steele, B.F., Droegemueller, N., and Silver, H.K. (1962). The battered child syndrome. *Journal of the American Medical Association*, 181, 17-24.

Kendall, P.R.W. (2000). *A report on the health of British Columbians*. Provincial Health Officers Annual Report – 1999. Victoria, BC: Ministry of Health.

Kendall, P.R.W. (forthcoming a). *Deaths of children and youth in care: What do the data show?* A report by the British Columbia Provincial Health Officer. Victoria, BC: Ministry of Health.

Kendall, P.R.W. (forthcoming b). *Children and youth in care: An epidemiological review of mortality, British Columbia, April 1974 to March 1999*. A Technical Report of the Office of the Provincial Health Officer. Victoria, BC: Ministry of Health.

Kotovich, P. (1998). *The doctor project*. Burnaby, BC: The McCreary Centre.

Kinjerski, V., and Herbert, M. (2000). *Child welfare caseload growth in Alberta: Connecting the dots*. Report prepared for the Minister of Children Services, Edmonton, Alberta.

Lee, M., Klein, S., and Murray, S. (1999). *Behind the headlines: A review of public policy in BC*. Vancouver: Canadian Centre for Policy Alternatives.

Leventhal, J.M. (1996). Twenty years later: We do know how to prevent child abuse and neglect. *Child Abuse and Neglect*, 20, 647-653.

Lockhead, C., and Shillington, R. (1996). *A statistical profile of urban poverty*. Ottawa: Canadian Council of Social Development.

MacLeod, J., and Nelson, G. (2000). Programs for the promotion of family wellness and the prevention of child maltreatment: A meta-analytic review. *Child Abuse and Neglect*, 24, 1127-1148.

Martin Spigelman Research Associates (1998). Unfulfilled expectations, missed opportunities: Poverty among immigrants and refugees in British Columbia. Prepared for the Working Group on Poverty, Ministry Responsible for Multiculturalism and Immigration. Victoria, B.C.

Mayer, M. (1998). Indicator mapping: From ecological analysis to community intervention. Proceedings of the First Canadian Roundtable on Child Welfare Outcomes, Bell Canada Child Welfare Research Unit, University of Toronto, pp. 152-157.

McCreary Centre Society (2001). *No place to call home: A profile of street youth in British Columbia*. Burnaby, BC: The McCreary Centre.

Mendelson, M. (1997). *A preliminary analysis of the impact of the Family Bonus on poverty and welfare caseloads*. Report prepared for the BC Ministry of Human Resources, Victoria, BC.

Merner, G. (1983). *Forecasting children in care counts*. Victoria, BC: Ministry of Human Resources.

Millar, J.S. (1993). *A report on the health of British Columbians*. Provincial Health Officer's Annual Report – 1992. Victoria, BC: Ministry of Health.

Millar, J.S. (1998). *A report on the health of British Columbians*. Provincial Health Officer's Annual Report – 1997. Feature report: The health and wellbeing of British Columbia's children. Victoria, BC: Ministry of Health.

Miller, J.L. (2000). Child welfare waivers: What are we learning? Policy Practice of Public Human Services. *Journal of the American Public Human Services Association*, December, 20-28.

Ministry for Children and Families (1997). *The first six months*. Victoria, BC: Ministry for Children and Families.

Ministry for Children and Families (1998). *Caring for BC's children: A community forum – Final proceedings*. Victoria, BC: Ministry for Children and Families.

Ministry for Children and Families (1999). *Strategic plan for Aboriginal services*. Victoria, BC: Ministry for Children and Families.

Ministry of Health (1997). *Health goals for British Columbia*. Victoria, BC: Ministry of Health.

Ministry of Social Development and Economic Security (2000). BC benefits – income support programs (*http://www.sdes.gov.bc.ca/programs/ispprog.htm*).

Ministry of Social Services (1992). *Protecting our children – Supporting our families: A review of child protection issues in British Columbia*. Victoria, BC: Ministry of Social Services.

Ministry of Social Services (1996). *BC benefits program: Renewing our social safety net*. Victoria, BC: Ministry of Social Services.

National Council of Welfare (2000). *Welfare incomes 1997 and 1998*. Ottawa: Minister of Public Works and Government Services Canada.

Ontario Child Mortality Task Force (1997). *Interim Report* (March); and *Final Report* (July). Toronto: Ontario Child Mortality Task Force.

Ontario Child Mortality Task Force (1998). A progress report on recommendations. Ontario Child Mortality Task Force. (*http://www.oacas.org/about/CMFT.html*).

Pallan, P. (2000). *Weighing the evidence: A report on BC's children and youth*. 1999 Annual Report of the Children's Commission, Victoria, BC.

Pallan, P. (2001). *The educational attainment of children in care*. Draft Report. Children's Commission, Victoria, BC.

Paliavin, I. (1993). The duration of homeless careers: An exploratory study. *Social Service Review*, 67, 576-598.

Pearson, L., and Gallaway, R. (1998). *For the sake of the children*. Report of the Special Joint Parliamentary Committee on Child Custody and Access. Ottawa.

Peirson, L., Nelson, G., and Prilleltensky, I. (2000). Family wellness and child maltreatment: An ecological perspective. *Canada's Children*, 7(Fall), 30-33.

Percy, A., Carr-Hill, R., Dixon, P., and Jamison, J.Q. (2000). Assessing the local need for family and child care services: A small area utilization analysis. *Child Welfare*, 79, 535-553.

Petch, H., and Scarth, S. (1997). *Report of the task force on safeguards for children and youth in foster or group home care*. Victoria, BC: Ministry for Children and Families

Picot, G., Zyblock, M., and Pyper, W. (1999). *Why do children move into and out of low income?* Business and Labour Market Analysis Division, No. 132, Statistics Canada, Ottawa.

Preston, J. (2000). *Not good enough*. 1999 Annual Report of the Child, Youth and Family Advocate. Victoria, B.C.

Reder, P., Duncan, S., and Gray, M. (1993). *Beyond blame: Child abuse tragedies revisited*. London: Routledge.

Roman, N., and Wolfe, P. (1997). The relationship between foster care and homelessness. *Public Welfare*, 55(1), 4-9.

Rosenfeld, A.A., Pilowsky, D.J., Fine, P., Thorpe, M., Fein, E., Simms, M.O., Halfon, N., Irwin, M., Alfaro, J., Saletsky, R., and Nickman, S. (1997). Foster care: An update. *Journal of the American Academy of Child and Adolescent Psychiatry*, 36, 448-457.

Ross, D.P., and Roberts, P. (1999). *Income and child well-being: A new perspective on the poverty debate*. Ottawa: Canada Council of Social Development.

Ross, D.P., Scott, K., and Kelly, M. (1996). *Child poverty: What are the consequences?* Ottawa: Canadian Council for Social Development.

Sauvé, R. (1999). *Trends in Canadian family incomes, expenditures, savings and debt*. Ottawa: Vanier Institute of the Family.

Save the Children Canada (2000). *Sacred lives: Canadian Aboriginal children and youth speak out about sexual exploitation*. Ottawa: Save the Children Canada.

Sedlack, A.J., and Broadhurst, D.D. (1996). *Third national incidence study of child abuse and neglect*. Washington, DC: US Department of Health and Human Services.

Silver, J. (1999). Starting young: Improving the health and developmental outcomes of infants and toddlers in the child welfare system. *Child Welfare*, 58(1), 148-165.

Sengupta, S. (2000). No rise in child abuse seen in welfare shift. *New York Times*, August 10, p. A-20.

Sinclair, M. (1997). *The historical relationship between the Canadian Justice System and Aboriginal people*. Paper presented to the Aboriginal Justice Learning Network, Ayliner, Quebec, April, 16-18.

Statistics Canada (1993). Language, Tradition, Health, Lifestyle and Social Issues: 1991 Aboriginal Peoples Survey. Statistics Canada, Ottawa.

Sullivan, P.M., and Knutson, J.F. (2000). Maltreatment and disabilities: A population-based epidemiological study. *Child Abuse and Neglect*, 24, 1257-1273.

Sullivan, R., (1998), Commentary. *BC Studies*, 118, Summer, 109.

Tajima, E.A. (2000). The relative importance of wife abuse as a risk factor for violence against children. *Child Abuse and Neglect*, 24, 1383-1398.

Thompson, A., and Newman, S., (1995). Mortality in a child welfare population: Implications for Policy. *Child Welfare*, 74(4), 843-857.

Trocmé, N., and Lindsey, D. (1996). What can child homicide rates tell us about the effectiveness of child welfare services? *Child Abuse and Neglect*, 20(3), 171-184.

Trocmé, N., Fallan, B., Nutter, B., MacLaurin, B., and Thompson, J. (1999). *Outcomes for Child Welfare Services in Ontario*. Bell Canada Child Welfare Research Unit, Faculty of Social Work, University of Toronto.

Trocmé, N., Fallon, B. , and MacLaurin, B. (1998). Canadian child welfare outcomes indicator matrix. In S. Ward and D. Finklehor (Eds.), *Program evaluation and family violence research*. Binghamton, NY: Haworth Press.

Trocmé, N., McPhee, D., and Tam, K.K. (1995). Child abuse and neglect in Ontario: Incidence and characteristics. *Child Welfare*, 24(3), 563-586.

Trocmé, N., McPhee, D., Tam, K.K., and Hay, T. (1994). *Ontario incidence study of reported child abuse and neglect*. Toronto: The Institute for the Prevention of Child Abuse.

Trocmé, N., and Wolfe, D. (2001). *Canadian incidence study of reported child abuse and neglect*. Ottawa: Health Canada.

Usher, C.L., Wildfire, J.B., and Gibbs, D.A. (1999). Measuring performance in child welfare: Secondary effects of success. *Child Welfare*, 78(1), 31-51.

Wade, A. (1996). Resistance knowledges: Therapy with Aboriginal persons who have experienced violence. In P.H. Stephenson, S.J. Elliott, L.T. Foster, and J. Harris (Eds), *A persistent spirit: Towards understanding Aboriginal health in British Columbia* (pp. 167-206). Victoria, BC: University of Victoria, Department of Geography, Western Geographical Series, Vol. 31.

Williams, C. (2001). Family disruptions and childhood happiness. Canadian Social Trends, Autumn, 2-4.

Wolfe, D.A. (1998). Prevention of child abuse and neglect. In *Canada health action: Building on the legacy. Determinants of health, Volume 1—Children and youth* (pp. 103-121). Ste. Foy, PQ: Editions Multimondes Inc.

Wolfe, D.A., and Jaffe, P. (1991). The psychosocial needs of children in care. In L.C. Johnson and D. Barnhorst (Eds.), *Children, families and public policy in the 90s*. Toronto: Thompson Educational Publishing, Inc.

Zlotnick, C., Kronstadt, D., and Klee, L. (1998). Foster care children and family homelessness. *American Journal of Public Health*, 88, 1368-1370.

Contradictions in Child Welfare

7

Fay Weller and Brian Wharf

Faculty of Human and Social Development, University of Victoria

INTRODUCTION

> *As we talked, Jane dug through her purse to pull out crayons and paper for Tanya, her three-year-old daughter, encouraging her to draw a picture for Gramma. Meanwhile her three-month-old continued to hungrily breastfeed* (Weller, 1997).

Jane was working. Her work was aimed at ensuring her children were fed, clothed, protected, and were filled with a sense of well-being. The work of caring for children, like other work in our society, requires time, energy, and resources to ensure the hoped-for outcomes.

Although Jane spent the majority of her waking hours carrying out the job of caring for her children, she was reported for child neglect and investigated by the Ministry for Children and Families. The investigation found that Jane's children were not neglected but the investigation process, however, left her feeling judged and invaded. For Jane, the interaction with child protection workers increased her isolation, established a distrust of the child welfare system, and increased her sense of hopelessness (Weller, 1997).

Isolation, hopelessness, distrust, and poverty have all been documented as risk factors for child neglect (Mosher, 1994). How then does a process that allegedly sets out to protect children from neglect instead increase the potential that neglect will occur? And, if the current approach doesn't prevent child neglect, what does?

This chapter turns the traditional approach to child welfare upside down and analyses it from the standpoint of those reported for neglect. The stories and analyses are based on research carried out by the authors (Weller and Wharf, 1995).

This chapter is organized in the following fashion. First, it reviews how the problem of child neglect has been named and how solutions have been established to correspond to the named problem. A view of child welfare is presented from the standpoint of the client—the mother being investigated for neglecting her children. It describes how the work of those reported for neglect is made invisible in the official documentation and discusses the disjuncture between the official child welfare process and mothers' experiences of that process. Next, the legislative and policy context of child welfare is presented. Alternative approaches that recognize the important work of caring for children and the need for sufficient support and resources for the job are discussed.

Finally, the chapter tackles the task of suggesting ways to prevent child neglect. It does not follow the approach of individualizing the problem of child neglect, but rather, identifies the underlying structural issues facing those caring for children in today's society. The stories of women reported for neglect form the starting point for both understanding and exploring the policy implications of preventing child neglect.

Throughout this chapter the word mother is used to describe the primary care giver of children. A positive trend in recent years is the growing number of situations in which the father has taken on that role. However, a single father is more likely to have sympathy from both community members and social workers because he is seen as doing work beyond the call of duty. In addition, single fathers are more likely to be raising older children who no longer require full time childcare. Unfortunately, in our society it is seen as the mother's duty to carry out the work of caring for her children. Therefore, when someone perceives that she is not carrying out the work successfully, there is no room for sympathy. The following quote from a child protection worker states this explicitly:

> *Mothers are traditionally responsible for raising those kids and caring for them, and we tend to be hard on them. We have expectations because they're mothers and they're supposed to protect and that is their role in life* (Krane, 1995).

DEFINING THE PROBLEM AND SOLUTION

Naming the Problem and Solutions

The power to name and define child neglect comes from those with power in our society. The official definition of the problem has been named by policy makers in provincial governments with support from professional groups and academics. With some exceptions, such as feminist academics, these groups have defined the problem as "bad or faulty mothers." In contrast to this focus on the individual as the problem, feminist academics have identified structural issues such as poverty, racism, powerlessness, and the lack of value placed on the work of caring for children.

The definition of child neglect is found in legislation, in policies, and in the prescribed practices of child welfare. The *British Columbia Child, Family and Community Service Act* states that a child needs protection if the child "has been, or is likely to be, physically harmed due to neglect by the child's parent." The *British Columbia Handbook for Action on Child Abuse and Neglect* defines neglect as follows: "Neglect involves an act of omission on the part of the parent or guardian that results or is likely to result in physical harm to the child" (Ministry for Children and Families, 1998). These official documents have defined the child neglect problem as faulty parents.

Solutions flow directly from the defined problem. If the problem is faulty parents then we must identify and fix them. The official process starts when school teachers, physicians, and other community members identify those parents they feel may be neglecting their children and report this potential neglect to the Ministry for Children and Families. After receiving reports from community members the Ministry's staff investigate to determine whether or not a child is being neglected and then either take no action if the investigation reveals neglect has not occurred or, if risk factors indicate neglect, provide family support or apprehend the children. These three components of the solution—reporting, investigation, and support/treatment—are outlined in more detail below with the corresponding experience of the parent reported for neglect. As evidenced in the following stories, there is a contradiction between the mother's experience and the official understanding of the problem and solution. To protect the women involved, the names used throughout this chapter are pseudonyms.

Reporting

Close to half of the reports to the Ministry for Children and Families are categorized as omission of care or neglect (Ministry for Children and Families, 1999; Wallace, 1994). As noted above, the broad definition of neglect includes a child who "has been or is likely to be harmed" because of neglect by the child's parent, as well as those children who demonstrate "severe anxiety, depression, withdrawal, or self-destructive or aggressive behaviour." Thus, reporting neglect is largely premised on perceptions of either a mother's parenting or on a child's behaviour. The following story provides an example of how assumptions may differ between a reporter and a mother:

> Jane: *This last summer I had gone to get groceries and when I came back there was a card in my door. It was from Social Services and it said to please phone them because someone had reported me for neglect because my kids were dirty when I went in to get the groceries. Lots of times if I go into town to pick up groceries I don't bother cleaning them to just go in and pick up a thing of milk. Whoever had reported me obviously doesn't have kids—kids like dirt. They go down to the creek and they play in the clay—they get just covered from head to toe in dirt.*

Jane's story illustrates how entry into the child protection system occurs. It is initiated by community members according to their standard of care, and it is their report that provides the first component of the official story. In addition, the anonymity of mandatory reporting allows members of the community to be absolved of any responsibility for assisting or supporting the parent before or after they make their report. Thus, a mother's experience of "community" is one of watchdogs (with the power of the child welfare system behind them) rather than supportive neighbours. One mother described the experience of anonymous reporting as "omnipotent invisible eyes who are everywhere and make you want to hide" (Weller, 1997). Statistics from the Ministry for Children and Families indicate that, for the 3 fiscal years 1997/98 to 1999/2000, more than three of every four reports is false (Table 7.1).

Table 7.1	Percent of false protection reports for 1997/98 to 1999/00
Fiscal year	*False reports(%)*
1997/98	75.6
1998/99	76.9
1999/00	81.9

Investigation

The second step of investigation assesses and then categorizes the mother so that child protection programs can be implemented according to the defined category of need. The assessment process involves child protection workers and other professionals in the community assessing the 'risk factors' of the mother in order to determine which programs or remedies are appropriate. Most jurisdictions have a formalized risk assessment tool that includes various risk factors. In BC, for example, the risk assessment instrument contains 23 categories of risk and most categories refer to the ability of the parent to care for a child without regard to such influential environmental circumstances as poverty, inadequate housing, and unsafe neighbourhoods (Table 7.2).

The child protection worker gathers information from other community members such as teachers or nurses, as well as the mother, then assesses the extent of risk for each risk factor. The results guide the child protection worker in recommending appropriate treatment or apprehension. These risk assessment procedures appeal to many involved in the child welfare enterprise. Administrators who want to control the work of staff can do so through computerized record keeping. When a risk assessment has been initiated, subsequent work can be monitored from head office. To line staff, risk assessment, while curtailing their discretion, contains the distinct advantage that if they follow the procedures outlined in the instrument their work cannot be criticized. Meanwhile, politicians can proclaim that they have taken action by establishing province wide assessment procedures to ensure that children will be safe. It is argued here that risk assessment has a contribution, but only a limited one and only if implemented with the family in a plan for action (Weller and Wharf, 1995; Sullivan, 1998).

Parents who have been investigated and assessed by child protection workers describe the process as demeaning and silencing. In interactions that are characterized by the power of the child protection worker, the mothers feel

Table 7.2   BC risk assessment criteria

Influence factor	Criteria
Parental	Abuse/neglect of parent as child
	Alcohol or drug use
	Parental expectations of child
	Parent's exceptance of child
	Physical ability to care for child
	Mental emotional ability to care for child
	Developmental ability to care for child
Child	Child's vulnerability
	Child's response to parent
	Child's behaviour
	Child's mental health and development
	Child's physical health and development
Family	Family violence
	Ability to cope with stress
	Availability of social supports
	Living conditions
	Family identity and interactions
Abuse/neglect	Severity of abuse/neglect
	Access to child by person accused of neglect/abuse
	Intent and acknowledgement of responsibility
	History of abuse/neglect committed by current parents
Intervention	Parent's response to identified need
	Parent's cooperation with intervention

Source: Ministry for Children and Families (1996). *The risk assessment model for child protection in BC*. Victoria, BC.

that every part of their life becomes open to invasion and they are powerless to prevent this from occurring. The experience of having other community members contacted is both embarrassing and invasive:

> Belinda: *The social worker phoned the school and the school said they are well looked after. I was embarrassed about him calling the school.*

They also describe the feeling of not being heard. "I felt invisible...like they didn't want to hear what I had to say" (Weller, 1997). Starting from the report from a community member the child protection worker's initial comments to a mother infer the assessment and decision has been made before she has had a chance to tell her story.

> Connie: *The first thing the social worker said to me was 'let me tell you something, you are in hot water.'*

For the most part the mothers feel that their context, their daily struggle of trying to care for their children without the needed resources, is not heard and not included as part of the official documentation. Instead, all their faults and potential faults are documented. These processes can lead mothers to a sense of hopelessness through realizing that they are not perceived as partners in the process of child protection, but rather as objects to be assessed, categorized, and treated with the appropriate solution, and that their voice relating to their context goes unheard in the process.

Support/Treatment

Support services may be provided to parents who request services, who voluntarily accept services after an unsubstantiated report, or who child protection workers decide 'require' support services. The provision of services is based on financial eligibility and proven risk factors. The child protection worker, knowing availability of services and eligibility requirements for each service, decides what is most appropriate for each family situation. To attain those services the child protection worker requires documentation regarding negative aspects within families. As described by Wallace (1994), this can leave a worker feeling uneasy:

> *There was a clear and distinctive boundary between ourselves as workers and the group called clients and carrying out my daily work seemed to maintain that boundary. I was outside the families I was working with passing judgement on them from a distance and referring to a policy manual to determine actions I would take to remedy their inadequacies as parents.... When I actually did make meaningful contact with a client, I could find limited means within my role to help them, other than referring them for personal counselling or parenting training.* (p.5)

The support practices that flow from defining the problem as parental fault can lead to differences between how the parent sees the problem and how the social worker or support worker responds to the problem. Mothers' stories demonstrate their travel down a path from positive anticipation of attaining help to a distrust and rejection of the Ministry for Children and Families and its approach to services. How does this happen? One mother reflected that it felt as if "her job is to spy on me" when trying to identify her discomfort with a worker contracted with the Ministry for Children and Families to support her in her parenting.

> Diane: *There is the fear of it coming back to you—I'm afraid of having Dawn (the support worker) mad at me because then she could turn around and say I'm not doing things right—my house isn't clean enough and stuff like that. And you also feel like they're all working for the same people and so they're all on the same side.*

> Joanne: *What would I change? I would have never gone in and asked for help. I would never have believed that it would have come to this where they are wanting to take my kids away.*

The mothers' own situations and strengths are not acknowledged because the entire enterprise is focused on fixing faulty mothers.

Different Views From Different Standpoints

The differing views of the so-called solutions are not about bad child protection workers or bad parents—they are about different standpoints (Smith, 1984). The child protection worker, while desiring to help the parent, stands within the administrative structure that has defined the problem as "faulty parents" and thus must conform to accountability systems and forms that ensure that the right "information" is captured. The mother, on the other hand, stands outside the official structure. There is an invisible line between the two: on one side is the power to name the problem, the solutions, and document the official reality of a mother's parenting and lifestyles; on the other side are the women doing the daily work of caring for their children, but without access to the resources required. Their world and work is *invisible* in the official systems and resulting documentation, except where that documentation captures information that points to the mother as "faulty."

How would the solutions change if the power to name the problem of child neglect were given to those who, with limited resources, must care for their children? Statistics regarding who is reported for child neglect and whose children are taken into care provide us with insight into how our systems and our current structures create systemic child neglect of children in certain families.

Those at the receiving end of reports, investigations, support/treatment, and apprehension are overwhelmingly poor, single mothers with young children. The following statistics present a picture of how reports against poor, single parents differ from the non-poor and those from two-parent families.

Table 7.3 demonstrates that neglect rather than sexual or physical abuse is the key reason for apprehending a child, usually a young child, from a single parent. It also shows how poverty plays a key role in whether a single parent is investigated and charged with neglect. Finally, the age of the child is crucial, as also shown in Table 7.3, which reflects the boundary age between when childcare is required and when it is not. It is also worth noting that physical/sexual abuse is much more prevalent for two parent families, and such abuse tends to occur to much older children.

Table 7.3   Apprehension, family make-up, and income

	Single parent (female) (%)	Two parents (%)
Reason for apprehension		
Sexual and physical abuse	17.4	52.0
Neglect	52.1	24.4
Other	30.5	23.0
Income assistance as source of family income	72.0	33.0
Income under $20,000	95.0	46.0
Age of child		
Adolescent	12.7	52.0
Under 11 years	77.3	48.0

Source: Campbell, J. (1991). *An analysis of variables in child protection apprehensions and judicial dispositions in BC child welfare practice.* Unpublished MSW Thesis University of BC, Vancouver.

The experience of all parents is that caring for young children, who need 24 hour supervision, is *Work*. This work requires a continual source of energy and labour. When there is a lack of labour due to only one parent being available and/or no money available for other labour (childcare) it follows that there is a higher potential for "omission" of care. In "job" terms there are insufficient human resources to carry out the job.

In addition to the financial resources required to enhance human resource capacity, financial resources are required to carry out the job itself. The financial resources required to raise a child from birth to 12 years of age were estimated at approximately $4,640 per year (not including childcare costs) (Vanier Institute, 1994). In 1997 the poverty rate for lone parent families with two children 0-18 years old was 65.8%, and 80.2% for children under age 7 (Doherty, 1997). The rate of deep poverty among children under age 7 in lone parent families was 58.8% (deep poverty is defined as incomes less than 75% of low income cutoffs established by Statistics Canada) (Doherty, 1997). The following choices facing single parents describe why these rates are so high.

In early 1999 in BC, a single parent on income assistance received a Family Bonus of approximately $1,200/year and the Canada Child Tax Benefit of approximately $1,000/year for each child. This works out to $2,200 per year per child—$2,440 less than the annual amount necessary to raise a child as esti-mated by the Vanier Institute. To make matters worse, any additional money or support earned or received by single parents on income assistance is clawed back from the income assistance cheque. This includes child support payments in most provinces, the majority or all of part-time earnings, and groceries paid for by someone other than the mother. On November 19, the BC government announced that a flat earnings exemption of $200 per month was being intro-duced for families on BC Benefits.

Women who head lone parent families are less likely than other mothers to have paid employment. In Canada in 1991, 52% of lone mothers with children under the age of 16 years worked at paid employment, compared to 65% of mothers in two parent families. Personal or family responsibilities are often reported by lone mothers as the reason they do not have paid employment, particularly in families with young children. Of Canadian lone mothers who were unemployed in 1991 and who had preschool-age children, 23% reported that they left their last job because of personal or family responsibilities. Such responsibilities were also cited as the reason they left their last job by 30% of those lone mothers not in the labour force and with preschool-age children (Lindsay, 1992).

A 1976 and 1993 comparison of the potential to raise one's income to the poverty line provides insight into the choice of many lone parents to stay out of the paid workforce. "In 1976, a single parent with one child needed to work 41 hours per week at minimum wage to bring the family up to the poverty line. In 1993, a single parent needed to work 73 hours a week to bring the family up to the poverty line" (Canadian Institute for Child Health, 1994). If a single mother finds work at double the minimum wage, she is caught in the high tax back position. At $30,000 a year, she is no longer eligible for full provincial childcare subsidies nor the full National Child Benefit. With child care costs for children under 6 years of age averaging $600/month, her income drops below the poverty line and she has the added stresses of maintaining work-related expenses, dealing with transportation costs, and responding to child care crises while working full-time.

Added factors in the choices facing lone mothers are the amount and reliability of child support payments. It is estimated that only 17% of single parents receive child support payments and the average payment is $350/month (Kennedy, 1995). There is a potential for moving out of the no-win situation through child support only for those lone mothers receiving the higher monthly amounts of $700 or $800/month per child. Of additional assistance are the new guidelines that ensure that the custodial parents are not required to pay tax on those payments (applicable only to those single parents with a child support agreement dated after May 1, 1998). However, for poor lone mothers who receive no child support payments (83%), who do not qualify under the tax change, and/or who receive only small and unreliable payments, the choices are not easy.

The stories of those who have been reported for neglect provide us with both short-term approaches and long-term sustainable approaches to addressing the issues of child neglect. The next section explores how child welfare practice could be reformed to acknowledge the daily lives of parents while the final section describes the structural changes required to stop the systemic neglect of children in poor, single parent families.

RESTRUCTURING THE RESPONSE TO CHILD NEGLECT

Philosophies, Policies, and Practice

The intent of this section is twofold: to place the preceding discussion within the philosophical and policy positions that govern child welfare in this and other provinces and to describe the policies and practices now in place in BC. Together with other observers of child welfare it is argued that two mutually reinforcing philosophical views prevail (see, for example, Armitage, 1993). Residualism holds that assistance from the state should not be forthcoming until all other forms of aid have been exhausted, and thus places the state as an agency of last resort rather than providing universal services for all citizens. Individualism places responsibility for personal and social problems in the hands of those experiencing problems. While individuals should take their share of responsibility, it is also patently wrong to attribute the failures of the state to individuals. For example, the mother who, along with her child, is forced to leave an abusive husband because of lack of appropriate police action, and as a consequence falls into poverty, should not be held responsible for this situation.

These philosophies are typically embraced by male and middle class policy makers who fail to recognize the difficulties many parents, and particularly single mothers, face in raising their children. In a very real sense, the combined effect of residualism and individualism consigns child welfare to a crisis-ridden and desperate enterprise that frustrates both clients and workers. While two reports on child welfare in BC (BC Ministry of Social Services, 1992) put forward a progressive vision for change, their vision has not been fulfilled. Indeed, in the view of one of the province's most astute observers of child welfare, "...we are now on the verge of a return to an Elizabethan approach to providing poor services to poor people" (Sullivan, 1998).

Ironically, a contributing factor for the failed vision was an inquiry into the death of a 5 year old boy (see **Chapter 8**) and the Ministry of (then) Social Services, which was supposed to put things right. The Gove Inquiry viewed the Ministry as a mismanaged and inadequately staffed enterprise (BC Ministry of the Attorney General, 1995). With the important exception that child welfare should be governed by communities, a recommendation that has been ignored, the Inquiry focused attention on organizational and staffing issues.

Thus, the Inquiry recommended: that child-related services provided by a number of different Ministries be brought into a single Ministry; that information and record keeping systems be improved; that case management arrangements and risk assessment procedures be put into place; that the work of the Ministry be monitored by both internal and external mechanisms; and, that the quality of staff be improved by requiring a Bachelor of Social Work as the minimum requirement for employment and by establishing a comprehensive in-service training program.

As critics of the Inquiry and of the new Ministry for Children and Families, which was created in September 1996, have pointed out as a response to the Gove Inquiry, such administrative changes may be necessary but they are scarcely sufficient (see, among other sources, Armitage, 1998; Sullivan, 1998; Wharf, 1998). Administrative rearrangements ignore the all important context of child welfare, poverty, poor housing, unsafe neighbourhoods, the absence of community involvement, the interminable delays that occur in courts related to family breakdown, and the volume of work faced by both the courts and child protection workers. Evidence supporting this view of the state of affairs in child welfare in BC can be gained from a number of sources. The prevalence of an investigative approach to practice and the absence of supports for parents has the inevitable consequence of more children being taken into care. And indeed this has occurred. "The ratio of children in care to all children fell in every year, from 11.5/1000 in 1981 to 7.5/1000 in 1993. This decline was reversed suddenly in 1994; by early 1998 the ratio was 10.5/1000" (Armitage, 1998).

A second source of evidence is the morale of staff. A survey conducted by the BC Government Employees Union (BCGEU) gave the Ministry for Children and Families a failing report card. "Over 1,200 BCGEU members said loud and clear that the new Ministry has failed on all counts—from consulting with workers and providing adequate resources and training, to improving service delivery and enhancing the quality of service" (BC Government and Services Employees Union, 1997).

Translating Philosophy into Practice: The Tyranny of the Case

The Gove Inquiry was anchored in the individualistic perspective noted above. In retrospect this lens was entirely predictable. Judges deal with individuals who have committed some wrong. They judge individuals, individual culpability, and individual responsibility. Individuals are of central importance in child protection work and perhaps in emulation of the legal profession we have framed and thought about individuals as cases. Indeed, the word case is embedded in our vocabulary. We talk about casework, caseloads, case reporting, and case management, but have rarely stopped to consider the impact of this language and this individualistic way of working on ourselves and our clients.

The impact of language is subject to interpretation and our interpretations may not be the same as all readers. Nevertheless, it is suggested that the word "case" has the unintended, but nevertheless powerful, effect of transforming people into objects. When talked, recorded, and conferenced about as "cases," individuals lose their uniqueness and their influence. Once individuals are assigned the status of a "case," it becomes possible for well-meaning professionals to organize case management conferences where "cases" have little ability to influence the discussion or the outcomes. A First Nations woman named Whitehawk made the telling observation at a child welfare conference that "case coordination is a conspiracy against my people" (Whitehawk, 1980). Whitehawk's concern was that when a number of "white" professionals get together to coordinate their efforts, the voice and the unique cultural factors of the First Nations clients are neither heard nor incorporated into the decisions. The same can be said about all case conferences unless deliberate attention is taken to ensure that the client is the most important person present and assisted to make her views known by a trusted friend or advocate.

The focus on individuals fits well with both the education and the inclination of practitioners. Most people enter social work and other helping professions to assist and counsel individuals. While they may be introduced in their formal education to theories that stress the impact of the environment, the legacy of these theories is fleeting if they are not reinforced in practice; and most often they are not, since the case orientation also fits very neatly with organizational imperatives. It is easy to count cases as the units of service and assign resources on the size of caseloads. It is also easy to monitor and control work organized on an individual basis. When a child is injured or dies or is removed from parental care for reasons that turn out to be insufficient, the individual social worker can be disciplined or fired. Disciplinary actions against individual workers have been taken recently in BC, and while there is a need for such action when individuals are culpable, the important structural factors are rarely singled out for attention.

The term "case" has helped child protection workers and administrators to see parents as objects to be inspected, judged, and monitored through risk assessment instruments and case conferences. Depending on the outcome of the risk assessment, parents will be punished by having their children removed, or counselled or trained to be better parents. In all situations the outcome is largely determined by the social worker, the supervisor, and senior bureaucrats with the consequence that the already fragile sense of self and confidence of clients is further eroded.

The focus on individuals has also had the consequence of excluding other approaches to practice. Clients are interviewed/counselled on an individual basis. The prevailing practice is for social workers to see clients in their offices, thus eliminating the need for staff to travel between the homes of their clients. While often viewed as an efficient way to practice and as emulating the example of the more prestigious professionals such as lawyers and physicians, office-based practice has a number of unfortunate consequences. First, and with the important exception that all initial contacts require a home visit, it allows staff to remain unaware of the housing and neighbourhood circumstances in which their clients live. Second, it reinforces the already unequal power balance between worker and client. Office visits let clients know in no uncertain terms that they are the "visitors." Office appointments and waiting rooms with controlled entry constitute a clear signal that the worker is in charge.

Finally, individual and office-based practice does not allow clients to get to know each other and to share their troubles and their solutions. All of these consequences reinforce the powerful message that one's troubles are one's own fault and can only be resolved by individual effort and professional help.

To summarize, it is argued that child welfare policy and practice focuses on the individual problems of individual clients and, as noted earlier, the problems and remedies are largely defined by professionals. Thus parents are referred to parenting or anger management programs even though these programs may not meet the unique needs of individuals. One parent expressed her frustration at this mismatch of program and needs by saying "What I need is a bus pass, what I get is a referral to a program I don't need and can't get to anyway" (Callahan, Hooper, and Wharf, 1998).

Reforming Practice

The discussion now turns to some suggestions for changing practice. The suggestions take the following form: individuals are important, but the re-framing of work with individuals emphasizes their unique needs and their strengths and which should be dealt with through an action plan developed by "client" and worker (Weller and Wharf, 1996). It is argued further that "clients" and "cases" should be seen as residents, and that group and community work approaches can make substantial contributions to practice. In order to be implemented on a widespread scale, these reforms require a supportive philosophical and policy context. Philosophies are deeply held and difficult to dislodge, but nevertheless, it is incumbent on those with different philosophies to argue their merits and to outline new modes of practice.

An action plan developed jointly by the resident and the worker turns the risk assessment instrument from a professionally driven investigation tool into a plan that looks for strengths as well as problems. The plan begins with the resident's statement of her problems and of the resources that would assist her. It continues with the assessment by the child protection worker and other professionals. Where disagreements occur time and energy is devoted to resolving them. Whenever possible the action plan attempts to use the resources of the Ministry for Children and Families to meet the particular issues facing residents. Such a tailored approach requires a global budget assigned to district offices rather than budgets for programs.

The other suggestions are based on an innovative project now taking place in Victoria where child protection workers from the Ministry for Children and Families are placed in neighbourhood houses. The intent is to ensure the safety of children by building a partnership between neighbourhoods and the Ministry. The approach is anchored in a philosophy of service embraced by neighbourhood houses whereby those receiving help are seen as residents rather than clients. The objective of the initiative is to assist child welfare staff to incorporate this philosophy into their day to day work.

Residents are welcomed into neighbourhood houses, treated with respect and dignity, and are expected to make a contribution by volunteering in one of the programs. Since neighbourhood houses provide a variety of programs, from libraries to day care to services for seniors, they are valued community resources. People coming to a neighbourhood house can do so without any sense of shame or failure; after all they may just as well be coming to the library as talking to a child welfare worker.

The aim of this project is to enable child welfare workers to become known in the neighbourhood as individuals who can be trusted, to discard the style of work captured by the labels of "baby snatcher" and "social cop," and to find ways to prevent children from being taken into the care of the state. Workers provide information about the field of child welfare, the legislation, and the resources that are available. They try to reduce the number of inappropriate complaints, thereby reducing the amount of time devoted to investigation. The initiative is concerned with neglect matters and with parents who require assistance, and have the capacity and desire to care for their children.

Including Group and Community Work

The essential contribution of group work is simple and straightforward. Group work brings clients together and provides a climate where they can talk about troubles and actions. Perhaps for the first time they learn that their troubles are shared by others, and that they should not shoulder the blame for inadequate income assistance rates, the absence of public housing, or the tortured arrangements necessary to secure day or respite care. They learn how others have managed to extract useful help from a service system that often seems designed to hinder rather than help.

Group work approaches can take a variety of forms. Mutual aid occurs when individuals who lack supportive relationships are included with a positive social network (Cameron, 1995; Fuchs, 1995). Mutual aid can be extended to encompass "structural empathy" (Carniol, 1990) whereby clients gain a comprehensive understanding of the societal factors that shape their lives. A third approach bordering on community work involves groups taking action on issues affecting them. In the Empowering Women projects in BC, groups of single mothers established a client run information centre on income assistance and a community garden and changed oppressive policies in a public housing project

(Callahan, Lumb, and Wharf, 1994).

A community work approach to practice seeks to embed practice in communities. It extends working with groups by its intent to transfer resources to communities, to build a knowledgeable constituency for child welfare and to pave the way for community governance. Community work is based on the assumption that neighbourhoods are well placed to care for the welfare of children. With adequate resources, neighbourhoods can provide daycare, family drop-in places, and centres for teenagers. Some of these resources are now located in the Ministry for Children and Families and handed out on a "case by case" basis in a most complicated and bureaucratic fashion. One long-range intent of the project noted above is to transfer resources for daycare to neighbourhood houses.

In addition and most importantly, community work uses the resources of the community in caring for children. Thus, workers find families who can become temporary foster parents, they solicit the help of older youths to help out in recreational and athletic activities, and they enlist parents as group leaders for young parent discussion groups. In a word, child welfare workers in neighbourhood houses become organizers for child welfare rather than child protection workers.

Without doubt, this approach runs counter to the prevailing thrust of individualism and investigation. Yet despite the inhospitable organization environment in both this and other provinces, some offices and some workers have managed to embed their practice in communities. A long-standing example of community work comes from the Metro Children's Aid Society in Toronto. Certainly, but not without a lot of difficulties, a unit of community social work has nevertheless existed in this agency for over 25 years and had a substantial record of achievement (see, for example, Barr, 1971; Lee, 1998).

Restructuring Systems to Prevent Child Neglect

The following recommendations require a fundamental rethinking of society's approach to the work of caring for children. If we are going to end systemic child neglect then we must treat the work of caring for children as work. As with other work the financial and human resources and the training and peer support opportunities for those doing the work must be adequate and readily available.

Increase Access to Financial Resources

There are two components to this recommendation. The first of these is to increase the financial resources to those caring for children; the second is to provide access to employment that is complementary to the work of caring for children.

Parents caring for young children should receive a parenting wage or family benefit that ensures that enough financial resources are available to the parent to provide "nutritious food, a safe place to live, and intellectual stimulation through exposure to a variety of activities" (Doherty, 1997). This benefit should not be tied to a monthly accounting of other income. Much like a guaranteed annual income, it could be provided directly to parents of young children. The income tax system could provide the income-testing required rather than the current monthly reviews and checks that are both demeaning to income assistance recipients and a costly, labour intensive approach.

Access to employment that supports caring work requires policies that encourage managing the balance between work and family responsibilities. In addition to provincial and federal policies, corporate policies are required to encourage job sharing, flexible hours, and supports for parenting responsibilities. In addition, provincial and federal policies to increase maternity, parental, and children's sick days would support parents' abilities to care adequately for their children while continuing their employment. For example, comparison between Canada and Sweden reveals that Swedish parents receive up to 60 days per year of paid leave to care for sick children under the age of 10, while there are no requirements in BC for employers to provide paid leave for care of sick children. Another support for parents is maternity and parental leave. Sweden provides new mothers and fathers up to 12 months of leave paid at 90% of previous earnings and an additional 3 months with a flat-rate allowance. In Canada a mother has only been able to take up to 17 weeks of paid leave at 60% of previous earnings if they have 20 weeks of insurable earnings. Additional parental leave has been available to either parent to a maximum of 10 weeks, again paid at 60% of previous earnings. The 2000/01 federal government budget increased to one year paid parental leave following the birth of a child.

In *addition* to the preceding family-friendly policies, there is the continued need for access to well-paying jobs and acknowledgement in the hiring process of the experience gained by those raising children. British Columbia does provide a higher minimum wage than the majority of provinces and has discussed potential increases. Acknowledgement, however, that child rearing experience is transferable to the labour market is not part of our culture yet, and requires promotion on all parts of society—both the public and private sectors.

Increase Human Resources

Accessible, affordable, quality childcare is the cornerstone for ensuring children are well cared for and their parents have access to paid work. The subsidy system in BC could be enhanced through ensuring that the subsidy can buy quality childcare and the income threshold is increased. In addition, quality childcare must be easily accessible. The development of a system of quality child care settings that provides a range of options from family to group set-tings for the parents within each community needs to be fully supported by all levels of government. The Ministry of Social Development and Economic Se-curity released a discussion paper on childcare entitled *Building a Better Future for BC's Kids* in the fall of 1999 and announced as part of its 2000/01 budget a major increase in subsidized childcare spaces, moving toward universal access over time.

As with any job, the job of child rearing requires breaks. Most of us can-not imagine working at our job 7 days a week, from morning to night, and being on-call through the night. Nevertheless many poor single parents must do exactly that. Opportunities for parents with limited resources to access qual-ity early childhood education programs such as preschool or flexible hours child care settings would reduce the stress levels for those working non-stop at child rearing, while at the same time providing a positive experience for the child.

Provide Access to Training and Peer Support

Provision of information to assist parents in their work plus opportunities for sharing on-the-job experiences and problem solving is similar to the career de-velopment opportunity most good employers provide. Information and access to peer sharing is needed in all phases of parenthood from prenatal through adolescence. Many parents currently access information and peer support net-works provided through the local public health centre/nurses, early childhood educators and local community programs. Continued support of these pro-grams and resources to ensure access is available to all parents is vital. This recommendation builds on the group and community approach to child wel-fare practice mentioned in the previous section.

Acknowledge Citizenship of Caregivers

In Canada, the support of children is regarded primarily as a private parental responsibility that has no value to society. In contrast, Sheila Kamerman notes "European countries have a long history of acknowledging that children are a major societal resource and that the whole society should share in the costs of rearing them" (Kamerman and Kahn, 1990). In Canada, raising a child in pov-erty, especially by only one person, can be discouraging and degrading. It is no wonder that depression and a sense of hopelessness is often found in par-ents reported for neglect. Acknowledging the importance of this job rather than treating parents as if they were out to swindle the government requires a different mindset, different ways of describing the work, and different resources. Changing our language, such as describing resources as pay for parenting, is a step in this direction. Group work as described in the preceding section is another. Including the experience of caring for children as relevant in paid employment is yet another. The impact of changing the way we view the work of women caring for children changes our treatment of them from one of "charity case'" to one of citizen.

SUMMARY

This chapter has dived below the surface solutions of child welfare and reflects on the root issues as described by those doing the work of raising children. The recommendations for restructuring child welfare as well as restructuring provisions for income and child care stem from the lack of recognition that raising children is work—work that needs to be acknowledged, and supported. Provincial, federal, and local governments, together with the community and corporate sectors, need to pull together to turn the current approach to preventing child neglect upside down and put into place policies and practices that acknowledge the citizenship of parents raising children and the societal value of their work.

REFERENCES

Armitage, A. (1993). The policy and legislative context. In B. Wharf (Ed.), *Rethinking child welfare in Canada*. Toronto: McLelland and Stewart.

Armitage, A. (1998). Lost vision: Children and the Ministry for Children and Families. *BC Studies*, 118, 112.

Barr, D. (1971). Doing prevention in Regent Park: Partnership can work. In B. Wharf (Ed.), *Community work in Canada*. Toronto: McLelland and Stewart.

BC Government and Services Employees Union (1997). *Report card on the Ministry for Children and Families*. Burnaby, BC.

BC Ministry for Children and Families (1998). *The BC handbook for action on child abuse and neglect*. Victoria, BC.

BC Ministry of Social Services (1992). *Making changes: A place to start*. Victoria, BC.

BC Ministry of Social Services (1992). *Liberating our children, liberating our nation*. Victoria, BC.

Callahan, C., Hooper, M., and Wharf, B. (1998). *Protecting children by empowering women*. Victoria, BC: University of Victoria, Child, Family and Community Research Program, School of Social Work.

Callahan, M., Lumb, C., and Wharf, B. (1994). Strengthening families by empowering women. A joint project of the Ministry of Social Services and the School of Social Work, University of Victoria, Victoria, BC.

Cameron, G. (1995). The nature and effectiveness of parent mutual aid organizations in child welfare. In J. Hudson and B. Gallaway (Eds.), *Child welfare in Canada: Research and policy implications* (pp. 66-81). Toronto: Thompson Educational Publishing.

Canadian Institute of Child Health (1994). *The health of Canada's children: A CICH profile*. Ottawa.

Carniol, B. (1990). Social work and the labour movement. In B. Wharf (Ed.), *Social work and social change in Canada* (pp. 114-143). Toronto: McLelland and Stewart.

Doherty, G. (1997). *Zero to six: The basis for school readiness*. Ottawa: Human Resources Development, Applied Research Branch Strategic Policy.

Fuchs, D. (1995). Preserving and strengthening families and protecting children: Social network intervention, a balanced approach to the prevention of child maltreatment. In J. Hudson and B. Gallaway (Eds.), *Child welfare in Canada: Research and policy implications*. Toronto: Thompson Educational Publishing.

Gove, T. (1995). *Report of the Gove Inquiry into Child Protection*. Victoria, BC: Ministry of Social Services.

Kamerman, S., and Kahn, A. (1990). Social services for children, youth, and families in the United States. *Children and Youth Services Review*, 12(2), 1-179.

Kennedy, S. (1995). *Family maintenance: Assessment, collection and enforcement*. Victoria, BC: Ministry of Social Services.

Krane, J. (1995). Least disruptive and intrusive course of action...For whom? Insight from feminist analysis of practice in cases of child sexual abuse. Paper presented at the *7th National Social Welfare Policy Conference*, "Re-making Canadian Social Policy: Staking Claims and Forging Change," June 26, 1995.

Lee, W. (1998). A community approach to urban child welfare in Canada. In L. Dominelli (Ed.), *Community approaches to child welfare: International perspectives*. Aldershot: Ashgate Publishing Ltd.

Mosher, C. (1994). *Neglect of children: A comprehensive review*. Unpublished manuscript, BC Ministry of Social Services.

Sullivan, R. (1998). Commentary on "Lost vision: Children and the Ministry for Children and Families." *BC Studies*, 118, 112.

Vanier Institute (1992).

Weller, F. (1997). *Child neglects from a mother's standpoint*. Unpublished master's thesis, University of Victoria, Faculty of Human and Social Development, Victoria.

Weller, F., and Wharf, B. (1995). *From risk assessment to family action planning*. Victoria, BC: University of Victoria, School of Social Work, Child, Family and Community Research Program.

Wharf, B. (1998). Child welfare: A personal reflection. *Perspectives*, 20, 2.

Whitehawk, M. (1980). *Taking control*, a video produced by the Taking Control Project. Regina, Sask.: University of Regina, Faculty of Social Work.

Plate 3 Living the future ▸

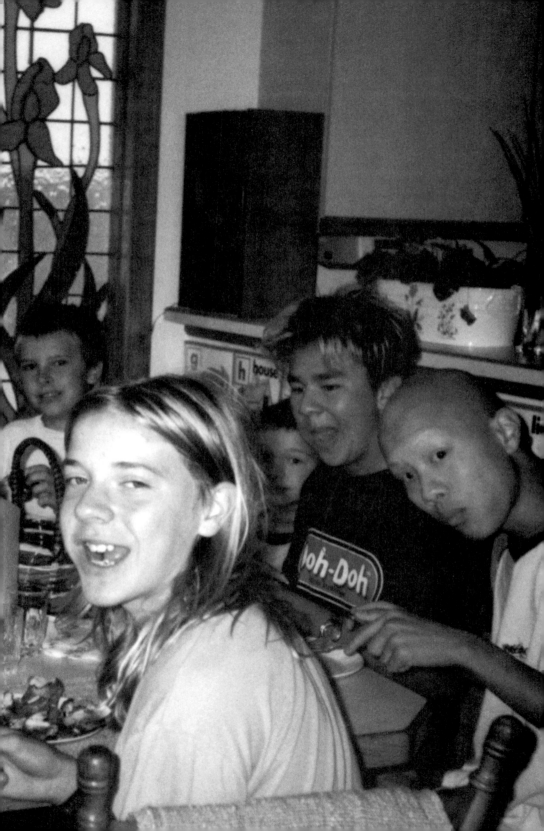

Learning from the Past: Improving Child-Serving Systems

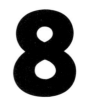

C. Morton

BC's first Children's Commissioner, 1996-1999

INTRODUCTION

The 1990s have been a decade of exploring change across BC's child protection, welfare, education, justice, and health care systems. This chapter will focus on these changes to determine whether these systems are meeting the needs of children more effectively today than a decade ago. The need to examine change across child-serving systems results from the "shared client"—the child whose complex needs should best be met by access to services from across the community.

This chapter's assessment of the changes to services and systems is based upon the author's experiences as the Transition Commissioner (Morton, 1996) responsible for the implementation of the Gove Report (Gove, 1995), and then as Children's Commissioner responsible for monitoring and evaluating the work of BC's restructured child-serving systems. The work of the Children's Commission is to assist in identifying necessary reforms to the services provided to children, make recommendations for system-wide and child-specific changes, and monitor their implementation.

This chapter will review and rely upon the information gathered by the Children's Commission since its establishment in September, 1996 through to the end of 1999. This information and data show that progress has been made in effecting positive changes for children in some critical areas, while in others the challenges are better understood and viable solutions have been identified but not yet implemented. The absence of full integration in service delivery or the funding of major new initiatives such as early intervention for children from birth through adolescence—a cornerstone of the change agenda not yet achieved—continues to result in critical weaknesses in how communities meet the needs of children. The information also indicates that change in policy, practice, and expectations is only achievable with a constant vision and a strong, shared, and visible commitment to these changes by leaders across the child servicing systems.

The population of children in BC in the 1990s is different in composition and need from the population of as little as a decade ago. The number of children whose first language is not English has tripled, placing challenges upon all systems to find new ways to reach out to these children and their families. Schools must find new ways to teach, public health must find new ways to connect with recently arrived families, and other support services must find new ways to be welcomed into homes to help with parenting and to overcome the effects of poor nutrition, poverty, and cultural isolation. As well, the number of Aboriginal children who are at risk and in care is known to be close to 40% of the 10,000 children in care. While First Nations struggle to achieve protocols and treaties for on reserve supports, children in these communities continue to suffer the effects of reduced and inadequate funding and a lack of qualified Aboriginal practitioners to meet their needs. For other Aboriginal children, their presence in the urban street life is growing at an alarming rate.

The rising number of children born to drug- and alcohol-addicted parents has created critical new challenges for all support systems. Services must now reach both parent and child to avoid the sometimes fatal, inter-generational consequences of drug and alcohol damage. Within the public school system, the dramatic rise in special needs children, especially with behavioural problems, has created daunting new challenges that cannot solely be addressed within a classroom. The lack of well trained medical practitioners, knowledgeable in the diagnosis and treatment of these special needs, creates huge gaps in service across the province.

Since the early 1990s, all child-serving systems in BC have undertaken sector specific reforms to address the emerging, large-scale needs of this complex child population. The Ministry of Education now funds additional school-based resources for special needs and Aboriginal children (Ministry of Education, 1999a). Community schools receive funding to support their broad-based approach to serving the needs of children and families that extend beyond the classroom. The Ministry of Health (1997) and Ministry for Children and Families (MCF) (1997) have created and monitor provincial public health goals and strategies for children at risk of poor health. The child protection and support system, largely funded and directed by the former Ministry of Social Services (now part of the MCF), undertook a major community consultation process with new legislation introduced to address the concerns about better services to children (see **Chapter 6**).

In the mid-1990s—after a period of fiscal restraint, changing leadership, and shifting philosophy—the former Ministry of Social Services, and those who worked with it, recognized that the child protection system and its related supports were lacking in a clear direction and a set of guiding principles about what constituted appropriate service for children and families. Beyond policy and legislation, practitioners had inconsistent approaches and philosophies as to what strategies most effectively engaged children and families in promoting healthy families and rigorous protection practices. Inconsistency, instability, lack of vision, and inadequate resources to upgrade technology or skill sets were recognized as the systems's barriers to meeting children's needs.

On July 9,1992, a 5-year-old boy named Matthew Vaudreuil was brutally killed by his mother. Both mother and child had been well known to both the Ministry of Social Services and the health care system throughout their lives. It was incomprehensible to many that this child, who had been the subject of so many reports of abuse to the Ministry of Social Services, who had been in and out of emergency wards his entire life, and who had been in child care facilities, nonetheless had remained in his mother's care with the risks he faced never adequately investigated nor understood. The media and politicians led a campaign to find out why this child had died and what needed to be changed in the child protection system to ensure such a case did not happen again.

A public inquiry was demanded and established. Judge Thomas Gove led this inquiry across the province and submitted a report to government that called for sweeping changes to the child-serving systems (Gove, 1985).

This chapter will examine the changes set out in the recommendations of the Gove Report, other reforms underway, and the process through which government assessed and acted upon those recommendations. Two key questions that British Columbia must continue to ask itself are whether the changes to the child-serving system are leading to improvements in the way children are served in BC, and if not, why not? Were the changes the wrong ones; has their implementation been inadequate or does the change agenda need more time to achieve its intended goals?

BACKGROUND

The public outrage and demand for change arising from Matthew's death has been faced in other provinces, where a child's death has propelled the child protection system into the public light for scrutiny and reform. In these reviews (see, for example: Ontario Child Mortality Task Force, 1997; Christianson-Wood and Murray, 1999), similar weaknesses have been identified in the child protection systems. In such cases, changes have been recommended and committed to by government, but none as extensively as in BC. As a result, the experiences of this province offer the most comprehensive opportunity in Canada to examine whether the systemic changes we have made are serving the best interest of children.

THE GOVE INQUIRY

After 18 months of public hearings, reviewing written submissions from diverse interest groups, and examining government documents, policies, practice manuals, and the files of individual children in government care, Judge Gove delivered his report to government in November of 1995. This report identified fundamental weaknesses in the child protection system that were not unique to Matthew's case, and concluded that many other children were equally at risk of physical harm and receiving poor service. Gove found the following shortcomings with the system:

1. Poorly trained social workers, often lacking in qualifications, were being asked to make difficult decisions about a child's risk, without adequate supervision or policy direction. Gove recommended that rigorous new recruitment criteria be adopted to ensure that staff with sound, consistent skills were hired who would then be trained continuously by the MCF. Management reform to ensure clear direction, feedback, and review of performance were to accompany the staff changes;

2. The system's veil of secrecy—born from a respect of individual client privacy but now the rationale for unnecessary refusals to discuss what was happening within the larger system—meant that the public had no effective, reliable means to measure how well children and families were being served. Gove proposed the creation of the Children's Commission, an office independent of the child-serving ministries that would monitor the work of those ministries, recommend change when necessary, and report to the public on these matters;

3. Policy and practice, both within and beyond the child protection system, failed to promote continuous planning or risk assessment throughout Matthew's life. Gove recommended the development of policies and practices, assisted by technology, that would follow a family wherever they lived, assessing risk over a continuous period of time This risk assessment and monitoring nwould be a responsibility of all child serving practitioners, to ensure all information about a child's risk was known (e.g., childcare facilities, emergency wards, schools, or reports to child protection);

4. There was no integration of decision making between practitioners within the Ministry of Social Services or with those who knew Matthew and his mother in the community (doctors, public health nurses, and childcare workers). Ministry social workers and other practitioners did not share information relevant to Matthew's risks because practitioners believed that confidentiality issues denied them the opportunity to inform each other of what was happening in this case. No single practitioner took the lead responsibility for ensuring this child was safe, no full assessment was made of Matthew's circumstances and risk, and all failed to engage in long-term planning for Matthew and his mother. The elimination of barriers between service providers was proposed through the creation of a single ministry to serve children, followed by significant reform to practice and policies that would promote integrated education, training, and service delivery across health, social services, education, justice, and policing services; and

5. The control of the child welfare system by the provincial government created a significant gap between what individual communities need and what the system delivered. The Gove Report recommended that a regional governance structure be established to empower communities to run their own child welfare systems, much like children's aid societies in other provinces.

RESPONSE TO THE GOVE RECOMMENDATIONS— THE TRANSITION COMMISSION

Judge Gove was concerned that the changes he had recommended to government would collect dust on a shelf in a ministry office. To reduce the likelihood of this, he recommended that government appoint a Transition Commissioner (Gove, 1995, p. 290) to oversee the implementation of the change agenda within 3 months of the delivery of his report. Gove also recommended that, once implemented, a Children's Commissioner be appointed to continue to oversee and evaluate the functioning of the new child-serving system (Gove, 1995, pp. 282-283). The Children's Commission was also to examine the death of all children known to the ministry, to ensure all such children received the benefit of a review and the system received an objective, thorough report on what it had done well and done poorly in serving that child so that further changes could be made as and when needed.

The government did agree to appoint a Transition Commissioner, but with different terms of reference than those contemplated by Gove (Gove, 1995). For Gove, the role was to oversee implementation of his proposed changes. For government, the role was to test the "doability" of the proposed changes and report back to the Premier with recommendations for implementation. The Transition Commissioner was to work within and outside of the government, testing the acceptability and effectiveness of the proposed changes and planning for their implementation where appropriate. In February 1996, this author was appointed Transition Commissioner with a 3 year term to complete the task.

The immediate task of the Transition Commission was to assess community and service provider response to the key recommendations and general direction proposed by Gove. (In all, a total of 118 recommendations were made.) While provincial politicians largely endorsed the changes, public servants, the medical and educational systems, the corrections and police system, and community agencies had mixed responses. In principle, most agreed that Gove had identified the key weaknesses in the delivery of services to children. Few discussed, however, how their areas of responsibility were prepared to affect the changes necessary to fix these weaknesses without assurances of new funding, job security, and the continued protection of traditionally defined professional status.

The absence of significant detail in "how" the changes would unfold created nervousness and apprehension, if not mistrust, in many service sectors where practitioners and providers were already fearing downsizing and consolidation. In agencies dependent upon government funding but accustomed to independence in management, a new collective employer association had been struck to find new ways to streamline human resources issues related to wages, standards, hiring, and competencies. Many feared that the subtext to these discussions was the elimination of funding to smaller agencies and the support of merging them into larger, more efficient organizations. This concern, in part, was related to an earlier study (Korbin, 1993) that led to the creation of the Community Social Services Employers Association. This was a single agency that oversaw the human resources issues of social services agencies in the province (Community Social Services Employee Association, 1999).

While senior management within the Ministry of Social Services endorsed the major changes necessary to implement the Gove recommendations, many ministry staff were concerned about job loss if they lacked the credentials and qualifications Gove had recommended. Much of middle management across the five child-serving ministries (Education, Attorney General, Health, Women's Equality, and Social Services) feared a loss of definition of programs and control over staff and budgets if integration between programs was to occur. In all ministries except Social Services, problems in the child-serving system were thought to reside elsewhere and many feared disruption of their "effective" services to address weaknesses they perceived to be largely housed within the child protection system.

Within government, the notion of creating a single ministry housing all of children's services was supported by the Ministry of Social Services, but none other. No other ministry saw the children's programs as severable from their larger agendas and all predicted a loss of expertise, identity, and culture within their systems that would follow a dismantling of the old and creation of a new, integrated system.

Outside government, communities were already struggling to implement a new regional health care delivery and governance system, and wondered where they would find the talent, energy, and resources to govern the yet to be designed child-serving system as Gove had recommended. Furthermore, Aboriginal communities did not see themselves reflected in the Gove model of service delivery and governance, despite their children being disproportionately represented among children in care (MacDonald, 1998).

It was the job of the Transition Commissioner to decide whether concerns expressed by those within and outside of government were resolveable, and to assess whether or not resistance to proposed changes in the system posed insurmountable barriers to the reform agenda.

The dialogue about how to implement and evaluate the usefulness of the proposed changes was one that few were prepared to enter into, fund, or expedite. This resistance was most apparent outside the Ministry of Social Services, in sectors which had traditionally served children in a way defined by the limits of a single profession, such as medicine, education, and the correctional system. Many in every sector presented their philosophical view of what they saw as meeting the best interests of a child, in ways which they felt were incompatible with the integration of other systems.

Medicine and public health in particular saw their role as dependent upon being welcomed into a home, whereas they saw child welfare as the heavy hand of the state, often feared by parents. Initially, the more traditionally minded in the education sector felt that they were already asked to do too varied a set of tasks to support at-risk children, and struggled with the notion of teachers, counsellors, and non-educators working as a community, rather than school-based, team.

In response to these reservations, the Transition Commission explored with stakeholders whether alternatives to the Gove model were viable and in the best interests of children. It was here that most participants in the policy development and consultation processes of the Transition Commission placed their energy. An approach to change for most was one that endorsed "incremental," tested models for change within the boundaries of one sector's definitions and culture. Once concerns and positions were tabled, the Transition Commission, ministries, and community agencies began a dialogue about instituting pilot projects to test the Gove reforms. These test sites were primarily intended to demonstrate whether the changes were possible, doable, and promising of better results for practitioners, parents, and children.

Barriers to both major and minor change could have been addressed with time and money. Unfortunately, neither was available in the summer of 1996 when the public, media, and politicians sensed that the child protection system was continuing to spiral downward and that children were increasingly placed at risk. Questions about how children in protective care had died and how many such children there were "known" to government went either unanswered or responses changed daily during the budget estimates debate in the Legislature. There was concern that the system was no longer functional. The "veil of secrecy" traditionally surrounding the world of child protection was creating confusion and anger among those seeking answers and reassurances, including Ministers responsible. In this vacuum of information, the public, media, and politicians concluded that nothing had changed since Matthew Vaudreuil's death. The public mood was intemperate and demanding action from government. The public mood was also largely correct—the resistance to real change was pervasive both within the public service and among government funded service agencies. Little had changed beyond the borders of the Ministry of Social Services and its implementation of the new *Child, Family and Community Service Act* in February, 1996 (Ministry of Social Services, 1994). The barriers between many doctors, public health nurses, teachers, social workers, police, and others serving children were as great as ever, with disjointed programs and inefficient spending.

As a result of the public's frustration with the lack of change almost 9 months after the submission of Gove's report to government, the Transition Commission was instructed by the Premier that its 3 year mandate was gone, and it had only weeks to decide what that change agenda should look like—the Gove model or something else. Ironically, the pervasive resistance to change met by the Transition Commission, coupled with compelling evidence of children not being well served by the status quo, was the most important factor that led the Transition Commission to recommend that sweeping change was in fact both necessary and urgent. The "doability" of this change, however, remained the largest question and required the most significant attention.

The Transition Commission's original goal to establish pilot sites in the fall of 1996, to illustrate to practitioners that integration and quality case planning were viable models for service delivery across sectors, was no longer possible. The models from other jurisdictions upon which these pilot sites were to be based became the source of advice and information to the Transition Commission as it developed its final report to the Premier. The Transition Commission had to assess the adaptability of these models that reflected the Gove model and had evidence of success in other jurisdictions—could they work in BC? Would they make the systems better for children? What were the prerequisites government and others must commit to if the changes were to be successful? Further, the newly introduced *Child Family and Community Service Act* was already the subject of extensive new policy and training design underway in the Ministry of Social Services.

The fall of 1996 provided a very rare and significant window of opportunity in BC to create a dramatically new approach to delivering services for children with the endorsement of the public and politicians. In other jurisdictions, the public demand for change had been blunted by divided political wills, fiscal constraint, or philosophical debates. In BC, the Transition Commission was given license to shape policy and program as it felt appropriate and in the best interest of children.

The Transition Commission's report to the Premier in September 1996 advised that there had been little success in engaging interested sectors in a dialogue about how to make significant change. Further, the resistance to a meaningful dialogue about change was symptomatic of the very large problems currently faced by many clients of these systems seeking help—a pervasive lack of coordination or trust between service providers, disjointed and inefficient approaches to funding a continuum of services, and the absence of a plan that engaged all family and service providers in its design and delivery. The same barriers children and families faced at the front line had been reflected in discussions between the Transition Commission and many in the professions, agencies, and ministries responsible.

The report to the Premier concluded that it was not possible to find piecemeal solutions to these fundamental problems, nor would the large solutions be pursued voluntarily. In addition, the Gove recommendations, coupled with the results of the community consultations of the early 1990s (Ministry of Social Services, 1992a; Ministry of Social Services, 1992b), all pointed to the public's vision of what it wanted to see for children—it was now the time to try to implement that vision, if possible.

The report also reviewed the work of scholars and the approaches of other jurisdictions. With some modifications, the Premier was advised that the fundamental principles underlying Gove's proposed new child welfare system appeared both sound and doable. While the development of pilot sites in BC would have provided information on how to run new families and children services, the Transition Commission concluded that pilots conducted around the world had provided considerable evidence of the success of these new approaches, and that adopting them without further pilots was feasible with training, leadership across all sectors, and management support.

The primary recommendations of the Transition Commission's report to the Premier, were:

1. Transfer all child, youth, and family services to a single, new ministry. This new ministry was to integrate programs formerly provided by the ministries of Social Services, Health, Education, Attorney General, and Women's Equality. The integration of these programs was to address matters of shared or complementary policy, practice, funding, and management.

2. The new ministry's mandate was to be established immediately and all programs were to be integrated fully within 6 months, with the Transition Commission setting out a schedule for what programs could be moved into the new ministry at what time.

3. Within the new ministry, a highly trained and dedicated child protection workforce was to be created and a new position, the Director of Child Protection, was to be appointed to ensure rigour, improved training, and accountability within this system. New tools were to be provided to this team to ensure consistent and appropriate decision making about a child's risk. This specialized team would have extensive practice connections to all other service providers within their ministry and communities, to ensure full and integrated planning for children who were brought into care.

4. The new ministry was to take over full responsibility for the implementation of those Gove recommendations endorsed by the Transition Commission and enumerated in its report to the Premier. Fewer than a dozen of the original 118 Gove recommendations were either amended or not adopted by the Transition Commissioner—it was felt that implementation or full adoption of these would be impossible without further experience. The only significant area of disagreement with the Gove report was in the proposal to establish a governance system that extended to regional authorities the power to run a newly defined child-serving system. The Transition Commission recommended that government not implement a community-based governance system for the child-serving system, until communities across the province had more experience in governing the recently devolved health care system.

5. A Children's Commissioner was to be appointed to review the death of all children as well as reviewing, streamlining, and overseeing all complaints processes across government that affected children. The Children's Commission was also to review the plans of all children in care, review the critical injuries of children in care and ensure public accountability and openness in the new system.

The Premier accepted the Transition Commissioner's report in its entirety and on September 23, 1996, both the Children's Commission and the new Ministry for Children and Families were created. This author was asked, and agreed, to become the Children's Commissioner. The Ministry of Social Services was immediately dismantled and its child-related parts became the first components of the new MCF.

IMPLEMENTING CHANGE: 1996 TO 2000

It is still the case, in 2000, that the implementation of the 1996 change agenda is far from complete. Progress has been made in some key areas, while other major initiatives—contemplated as cornerstones of the new system—have not yet been fully designed nor implemented. Since September, 1996, the Children's Commission has issued regular reports on the state of change (see, for example, Pallan, 2000). The Children's Commission has identified key initiatives and principles required for change, and wherever possible developed a means to assess the extent and effectiveness of change.

The Children's Commission's public reports and recommendations for policy or practice reform were, for the first year of its existence until the end of 1997, largely based upon the individual and collective review and release of reports on the deaths of all children who received services from someone in their communities (doctors, public health nurses, schools, probation officers, or social workers). In addition, the hearing of complaints of children seeking or receiving services from the new ministry was another early and important source of information for the Commission about the state of change and front line practices.

In the summer of 1997, the *Children's Commission Act* (Ministry of Attorney General, 1997) was passed in the BC Legislature, establishing a wide scope of responsibilities for the office that extended beyond the review of deaths and hearing of complaints to include review of the plans of care for all children in the continuing custody of government, and a general oversight and monitoring role. By the spring of 1998, in an effort to gather information of a systemic nature to help understand the state of change, the Children's Commission had established protocols and information systems links with many agencies and the new MCF to gather information on the services they, staff or agencies had provided to children. This included protocols with the Coroner's Office, the College of Physicians and Surgeons, Vital Statistics, Pharmacare, police forces, and various provincial government ministries.

Where protocols have not succeeded in removing barriers to information gathering, the Commission has exercised its ability to summons documents and persons to ensure a thorough investigation. As well, the Commission conducts extensive consultations yearly with youth, Aboriginal representatives, and service providers. These are the sources of information upon which the

Commission bases its analysis of an individual case as well as its conclusions about systemic problems and solutions.

In the spring of 1998, 1999, and 2000, the Children's Commission issued annual reports (Morton, 1999a). In these reports, information gathered in the previous year is analysed and, where available, data from prior years has also been used. These sources of information consisted of the following:

- over 400 completed and released fatality reports covering the deaths of children (principally between 1996 and 1999);

- the review of a sample of 700 plans of care for children in the continuing custody of government for 1998 and 1999;

- assistance to nearly 800 children and their advocates in resolving complaints with the MCF through 1999 including independent complaint tribunal panels (in the years 1996 and 1997, no internal ministry complaint process existed but the Children's Commission had jurisdiction to hear and resolve a child in care's complaint; in the fall of 1997, the MCF implemented a formal complaint process) (MCF, 1997);

- critical injury reviews, where a child could have died or where the injury resulted in serious impairment of the child's physical health;

- a review of the MCF's internal complaints process (Morton, 1998a) and its adherence to an agreed set of child-centred principles negotiated between the Children's Commission and the MCF;

- the results of continuous consultations and focus groups across the province with youth and service providers;

- the conclusion and recommendations of numerous "special investigations" at the request of the Attorney General, including those conducted into the apprehension of dozens of children in Quesnel (Morton, 1998b), the death of Mavis Flanders (Morton, 1998c), and the severe shaking of several infants in the Capital Region (Morton, 1998d).

CHILDREN'S COMMISSION FINDINGS

In this section of the chapter, the Children's Commission reports will be used to examine the success of the MCF, the health and education systems, and other community-based partners in achieving real change for children. Only the most significant components of the change agenda will be reviewed, as the detailed and sector-specific reforms required to achieve full integration and a high quality of service are too extensive to address in this chapter. The Children's Commission's detailed recommendations for change, which are both sector-specific and across sectors, are set out in the "recommendations tracking" documents (Table 8.1 and Table 8.2) available from the Children's Commission (Morton, 1998e; see also, Pallan, 2000).

Table 8.1   Children's Commission recommendations by category, 1996-1999

Category	Number of recommendations
Integrated case management	117
Safety and injury prevention	116
Information sharing	115
Prevention and early intervention	98
Services to youth	95
Risk assessment	68
Education and training	76
Services to aboriginal children and youth	27
Public education	10
Commendations	5
Total number of recommendations	**727**

Source: Based on Pallan (2000).

In the three annual reports released by the Children's Commission, the same key findings as to what works for children and what does not have been reaffirmed from one year to the next and from one subject area to the next. The work of the Commission continues to confirm that the principles upon which the new system are based remain the correct ones. The work also confirms that progress has been made in introducing a new rigour to the child protection decision making process, but in other areas less familiar to a traditional child welfare system, such as early intervention or more relevant and accessible services to at-risk youth, much is still to be done to translate the principles of prevention, integration, and hearing the voice of the client into a new way of serving children and their families.

While the MCF has a significant leadership and funding role to play in shaping and implementing much of this change, the Children's Commission has identified serious gaps in leadership across other related sectors that compromise that ministry's ability to achieve the agenda of integration and removal of barriers between service providers. For those areas of change outside of the MCF's mandate, such as policing, mainstream education, and health care, the Children's Commission has found that system-wide change is difficult to achieve and a focus on children's needs is diminished by a myriad of other issues and demands. When leaders are found—usually front line practitioners —they are the key factor in affecting change within a community, a region, or across a sector. The importance of these leaders cannot be underestimated in affecting major change, and will be discussed later in this chapter.

Table 8.2   Children's Commission recommendations by agency type, 1996-1999

Agency type	Number of recommendations assigned
Ministry for Children and Families	351
Other provincial ministries	170
Hospitals/community health boards	79
Other medical organizations	41
Aboriginal agencies/bands/councils	38
Federal ministries/departments	34
School boards/districts	23
Crown corporations	23
RCMP detachments	22
Provincial coroner	16
Municipalities	15
Community agencies	11
Sub-total	823
Other agency types (media, recreational organizations, post-secondary institutions, etc.)	58
Total number of recommendations	**881**

Source: Based on Pallan (2000). The total recommendations in Table 8.2 are higher than those in Table 8.1 because the same recommendation was made to more than one agency type.

The Children's Commission's work to date has examined the detailed components of a change agenda, and has also wrapped these detailed components into larger themes of change—many reflective of Gove and others which have proven relevant in the work undertaken since the initial Gove report. The need for rigorous and continuous training, policy development, and the use of technology, for example, are all detailed components of a larger agenda to ensure full information sharing and case planning.

What follows are the most significant, broad components of a successful change agenda. What is apparent is that this agenda is the same as that called for by the consultations of the early 1990s, the Gove Inquiry, and the Transition Commission already discussed. The responsibility of the Children's Commission is to try to ensure that the recommendations remain relevant and are adapted as times and constraints change. As well, the Commission's work has proposed new components of an agenda that will achieve the broader principles.

Planning for High Risk Children: Apprehension of Children at Risk

A fatal flaw in the child protection system throughout much of the 1990s has been its inability to consistently assess the risks children face in their homes. These critical weaknesses included inexperienced staff with too much responsibility and a lack of training, decision makers with an inadequate focus on supervision, little policy direction, and increasingly complex caseloads (Petch and Scarth, 1997; Weller and Wharf, this volume).

The Children's Commission has found and reported that the new ministry's response to this need for assessing risk accurately has been one of the most significant and successful initiatives undertaken since 1996 (see **Chapter 7** for a list of factors now taken into consideration in determining risk). Better training of staff, the requirement of enhanced credentials for child protection workers, the implementation of technology-based planning, and new tracking and risk assessment tools have ensured greater safety for children at risk. While the Children's Commission continues to witness ministry staff struggling to use these new tools effectively, the initial decision making about when to remove a child, and when supports can be offered more effectively while the child lives at home, appears in the cases examined to be better made and better managed. Risk is more clearly understood, identified, and responded to, thereby reducing, although not eliminating it. It may be the case that more thorough risk assessment, coupled with inadequate community based services for families has resulted in an increased number of apprehended children. Once in care, the data indicates their time in care is unnecessarily long and not adequately planned. However, the statistics of the Children's Commission also show that fatalities resulting from child abuse or neglect are declining (Kendal, 2001).

It would also appear that a greater public, media, and practitioner awareness of the duty to report suspected abuse or neglect since the Gove report has largely assisted the system in honing its decision making about whether a child needs help. This willingness to collaborate between the public, the practitioners, and the MCF is a model of success that is assisted by continuous public discussions and heightened expectations about recognizing and responding to a child's risks. Some of this is undoubtedly related to the regular release of fatality reports by the Children's Commission, and the associated reporting by the media (see, for example, Ontario Child Mortality Task Force, 1998, pp. 14-15).

It is the conclusion of the Children's Commission that the use of the risk assessment tool is progressing with experience and training, and children's risks are being more accurately assessed and addressed. Issues of immediate safety are better addressed today than in the past. However, once children are brought into care, the continued inadequate level of planning makes their futures unnecessarily uncertain. The challenge for the child-serving systems is what to offer these children either to avoid the need to remove them from their homes through a renewed commitment to early intervention programs, or once they are removed from their homes, what planning is done to either return them home safely or create a new, stable home for them elsewhere. Both of these challenges must be addressed before the fundamental shift in the child-serving system occurs—the shift away from the need to apprehend children to a society that supports the development of healthy families from the time before a child is born through to adulthood. How to respond to both of these challenges has been the subject of extensive analysis by the Children's Commission.

Planning for Children in Care:
The Cornerstone of Integration, Information Sharing, and Inclusion

Both Gove and the Transition Commission called for a new approach to planning for children. To avoid a child's drift through the foster care system, adequate knowledge and planning by caregivers and service providers about how to meet that child's long-term needs is critical. The work of the Children's Commission continues to identify planning as a child's most important need, the system's most critical weakness, and the true test of whether integrated service delivery is working.

Since the MCF was established, it has committed to a new approach to planning that embraces a case management modelled by ministry staff but engaging all relevant practitioners, family, and foster parents where appropriate, in designing and delivering services to a child. Efforts to design this new approach began in 1997, with models proposed and nondirective policies delivered across the province. In some regions, integrated planning and case management is used well, although ministry policy states such planning is expected in all areas of the province.

This most significant change in services to children in care was initiated in 1999 across the province with the introduction of a new tool for planning called "Looking After Children" (LAC). This initiative was based on work developed in the UK (Dartington Social Research Unit, 1995) and includes principles of integration, sharing of information, rigorous monitoring of the usefulness of the plan and the effectiveness of services delivered, and the inclusion of children, youth, and their families in the plan's development and implementation. It is the conclusion of the Children's Commission, based upon a review of many plans of care, that the appropriate and extensive use of LAC is urgently needed across BC. Planning forms the hub of our service delivery system to the most vulnerable children, and experience in other jurisdictions and in the LAC pilot sites across BC demonstrate that, when done well, it is consistent with the fundamental shifts expected of practitioners since the Gove Report.

While it is the MCF that must take the lead for the introduction of LAC, its effect should be felt across all child-serving systems as social workers interact with doctors, public health nurses, teachers, police, probation officers, and agencies to meet the needs of children and youth. It is clear that LAC is not capable of affecting the way we plan and deliver services to children unless it is accompanied by a commitment to working together, differently, and well beyond the borders of the MCF.

The work of the Children's Commission has disclosed serious deficiencies in the quality and recording of plans for children in care which must be the focus of training, supervision, and integrated service delivery.

1. Compliance with the legislative requirements for the development of a plan of care within the last 6 months was adhered to in 130 of the 294 plans of care reviewed in 1998. Of the 130 current plans of care, only 8% were in full compliance with the legislative and policy requirements for all areas of a child's needs to be assessed and a plan to address them mapped out. Compliance ranging between 0% and 86% (average 35%) was recorded in the remaining 92%. In 1999, a review of 437 initial care plans showed that full compliance had grown to 20% from 8% the year before, indicating a growing commitment to, and familiarity with, effective planning.

2. In all of the LAC pilot case plans, the quality and thoroughness of the plans' assessment of a child's needs exceeded all other plans reviewed. What continued to be lacking in these LAC plans of care was a thorough response to the needs identified. For example, while behavioural issues at home or school may be identified in the LAC plans more regularly than in the other plans of care, a strategy in the plan on how to address these behavioural issues through medical or educational interventions was frequently lacking. This indicates that the LAC plans assist staff in establishing what a child's needs are, but to meet these needs practitioners beyond the child protection system must become engaged and lend their expertise and services as part of a planning team.

3. The review of the deaths of children to date has included children who were in care and those who were known to the MCF or its predecessor, the Ministry of Social Services, or who were part of the general population (Morton, 1999a, p. 72). The Children's Commission assessment is that most of the planning done for children known to the former Ministry of Social Services who died of abuse, neglect, or under violent circumstances was woefully inadequate and, as a result, the risks many children were exposed to, resulting in their deaths, were much greater than would have been the case with interventions. Since the creation of the MCF, the frequency of such deaths has lessened, and the overwhelming majority of children known to the ministry who die are medically fragile (Morton, 1999a, pp. 47-73).

While the Children's Commission has concluded that this reduction in the number of violent or abusive fatalities is likely due to better risk assessment and apprehensions, the quality of planning for those children in care who died before and after the creation of the MCF does not yet show an improvement in quality. While testing the pace of change is difficult to do when viewing the most difficult of cases—such as those reflected in the fatality reports—these cases are also the most critical test of a system's capacity to cope with the complex, high risk child. As a result, while they are the hardest cases by which to judge a system, they also offer the most revealing evidence by which to assess whether change for those who need it most is really happening. The Children's Commission has concluded that fewer children are left in life threatening situations, but those who are left in these circumstances remain because their needs are not fully understood nor their risks adequately assessed. Planning and its required collaborative and multidisciplinary assessment and decision making is still the major challenge to achieving a truly responsive child serving system.

In exploring the reasons for inadequacies in planning the care for children known to the ministry who have died, the following shortcomings were identified frequently across these cases:

- the available tools are not being used effectively because workers lack experience or training;
- workers need more access to the time and advice of experienced supervisors;
- workers are often uncertain about how to approach other service providers to gather information and undertake joint planning; trust is a major issue and the confidentially rules remain either unclear or not well understood; and,
- workload is identified by workers as the major reason plans are not written, are not updated, and are not reflective of the advice and information from other practitioners involved in the child's life.

These problems disclose systemic issues in the implementation of this significant new expectation.

4. The most prevalent source of complaints received by the Children's Commission is from the child, youth, or their advocate about the adequacy of planning for the child's future. Next is the lack of information sharing with family and youths about services and placements. Third is from Aboriginal children, youth, and their advocates about Aboriginal placements not being pursued rigorously in making or implementing a plan of care. The loss of family and community contacts while a child is in care is also noted (Morton, 1999a, p. 37). In 1999 there was a growing number of complaints about access to special needs services while in care (Pallan, 2000, p. 12).

The ability to develop a relevant, comprehensive plan of care is a very important step in meeting the needs of a child at risk. However, until more specialized services exist across the communities of BC, many of these needs may be identified in planning, with no response available.

Integration Across Systems that Serve Children

The ability of workers to plan for children in care is directly related to the introduction of a fundamental shift in service delivery that goes well beyond the borders of either the child protection system or the MCF. It is the establishment of a new way of meeting the needs of children by practitioners and professionals undertaking joint planning and coordinated service delivery. It is the complementary approach for services to all children to the use of LAC for children in care. It must engage teachers, health workers, community and volunteer agencies, police, probation, and family. It relies upon the open, shared understanding of what a family and child's needs are and how each involved member of that community can assist in meeting those needs. For children in care or those receiving services from the MCF, it is taking this model of community service delivery and applying it to an individual child's plan. This is called integrated case management (ICM) and has been the focus of over 16% of all recommendations made by the Children's Commission (see Table 8.1).

Data show that the improvements to be found from the use of this approach, from a client's and funder's perspective, are significant. The work of the Children's Commission—whether in the fatality reviews, the analysis of plans of care, or the hearing of a child's complaint—has identified the client's repeated desire for coordination, clarity, frequency of contact with one person responsible for managing all services provided, and the right to participate in planning and assessing services received.

The MCF instructed all regions to put an ICM model in place, but allowed each region to have an operational approach which recognizes the diversity throughout the province. In October 1999, the MCF issued its training guide for staff (MCF, 1999a). In some regions, ICM is seen as a tool solely to be used in the child protection stream. In other regions, the model is adopted more broadly and encompasses all services to children that are funded by the MCF, which includes (at least in part) infant development, childcare,[1] education, youth justice, and health care.

The barriers to implementing integrated case management stem largely from the need to coordinate time between practitioners, the acceptance of a joint assessment as to what the child's needs are and how best to meet them, and the willingness to share information. While these may sound insignificant, they have proven the most difficult barriers to overcome and the fundamental challenge to moving from a "stove pipe" system of separate services to an integrated one where the child is viewed holistically.

In the Children's Commission fatality reviews, those children who received services from more than one practitioner in their community (i.e., the school, a doctor, a community agency, or counsellor) had a higher likelihood of a child and family's needs being addressed when services were integrated, coordinated, and monitored. For example, medically fragile children were most often provided with the most effectively integrated services, usually coordinated by a health care practitioner or a staff person from MCF outside the child protection system. When services were not coordinated, cases consistently demonstrated children wandering from one piecemeal solution to the next, with no long-term benefits and substantial harm.

In the Commission's 1998/99 review of plans of care (Morton, 1999a), the frequency and quality of consultation amongst practitioners and the delivery of integrated services was as follows:

- For school aged children in care, 75% who had plans of care were identified in the plans as having educational difficulties. However, in two thirds of these plans of care, there were no recorded plans nor consultations with teachers to address these educational needs. This was particularly the case for older children in care.

- Primary health care status (immunizations, optical, hearing, etc.) was identified in 30% of the plans of care. An additional 10% of the plans identified dental needs and status. For the remaining 60% of children in care with written plans, there is no record of their medical history.

- Planning for reconnection with family was contained in 40% of the current plans of care, although in 80% of all plans family and significant relationships were recorded.

- Sixty percent of the plans indicated plan of care meetings had occurred, which typically involved the social worker and foster parent. Children were involved 55% of the time in such meetings.

The Children's Commission has concluded that LAC, coupled with a rigorous commitment to ICM, must be implemented concurrently and across all child-serving systems. Further, it is the opinion of the Children's Commission that the MCF, and those with whom they work, is one to two years behind in the implementation of these agreed to initiatives, which have so much impact on the implementation of more relevant and effective services for children.

While scarce funding is always a barrier to full scale change, it is the case that a shift to ICM is more about leadership across numerous sectors, both provincially and regionally. It is about a common vision of serving children and the dedication of leaders to ensure it happens. Once again, this leadership has been erratic.

By early 2000, the use of ICM remained incomplete. While assistance and models are available centrally, each region has been asked to create its own definition of what ICM is to look like for their area of the province and develop an implementation process. The absence of clear expectations through policy and practice guidelines provided centrally and acceptable at a provincial level by the education and health care systems is a different approach than what has been endorsed and recommended by the Children's Commission. The regional variations may create an integrated approach to service delivery that is better tuned to community expectations and needs, or it may have the negative consequence of confusion and delay. It is still too soon to evaluate this, and a users guide for ICM will only be finalized by the MCF in 2000 (Pallan, 2000, p. 20).

Early Intervention

As noted previously, the cornerstone of the new child-serving system was to be the development and delivery of a provincial, early intervention strategy. This recommendation from the Transition Commission was based upon the review of the successful experiences of other jurisdictions and the evidence which confirms the need for quick responses to family's at risk. In Hawaii, the delivery of services to at-risk families at a very early stage had shown success in reducing the risks to a child staying with that family, as well as a substantial savings in services to, and interventions for, that family and child throughout the following decade (Fuddy, 1992).

In the Perry Preschool Project in the US, at-risk children were offered extensive supports when very young (Schweinhart, Bames, and Weikart, 1993). These same children were followed and found not to have become clients of costly support systems one could have expected had the risks in their young lives continued. Investment in these children at an early age was found to be seven times less than the cost associated with being wards of the state, welfare recipients, mental health patients, or incarcerated in the corrections system (Table 8.3). In addition, the human cost of failing to intervene and allowing children the opportunity to grow feeling loved cannot be quantified.

Table 8.3   High/Scope Perry Preschool Project—Major findings at age

Factor	With Program (%)	Without Program (%)
$2,000 or more monthly earnings	29	7
Homeowner	36	13
High school (or equivalent) graduate	71	54
Social services needed in last decade	59	80
5 or more arrests	7	35

Source: Based on Schweinhart, Barnes, and Weikart (1993).

Contemporary research reinforces the value of early supports to parents and children, when a child's nervous system and brain are developing in ways that determine their behaviour, social skills, and physical conditions (Hertzman, 1997; Keating and Hertzman, 1999; Steinhauer, 1999). For example, if a child is not loved, held, or nurtured at a very young age, devastating behavioural consequences can result when that child grows and exercises the freedoms of adolescence. Many parents are the product of neglectful or abusive parents themselves, and have little skill or knowledge in how to parent infants. The Children's Commission has been vigorous in its plea that communities engage in a coordinated and extensive commitment to new families through early intervention programs (Morton, 1999a, pp. 6-7; Pallan, 2000, pp. 23-24). Failure to do so will result in the continued cycle of children being apprehended, demonstrating such risk behaviours as school drop out, runaways, violence, drug and alcohol abuse. It is the Children's Commission conclusion, as reflected in its annual reports, that if BC is to achieve the kind of fundamental change to services for children which will improve their health and social status, the development and introduction of a multi-system, early intervention strategy cannot be delayed.

The Children's Commission first annual report (Morton, 1997) noted that two thirds of the 40 children under 1 year of age whose lives and deaths were examined were exposed to alcohol and drugs *in utero*. One third were known to have been assessed as high risk at birth due either to the infant's medical condition or the mother's alcohol or drug use during pregnancy. Some of these are infants that could have been saved by intervention in their new homes of lay or professional supports, to ensure the child's medical, nutritional, and emotional needs were being met while the parents received the help they needed in order to reduce the risks in that home. Many of these children died from Sudden Infant Death Syndrome, where alcohol and drug use by a mother is a known risk factor, yet very few foster care providers or mothers understood the elevated risks of these infants and how to reduce them when they took them home (see **Chapter 4**). Recent estimates put the rate of Fetal Alcohol Syndrome (FAS) in the general population at 33 per 100,000, and between 200 and 300 infants are born each year with full features of FAS (Pallan, 2000, p. 29-30).

Effective early intervention should envision supports to persons who may become parents, but whose at-risk behaviours predict serious consequences for any child. In many fatality cases, women with drug and alcohol abuse problems or young women not living in a safe environment were having multiple children with some supports from community agencies, but no monitoring of whether services were making a difference.

Acceptance of the Transition Commission report meant government was to implement a provincial early intervention strategy as part of a core delivery system. The long-term effect on reducing the number of apprehensions, coupled with the cost saving of investing early in children, was to justify the initial investment required for such a program. Unfortunately, the province has not yet developed a fully comprehensive early intervention strategy nor provided a funding commitment through the budgetary process beyond some successful pilot projects in selected communities, known as Building Blocks. In these pilots, preliminary evaluation points to significant issues to be addressed in a successful early intervention scheme, including links to an overall provincial strategy, to other provincial initiatives such as childcare, and to the National Children's Agenda; security of ongoing or new funding to sustain or expand service delivery; and consistency of data gathering related to outcomes, to provincial health goals, and to the reporting of results (Pallan, 2000, pp. 23-24).

The Role of the Health Care System

Beyond the MCF is the need for the health care and education systems to change their approaches to early intervention, prevention, and overall service delivery to children and youth. This includes the hospitals, public health, private medical practitioners, the British Columbia Medical Association, and all partners in the school system. Better knowledge of paediatric illness and its treatment, more accessible services at the times and places where at-risk families and children can be found, and an increased willingness to engage in long-term planning for the care of these children and families is required. The reasons for these existing shortcomings are frequently cited as financial, but consultations with many leading practitioners in the field of paediatric medicine suggest the greatest barriers relate to trust between practitioners and lack of familiarity with the special needs of children and youth. Hopefully, the building of trust and sharing of expertise across fields of practice will emerge as ICM becomes more accepted and adopted throughout the province.

The health care model of "prevention" has consistently proven to be very cost effective, but is not always the one that communities see reflected in the nature and quality of medical care provided to children or new parents. To "prevent" a child from being at high risk requires, among other things, thorough and early sex education, adequate prenatal care to high risk mothers, screening of newborns for environmental and physical risk factors, and delivering services to these mothers and infants to reduce risks once they return home. This preventative model of early intervention is based on a health model, but can only be carried out with a fully integrated delivery system between health, education, social services, and community-based agencies.

It is also often the case that the first practitioners to detect risk in the behaviours of parents or the health of a child is the family medical practitioner, the doctor at a clinic, the hospital in which a child is born, or the public health nurse who visits a newborn and parents (Health Canada, 1999). A number of factors have been identified in the fatality cases reviewed by the Children's Commission as contributing to the lack of appropriate early intervention or integration of services. A key weakness is that public health nurses are no longer able to consistently conduct home visits, given resource constraints and competing priorities. In some communities, a single public health nurse visit no longer occurs and in most other communities there is only one visit. In an effort to find new ways to reach the parents of newborns, infants, and toddlers, efforts are made by public health units to have new parents come forward voluntarily to self identify for support or child immunizations. Placing the onus on often isolated, high risk parents creates an obvious barrier to reaching the most vulnerable of young children.

The Hawaii Healthy Start model, already mentioned (Fuddy, 1992), offers an alternative to the need for public health nurses to attend at homes where high risk parents and infants live. Instead, trained lay persons attend the homes of all infants determined to be high risk at birth by hospital staff. These lay supports—often women from the same community—are trained to connect the family with practitioners and services. It is the concern expressed by some nurses in BC that to alter the public health nurse's responsibility is to erode the quality of care provided to newborns and their parents. These concerns may be legitimate, but a refusal to endorse a new way of meeting a family's needs—

when the alternative is no service at all —is not child focused. Such resistance poses one more barrier to the implementation of cost effective early interventions desperately needed by families and no longer paid for nor available from the health care system.

Another barrier to the implementation of a prevention-based medical strategy for children is that many medical practitioners continue to struggle with their loyalty to adults in a family versus the needs of a child. A physician's desire to assist the family is complicated by their oath of confidentiality and their frequent distrust of the child welfare system. While it has often been the case that family physicians will be the greatest advocates for children they feel are at risk, some cases examined by the Children's Commission also demonstrate that physicians continue to try to manage issues of alcoholism and drug abuse within their treatment of a family to the exclusion of others who may also assist in weighing and responding to a child's risks. This stressor between treating the adult and "protecting" the family versus protecting the child is also seen in the approaches of other adult-oriented community agencies, which are reticent to disclose "confidential" patient information that may suggest a child is at risk due to addictions of parents.

A more prominent issue, however, is the physician's frequent inability or unwillingness to engage in case planning for a child in need of interventions, whether they be early interventions or at the time of crisis. The cause of their absence appears to be twofold—a lack of time and money available in the Medical Services Plan budget of the Ministry of Health for the physician to participate in time consuming planning meetings, and a reluctance of some physicians to be seen as participants in the possible apprehension of children. The Children's Commission has made several key recommendations to government and the medical profession to encourage a review of funding practices, as well as enhanced physician training on the value of case planning with other practitioners.

For early intervention and prevention to be effective, it must ensure accessible and well informed medical care across the province. The early diagnosis and treatment of conditions such as Fetal Alcohol Syndrome/Partial Fetal Alcohol Syndrome, Attention Deficit Hyperactivity Disorder, and other complex conditions can make the difference between a lifetime of success for a child or despair. The need for medical practitioners across the province to acquire new skills in diagnosis and treatment, coupled with good access to tertiary sources of expertise, remain challenges in BC today. Progress has been made under the leadership of the BC Childrens Hospital Services Centre and the University of British Columbia medical school. More is required.

The health care system's distance from the other parts of the child-serving system and funding constraints affecting the physician's ability to engage in complex case planning are perhaps the most significant barriers to integration and early intervention notwithstanding the existence of written protocols between the MCF and the College of Physicians and Surgeons.

There are signs of important change. The Children's Commission recommended that new discharge procedures be developed and used by all hospitals across the province when a child is leaving the hospital after birth or treatment and is considered at risk medically or because of the environment in their home. These discharge procedures were to address repeated instances of newborns and children returning to homes without supports for parents, seen in case after case struggling with poverty, acoholism, and isolation. These procedures, which were finalized in November 1999, and distributed by the BC Reproductive Care Program (1999), will ensure that case planning occurs between medical practitioners, child welfare workers, and community-based agencies. The follow-up to these case plans will be of critical importance to ensure that what the family needs is actually delivered.

Access to qualified physicians and nurses for at-risk parents—before and after a child's birth —can make a life or death difference to a child. In addition, a cornerstone of effective early intervention is to quickly identify and treat children suffering from physical and emotional disabilities or trauma. The training and accessibility of qualified physicians in remote areas remains a challenge in most parts of BC, despite the best efforts of the Children's Hospital to provide this training and outreach. In the last 3 years, new centres of expert medical care have been designed between the MCF and paediatric health care leaders and have been implemented in Victoria for children at risk who live on the island, in Surrey for parts of the lower Fraser Valley, and others are being planned for Prince George for the Northern region. These centres have been motivated by a better understanding of the need for expert, accessible care—informed, in part, by recommendations of the Children's Commission contained in numerous fatality reviews.

The Role of the Education System

It has become very clear to many educators that the need for multiple services to children can only be met by the invitation of the community into the schools. The high increase in the number of special needs children over the last 5 years, coupled with the 75% increase in the number of English as a Second Language (ESL) children over the last decade, make the school environments both complex and difficult to manage without outside assistance.

The introduction of new school programs and funding for special needs and ESL children over the last few years has not and cannot keep up with the needs of these children. Services and expertise in community agencies, health care, and adult supports for parents must also be part of a school's support system. While in principle the school system accepts the need for community agency support, there still remain issues of trust and working protocols which often preclude such integration and case planning from occurring. Teachers are frustrated by a lack of information about a child in their classroom from doctors or social workers. Counsellors cannot get children into community programs, and child welfare workers wonder why children clearly exhibiting signs of risk are not identified to them by teachers. While these barriers are not new ones, their presence becomes more apparent when the number of at-risk and special needs children increase so dramatically over a short period of time.

The introduction of Community Schools and At Risk programs across the province has made a difference because these models of service delivery integrate education with other supports and services available within their communities. While many school boards complain funding for special needs is inadequate and have made reductions to meet legislated balanced budgets, they must be challenged to find a new approach to serving children that places their resources on the table with those available from other community-based child service providers. Effective, efficient, and integrated models of educating and supporting children are tested and available, yet there is inadequate take-up across the province.

At the request of the Children's Commission, the Ministry of Education is preparing a best practices manual to share with school boards on such opportunities for integration. As well, in May 1999, the ministry prepared and sent to all schools across the province a manual on alternatives to out of school suspensions, which are often the last tie between a troubled youth and their community (Ministry of Education, 1999b). Once broken, that child or youth may never return to his peers, home, or community again. The Commission called for a "non suspension" policy in all schools until the child or youth receives a special needs assessment and a plan that engages other community practitioners is developed and put in place to respond to their needs. This model has not been prevalent in BC and the Ministry of Education has resisted imposing this requirement on school boards. As children's deaths are examined by the Children's Commission, individual schools and school districts are approached and encouraged to implement such "no suspension" policies. In these cases, the Children's Commission has had success in affecting change at a local level, but sadly only after a child has died, and the death subsequently reviewed by the Commission. What is required is systemic change to prevent further isolation and death of adolescents by removing a child from school—their last safe harbour—before best efforts have been made to understand and address their problems.

Services to Aboriginal Children

In the Children's Commission examination of the fatality of all children across BC, Aboriginal children were over-represented and their deaths more frequently occurred in the most violent of circumstances (Foster, Macdonald, Tuk, Uh, and Talbot, 1995). For example, compared to non-Aboriginals, Aboriginal SIDS deaths are 6 times higher, the youth suicide rate is more than 8 times higher for Aboriginal males, and 20 times higher for Aboriginal females (Pallan, 2000, p. 28). In examining the lives and deaths of these children, the most pervasive difficulty they and their families faced was the absence of adequate, accessible services to address such complex issues as inter-generational alcohol, substance, and sexual abuse (see **Chapter 6**). Further, many of these children and youth faced lives of boredom and exclusion, often suspended or departing from school at an early age with little else to do but find a new community on the streets, often far away from their homes.

In more than a dozen cases, the Children's Commission has attempted to assist bands in having the provincial and federal governments clarify who is responsible for bringing services to these isolated, poor communities. The Commission, together with bands, has also proposed service delivery models for these communities to be funded by the various levels of government. In most cases, the responsibility has not yet been accepted for either enhanced funding or policy leadership. In other cases, the Children's Commission has shared its concerns with the band and the governments that children were not being adequately cared for nor protected in certain communities, often due to a shortage of resources coupled with the absence of a clearly defined child protection presence.

These cases have prompted frequent recommendations from the Children's Commission relating to clarifying accountability, enhancing the quality of training and service delivery and funding. The provincial government's responsibilities are being addressed in part through the implementation of an Aboriginal Strategy (MCF, 1999b), developed with and agreed to by the MCF and bands across the province. However this strategy does not bind nor define the federal government's roles and responsibilities, nor does it clarify how the provincial government will ensure children are safe pending the implementation of the sweeping changes contemplated.

For children in government care, agreements exist between the provincial government and many tribal councils or bands to deliver services on behalf of the province, within their own communities. These services may or may not include child protection decisions. In one instance, the province entered into an arrangement that devolved all responsibilities to a band. A panel of the Children's Commission determined, however, that this arrangement was inappropriate and that the MCF retained ultimate responsibility to ensure the safety of the children in the band's care.

In reviewing the planning for Aboriginal children in care, the Children's Commission determined little difference in the quality or frequency of plans between Aboriginal and non-Aboriginal children, whether under the care of a delegated agency (an Aboriginal agency delegated by the Director of Child Protection to provide all or some child welfare services) or under the care of a provincial ministry office. In a large majority of both cases, the adequacy of planning was poor and did not reflect the needs of the child. In addition, in reviewing the data for all children in care, a discrepancy was identified by the Children's Commission that suggests that the MCF's data may be inaccurate. In examining individual plans of care in 1999, 12% of the children who were identified on the plan as Aboriginal were not identified in the ministry's data systems as Aboriginal. In addition, 59% of the Aboriginal children in care are under age 12, compared with 38% of non-Aboriginal children. This statistic suggests the proportion of Aboriginal children in care is likely to increase as these under age 12 year olds grow and remain in the system while new ones enter. Indeed, Foster and Wright in their chapter in this volume have shown a major increase in the number of Aboriginal children in care over the last 2 years.

The *Child, Family and Community Service Act* requires that a child's connection with and education about their culture be addressed within all plans of care. This occurred in 30% of the care plans of Aboriginal children reviewed in 1998, with other plans establishing family contact in the summer or on other occasions and some plans indicating that the child did not wish contact. An additional responsibility exists towards Aboriginal children to retain their cultural and community links wherever possible. In the plans examined, 13% of Aboriginal children are in the care of a relative or parent. There are no data to show whether additional Aboriginal foster homes exist beyond this 13%, putting Aboriginal children in care at increased risk of losing their cultural identity.

Indeed, approximately 24% and 32% respectively of the 1998 and 1999 complaints about the adequacy of service reviewed by the Children's Commission have related to the care of Aboriginal children. The key issues raised in these complaints involve maintenance of their Aboriginal heritage and their family's desire that a child be placed in an Aboriginal home.

The Needs of Our Youth: The Bigger Picture

As indicated earlier, the scope of the Children's Commission work extends well beyond the child protection system and reviews the lives and deaths of all children in the province. Matters of public safety, the appropriate treatment of disease, and the design and manufacture of child and youth care and recreational products have all been addressed in one or more cases. While many of our findings and recommendations are unrelated to the main purpose of this chapter, some linkages not apparent at first have been identified and must be pursued. For example, the leading cause of death for youth in BC is motor vehicle accidents. Drinking, speed, and recklessness are key contributing factors (Morton, 1999a, p. 64).

In many cases, a youth's drinking habits are directly related to deep-seated and unresolved issues of depression and abuse. Drugs and alcohol are often turned to by youth to "self medicate" depression or mental health concerns. By understanding the life of that youth and the circumstances of their death, we are better able to target our anti-drinking and driving initiatives to the relevant audience. As well, it is often the case that drinking and parties in isolated locations are a result of bored youth lacking alternatives within their home communities (see **Chapter 10**). Too often, alcohol and drugs are more accessible than places for youth to drop in and hang out safely. These youth often share the same needs of youth in the child protection system, and our consultations with both groups confirm a common request—places to go that don't cost money, aren't exposed to alcohol and drugs, where they can meet each other and caring adults (Morton, 1999b).

In 1997 the Children's Commission called upon MCF to develop a Youth Strategy that would respond to the complex needs of the youth population. In May 2000 a youth policy framework was finally completed (MCF, 2000) following a consultation process with the broader community. This area of needed reform has preoccupied the Children's Commission due to the large number of youth whose deaths come after years of drift, unresolved issues of abuse or neglect, and erratic interventions before life on the streets kills them.

Announcements of new mental health services, addictions treatment services, and street level supports are good news and can assist in forming the foundation of a desperately needed community level system of accessible, safe, and affordable services. These services for youth must include housing, job readiness, income assistance, and mentoring. These services must be placed in a larger, comprehensive youth strategy to allow us the ability to ensure all of the pieces are being developed and delivered effectively.

The child welfare system has adopted a new approach to determining when a youth will be taken into care. It assumes, correctly, that too often children in care do not receive the services they need and do not need to be in care but rather need access to more and better services. The system's solution is to develop "Youth Agreements" (MCF, 1999c) as an alternative to placing at-risk youth in care. The Children's Commission has consistently endorsed the need for agreements with youth, due to a lack of consultation with these clients about their needs, goals, and willingness to engage in services.

The Commission has advised the MCF that Youth Agreements are workable if a new set of extensive supports targeted at youth's needs are created in all communities. These supports do not yet exist, and the Commission has cautioned the MCF not to remove the availability of a safe place to live for many of these youth (foster homes or group homes) without alternatives in place. The Children's Commission has received assurances from the MCF that youth will remain in, or be brought into, care until the new services and supports exist to replace it. By the end of 2000, more than 100 youth had entered into special, supported youth agreements. This initiative will be carefully monitored.

Leadership

As has been noted throughout this chapter, leadership within and across the child-serving system is the most significant determinant of whether the change agenda will be successful. Only when those responsible across the child welfare, education, health, youth justice, and community-based systems make every effort to work with a shared vision of family and child's needs will the change agenda be implemented as intended first by Gove, then by both the Transition and Children's commissions. Until that time, it is impossible to conclude whether the changes are doable. It is, in this author's opinion, and that of the recently appointed Children's Commissioner (Pallan, 2000), possible and correct to conclude that the changes are the cornerstones of a new system for children that will serve their best interests, based upon the consistently identified weaknesses of the old and still partially intact child-serving systems of the 1980s and first half of the 1990s.

While the public holds the MCF largely responsible for this leadership role, there are other critical players that must also be held accountable for their role in changing how the needs of children are met. These leaders reside in the education and health care systems, the taxation system, those responsible for Indian Affairs federally, and those who lead community-based agencies and municipal governments. In addition, the media has a large responsibility to ensure that the public has a balanced understanding of the need for change and what can and must be done at a community level to achieve it. The media's willingness to profile the needs of, and educate the public on children and families on a consistent basis, can assist in maintaining the change agenda as a political priority of all governments. Unfortunately, the frantic, sometimes exploitive coverage of one child's death in the media cannot accomplish this same long-term public awareness of the need to invest in children.

Leadership must be constant and commitments must reflect a multi-year, long-term approach to setting priorities for policy development, funding, and changes to practice. We have yet to determine how to ensure that this multi-year, multi-sectoral approach will be consistently adopted across the province, and this is the lesson we have not yet learned from the past.

CONCLUSION

It is the belief of the Children's Commission that the MCF continues to offer the best opportunity in which cultures can be changed, funding realigned, and policies and practices integrated. Structure alone, however, is not a recipe for success. Structure can enhance or reduce bureaucratic barriers that separate ministries from shared planning, funding, or operations. A long-term and unwavering commitment to the key components of the provincial change agenda, strong leadership within and outside government, continued public demand for change, and community-based supports for families, children, and youth are the factors for the success of the change agenda. While the substance of the change agenda envisioned by Gove remains sound, the principal lesson learned by the Children's Commission, and communicated continuously to the child-serving systems, is that we must not allow the sectors who serve children to drift back to their separate corners and deliver services in isolation from each other and often in isolation from their clients.

From the point of view of the Children's Commission, what has already been learned from the past is significant and has affected positive change. What has been learned is that children need a voice and children need advocates to speak on their behalf and require action when necessary, to ensure effective service from complex and mysterious systems that are funded to serve them. While such agencies as the Children's Commission continue to meet resistance in some quarters, a growing credibility with the public, youth, advocates, service providers, and the MCF will ensure that the Gove recommendations and the work that evolves from them will not collect dust on the shelf of any ministry office.

If the change agenda is not implemented, it is because public interest does not demand that it occur, politicians and the media move away from their support of children, and that practitioners reject the work of such offices as the Children's Commission. Mental health, public health, education, and social services cannot be allowed to resurrect the more comfortable definitions of role, mandate, and client. Change must be focused, commitment firm, and evaluations the basis of further change. If the change agenda is rejected before fully implemented and evaluated, it is the responsibility of the Children's Commission to acknowledge this failure. To date, response to the work of the Children's Commission has been to accept the recommendations for change and reform in over 90% of the cases. These responses are set out in their entirety in the recommendations tracking document of the Children's Commission. While approximately 40% of these recommendations pertain to the MCF (Pallan, 2000), more pertain to other child-serving systems, agencies, and practitioners and should not be overlooked.

It is believed by this author that if these positive responses to the recommendations are carried through to full implementation—as committed to by the affected agencies—then the cornerstones of the change agenda will take hold provincially, regionally, and locally. While some calls for change have not received as rapid a response as considered warranted, especially in the areas of early intervention, ICM, special needs services, and services to youth, the commitment to act in the near future has been made. If such a commitment to act fails to occur or garner the expected results, the ongoing fatality reports, reviews of plans of care and complaints of children to the Children's Commission will likely tell us the disasterous results. Future annual reports of the Children's Commission will need to revisit whether we have indeed learned our lessons from the past.

Editor's Note: In late July, 1999, the childcare subsidy program was transferred to the newly created Ministry of Social Development and Economic Security.

REFERENCES

BC Reproductive Care Program (1999). *Guidelines for perinatal care of substance-using women and their infants.* Vancouver, BC: BC Children's and Women's Health Centre.

Christianson-Wood, J., and Murray, J.L. (1999). *Child death reviews and child mortality data collection in Canada.* Ottawa, Ontario: Health Canada, Child Maltreatment Division.

Community Panel, Family and Children's Services Legislation Review in BC (1992a). *Making changes: A place to start.* Victoria, BC: Ministry of Social Services.

Community Panel, Family and Children's Services Legislation Review in BC (1992b). *Liberating our children—Liberating our nations: Report of the Aboriginal Committee.* Victoria, BC: Ministry of Social Services.

Community Social Services Employee Association (1999). About CSSEA. *http://www.cssea.bc.ca/about.htm.*

Dartington Social Research Unit (1995). *Looking after children.* Department of Health, HMSO, UK.

Foster, L.T., Macdonald, J., Tuk, T.A., Uh, S.H., and Talbot, D. (1995). Native health in British Columbia: A vital statistics perspective. In P.H. Stephenson, S.J. Elliott, L.T. Foster, and J. Harris (Eds.), *A persistent spirit: Towards understanding Aboriginal health in British Columbia* (pp. 43-93). Victoria, BC: Department of Geography, University of Victoria, Western Geographical Series, vol. 31.

Fuddy, L.J. (1992). Hawaii healthy start successful in preventing child abuse. As referenced in J. Millar (1998), *A report on the health of British Columbians: Provincial Health Officer's Annual Report – 1997.* Victoria, BC: Ministry of Health.

Gove, T. (1995). *Inquiry in to child protection. Report of the Gove Inquiry in child protection,* 2 volumes. Ministry of Attorney General, Victoria, BC.

Health Canada (1999). *Child abuse: Reporting and classification in health care settings.* Ottawa, Ontario: Health Canada.

Hertzman, C. (1997). The case for child development as a determinant of health. *Canadian Journal of Public Health,* 89, Supplement 1, 514-519.

Keating, D.P., and Hertzman, C. (Eds.) (1999). *Developmental health and the wealth of nations: Social, biological and educational dynamics.* New York, NY: The Guildford Press.

Kendal, P.R.W. (2000a). *Deaths of children and youth in care: What do the data show?* A report by the BC Provincial Health Officer. Victoria, BC: Ministry of Health.

Korbin, J. (1993). *Commission of Inquiry into the Public Service and the Public Sector.* Victoria, BC: Ministry of Attorney General.

MacDonald, K. (1998). Commentary. *BC Studies,* 188, 114-119.

MCF (1997a). *Measuring our success: A framework for evaluating population outcomes.* Victoria, BC: Ministry for Children and Families. A second, updated edition was published in early 2000 with the same title.

MCF (1997b). *First six months and 1997/98 priorities.* Victoria, BC: Ministry for Children and Families.

MCF (1999a). *Integrated case management: A training guide.* Victoria, BC: Ministry for Children and Families.

MCF (1999b). Strategic plan for Aboriginal services. Victoria, BC: Ministry for Children and Families.

MCF (1999c). Amendments to the *Child, Family and Community Service Act (1994).* Victoria, BC: Ministry for Children and Families.

MCF (2000). Youth policy framework. Victoria, BC: Ministry for Children and Families.

Ministry of the Attorney General (1997). *Children's Commission Act*. Victoria, BC: Ministry of Attorney General.

Ministry of Education (1999a). *How are we doing? An overview of Aboriginal education results for Province of BC*. Victoria, BC: Ministry of Education.

Ministry of Education (1999b). *Focus on suspension: A resource for schools*. Victoria, BC: Ministry of Education.

Ministry of Health (1997). *Health goals for British Columbia*. Victoria, BC: Ministry of Health.

Ministry of Social Services (1994*)*. *Child, Family and Community Service Act*. Ministry of Social Services, Victoria, BC. The Act was ammended in 1995, before implementation.

Morton, C. (1996). *Morton Report: British Columbia's child, youth and family serving system— Recommendations for change*. Report to Premier Glen Clark. Transition Commissioner for Child and Youth Services, Victoria, BC.

Morton, C. (1997). *Annual report of the children's commission – 1996/97*. Victoria, BC: Ministry of the Attorney General.

Morton, C. (1998a). *Review of Ministry for Children and Families complaint process*. Victoria, BC: Ministry of the Attorney General, BC Children's Commission.

Morton, C. (1998b). *A report concerning the relationship between practice audits in the Quesnel office of the Ministry for Children and Families and the removal of 65 children from their families*. Victoria, BC: Ministry of the Attorney General, BC Children's Commission.

Morton, C. (1998c). Review of the circumstances surrounding the death of Mavis Flanders: Report to the Honourable Ujjal Dosanjh, Attorney General. Victoria, BC: Ministry of the Attorney General, BC Children's Commission.

Morton, C. (1998d). *The investigation of Baby M*. Victoria, BC: Ministry of the Attorney General, BC Children's Commission.

Morton, C. (1998e). *The Children's Commission's and Responses Summary Document*. September, 1996 to December, 1998. Victoria, BC: Ministry of the Attorney General, BC Children's Commission.

Morton, C. (1999a). *1998 Annual report of the Children's Commission*. Victoria, BC: Ministry of the Attorney General.

Morton, C. (1999b). *The youth report*. Victoria, BC: Ministry of the Attorney General, BC Children's Commission.

Ontario Child Mortality Task Force (1997). Final Report. Toronto, Ontario: Ontario Child Mortality Task Force.

Ontario Child Mortality Task Force (1998). *A progress report on recommendations*. Ontario Association of Children's Aid Societies. *http://www.oacas.org/about/CMTF.html*

Pallan, P. (2000). *Weighing the evidence: A report on BC's children and youth*. 1999 Annual Report of the Children's Commission. Victoria, BC: Ministry of the Attorney General.

Petch, H., and Scarth, S. (1997). *Report of the Task Force on Safeguards for Children and Youth in Foster or Group Home Care*. Victoria, BC: Ministry of the Attorney General, BC Children's Commission.

Schweinhart, L.J., Barnes, H.V., and Weikart, D.P. (1993). *Significant benefits: The High/Scope Perry Preschool study through Age 27*. High/Scope Educational Research Foundation Monograph, No. 10. Ypsilanti, Michigan: High/Scope Press.

Steinhauer, P.D. (1999). The brain and child development: How a child's early experiences affect development. *Interaction*, 13(Spring), 15-21.

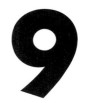

Toward Evidence-Based Child Policy: What Money Can't Buy

Rebecca N. Warburton

School of Public Administration, University of Victoria

William P. Warburton

Economic Analysis Branch, Ministry of Social Development and Economic Security

It ain't so much the things we don't know that get us into trouble, it's the things we know that ain't so.

> — unknown; attributed to Artemus Ward, Mark Twain, Josh Billings, and others

INTRODUCTION

A society's future is in its children. To maximize the well being of our society in the future, we must ensure that all children can achieve their full potential. Unfortunately, many do not. In terms of work, education, health, and other outcomes, low-income children have worse prospects than more affluent ones. Quite apart from outcomes for children, we may be concerned with children's access to goods and services. Even if their essential material needs are met, low-income children clearly have less access than others to the cultural and social opportunities of our affluent society.

In this chapter we seek to identify both strategies that will increase the material well-being of children, and strategies for which there is "sufficiently good" evidence that government action would be likely to improve the outcomes for disadvantaged children. The chapter has four parts. First, we discuss the income gradient in children's outcomes, that is, the extent to which children's successes are correlated with the incomes of their parents. Second, we briefly discuss the criteria that we use to determine whether the evidence is "sufficiently good." Third, we discuss strategies to raise standards of living or improve outcomes for poor children. Fourth, we discuss implementation issues that indicate that government's task does not end with adopting policies and programs that have been shown to be effective elsewhere. We conclude with a summary of the evidence and a call for action.

The Outcomes Gap: Differences Based on Income

The correlation between childhood poverty and life outcomes is well documented. This chapter cites a small selection from this very large literature. Given the wide range of outcomes discussed in the literature, this chapter will not attempt to be exhaustive, but instead will briefly examine the gap between outcomes for high-income and low-income children in the areas of:

- educational attainment and work income;
- public assistance income;
- physical and mental health;
- becoming a child in care; and
- teenage childbearing and lone parenthood.

As we will discuss later, these raw gaps give a clear idea of the magnitude of differences in outcomes between low-income children and others, but the causal pathways through which these gaps are produced are less clear.

Educational Attainment and Work Income

The poorer educational attainment by children in families with low socio-economic status shows up early and persists. The Peabody Picture Vocabulary Test (PPVT) was administered to more than 3,000 children aged 4 and 5 years as part of the Canadian National Longitudinal Survey of Children and Youth (NLSCY). Willms (1996, p. 79) reports that each standard deviation increase in socio-economic status (SES) is associated with more than a third of a standard deviation increase in PPVT scores. Similarly, mathematics scores for children in grades 2, 4, and 6 were statistically significantly related to SES. Each standard deviation increase in SES was associated with 20%, 23%, and 22% of a standard deviation increase in math scores (Willms, 1996). Ross, Scott, and Kelly (1996) report that in 1993, 5% of 16-17 year olds from families above the Statistics Canada low-income cut-off drop out of high school, versus 8% from families below the cut-off.

This is not just a Canadian phenomenon. Haveman and Wolfe (1995, p. 1870) reviewed more than 100 US studies of the determinants of children's attainments, and concluded that: "Children who grew up in a poor or low income family tend to have lower educational and labor market attainments than children from more affluent families." Mayer (1997) shows outcomes for young adults with parents in the top and bottom income quintiles, and reports that:

- US male workers from families in the top income quintile earn 56% more than those from the bottom quintile;
- young adults from top-quintile families have an average of 2 more years of schooling by age 24; and

- bottom-quintile 24-year-old men are twice as likely (16.7% versus only 7.7%) as those from the top quintile to be "idle," that is neither working nor in school.

Public Assistance Income

Mayer (1997) reports that US children with parents in the bottom income quintile are 20 times as likely as children from top-quintile families to receive welfare as adults (10.8% versus 0.5%). Haveman and Wolfe (1995) also found that: "Growing up in a family that has received welfare increases the probability that a girl, if she becomes a lone mother, will choose welfare recipiency."

Physical and Mental Health

Ross, Scott, and Kelly (1996) report several health differences in Canada based on income. Infant mortality rates are 50% higher in neighbourhoods in the bottom income quintile than in those in the top quintile; low birth weight (<2500 g.) is 40% more prevalent in bottom-quintile than in top-quintile neighbour-hoods; and disability rates are more than twice as high for children in bottom-income-quintile families as for those in top-income-quintile families (7.7% versus 3.6%). The same paper reports (based on a 1983 survey of Ontario school children) that children from families below the StatsCan low-income cutoff were much more likely than other children to display hyperactivity (13% versus 5%) and emotional disorders (11% versus 5%). Wilkins (1995) reported that 1991 infant mortality was 64% higher in lowest-quintile neighbourhoods in Canada than in highest-quintile neighbourhoods (7.5/1000 versus 4.5/1000), a narrowing of the gap from 1971 and 1986 (97% higher and 82% higher, respectively) (see also Wilkins, Adams, and Brancker, 1989; Wilkinson, 1996 and 1997).

Becoming a Child in Care

The Provincial Health Officer of BC (PHO, 1998) reports that low-income and aboriginal children are more likely to be in care of the Ministry for Children and Families than other children. One-third of children in care are aboriginal (versus 6% of all children); 60% are from families in receipt of welfare (versus 8 to 14% of all children[1]); and 60% are from one-parent families (versus less than 20% of all children) (see also **Chapter 6**).

Teenage Childbearing and Lone Parenthood

Ross and colleagues (1996) report that among Ontario females 16 to 19 years of age, 18% of those from households with less than $30,000 in annual income in 1990 had been pregnant in the last 5 years, versus only 4% of those from families with higher incomes. Mayer (1997) reports that 47.4% of women with parents in the bottom income quintile were lone parents by the age of 24, versus 7.5% for women with parents in the top quintile. Compared with children of two-parent families, children of one-parent families are twice as likely to drop out of high school or to become teenage parents themselves (McLanahan and Sandefur, 1994).

PROMISING STRATEGIES TO INCREASE STANDARDS OF LIVING OR IMPROVE OUTCOMES

Policy cannot await perfect information; but evidence-based policy should use whatever research evidence is available as a guide. In particular, it is useful to target policy on areas where beneficial effects seem most likely to be achieved at reasonable cost, whether or not the causal mechanisms are fully understood. Several key areas of child policy will be discussed, with a view to presenting the evidence that suggests some more (and less) promising avenues for policy change in British Columbia and Canada. First, we discuss policies to raise standards of living for low-income families directly (social assistance, in-kind assistance, work income, and maintenance payments). Next, we discuss policies to improve children's outcomes.

Social Assistance Payments

With children's outcomes consistently associated with higher family income, it is not surprising that many researchers and policy-makers call for increases in family income to improve the life chances of children. Government can directly control the level of social assistance payments, so it is often suggested this is where action should be taken. However, policy makers must take the cost-effectiveness of direct transfers into account. There are two key problems that make it impractical to rely on increases in social assistance payments to improve outcomes for vulnerable children: the costs (disincentive effects) are large, and the benefits (for children) are small.

Using our tax system to redistribute income has been compared to transporting water in a leaky bucket; the more you try to carry, the faster it leaks (Moffitt, 1992; Mankiw, Kneebone, McKenzie, and Rowe, 1999, p. 435). Higher social assistance payments must be financed with higher taxes, and both higher taxes and higher social assistance payments result in "leaks" in the form of reduced work and investment (Feldstein and Feenberg, 1995). Taxes on high income earners reduce work effort and (by reducing after-tax income) also reduce savings, investment, and growth in the long run (Frenze, 1996). In addition, social assistance payments directly reduce work effort. Killingsworth (1983, p. 398) reviews a series of large random assignment experiments that showed that people who were eligible for higher transfer payments worked less on average than people who were eligible for lower transfer payments. These results were robust over a large number of studies conducted in different locations. Moffitt (1992) reported that in the US, for every $1 of welfare paid to lone mothers, 37% is "consumed" in the form of reduced earnings. An increase in welfare payments of $1 therefore increases a lone mother's income by only 63 cents.

If money income on its own is genuinely beneficial to children, then increasing any component of family income would improve outcomes for children. The competing hypothesis, expressed by Mayer (1997, pp. 2-3) is that the correlation between income and outcomes is seen:

> ...because the parental characteristics that employers value and are willing to pay for, such as skills, diligence, honesty, good health, and reliability, also improve children's life chances, independent of their effect on parents' income. Children of parents with these attributes do well even when their parents do not have much income.

If Mayer is correct, then we would expect a positive correlation between earned income and children's outcomes, but a negative correlation between transfer income and children's outcomes (since earned income is correlated with unobserved beneficial parental characteristics, and transfers correlated with unobserved negative parental characteristics).

Corak (1998) addresses this issue head on, looking at four different types of income. He finds that $1 of income from assets appears to improve the life chances of children more than $1 from self employment which in turn has a bigger "impact" than employment income. In the same analysis, each additional $1 of transfer income *harms* the children. The conclusion to draw from this is not that inheriting money helps children or that giving more money to people on welfare hurts their children, but rather that the data that we, as a society, collect is not sufficiently detailed or accurate to adjust for the individual and family characteristics that affect children's outcomes, and that act as confounders when we try to measure the impact of money income on the outcomes of children.

In-kind Assistance

If higher transfer payments are not the answer to improving the outcomes of children, direct programs to supply some of the environmental deficits encountered by low-income children may be. One alternative to providing cash transfers is to provide transfers in kind. Historically, economic theory was used to support cash transfers as being more efficient because they enabled individuals to choose the items that they most needed. In addition, the administrative costs of in-kind transfers are expected to be higher. The preference for cash transfers is consistent with the economist's notion of consumer sovereignty— the idea that each consumer is the best judge of what they want and what to pay for it. However, when it comes to assisting vulnerable children, who typically do not make their own consumption decisions, in-kind transfers may deserve another look.

Currie (1994) has completed an empirical study of the relative effectiveness of cash and in-kind programs in the US. She compares results from negative income tax experiments (cash transfers) with results from food stamps, housing, Medicaid, school nutrition and Head Start programs. She concluded that "Programs that target services directly to children have the largest measured effects, while unrestricted cash transfer programs have the smallest" (p. 32).

Low-income Canadian children probably already have better access than similar American children to public programs such as Medicare, housing subsidies, and child care subsidies. Where Canadian children lack basic material needs, however, targeted in-kind assistance (such as school lunch programs or food stamps) could well be a better solution than increased cash transfers. Better access to preschool and child day care could also improve school readiness for many low-income children. More investigation is needed into the characteristics that might be used to identify sub-populations of children in Canada who may be lacking basic physical or environmental needs (e.g., small height for age, developmental delays) and who might therefore benefit from appropriate in-kind assistance.

Parental Earnings

Discouraging results from transfer-payment programs have led to renewed interest in programs to raise earnings. The Self-Sufficiency Project (SSP) was begun in 1992, to investigate whether offering financial incentives to welfare recipients could induce them to begin working. Long-term single parent welfare recipients in BC and New Brunswick were offered large income supplements if they found full-time (>30 hours/week) employment. The supplements amounted to one-half of the gap between the participants' actual earnings and the "target" income, which was $37,000 per year in BC, and $30,000 per year in New Brunswick. Eligibility was limited to single-parent recipients who had been on welfare for 11 or 12 of the past 12 months. The supplement could be paid for up to 3 years. Participants and controls were selected by random assignment to facilitate rigourous evaluation, and the results after 18 months of experience (Lin et al., 1998) are encouraging. Comparing participants to controls reveals that SSP:

- doubled the rate of full-time employment (from 14% to 29%), mostly by moving participants from no employment to full-time employment;
- reduced receipt of welfare (from 80-83% to 66-70%) and lowered average benefits;
- raised earnings substantially; participants gained more than $2 in additional earnings for each $1 spent on SSP benefits (i.e., $1 in public spending brought

participants more than $3 of additional income; instead of 63 cents as with direct increases in welfare payments);

- increased employment rates even for recipients who had reported barriers to work such as lack of Grade 12 (from 10.1% to 23.6%), lack of child care (from 8.5% to 21.9%), or having a physical activity limitation (from 9.2% to 21.3%);

- produced similar results in both BC and New Brunswick, though New Brunswick's unemployment rate was higher than BC's at the time of the study;

- lifted 12% of participants above the Statistics Canada Low-Income Cut Off (LICO[2]; 90% below LICO in the control group versus 78% for SSP);

- moved 3% of participants from below 50% of the LICO to 50-100% (22% below 50% of LICO in the control group versus 18% for SSP); and

- helped families meet basic needs (food, children's clothing, and housing), reduce their use of food banks, save (more had savings accounts or RRSPs), or have a car.

SSP has clearly been successful in increasing both employment and income, and may be able to modify some of the unobserved parental characteristics that both influence earned income and benefit children directly. Naturally it did not affect pre-existing differences between those who worked or did not work, so it was an excellent project for looking at the impact of parental employment on the outcomes of children. In addition, measuring impacts on children was one of the stated goals of the SSP, and considerable data was collected so that the impacts on children could be measured. Disappointingly, the impacts thus far on children were small and not uniformly positive. Morris and Michalopolous (2000) found that:

- SSP had no effects on the youngest children's functioning. For children in the younger cohort, who were infants and toddlers at the beginning of the program, SSP did not affect test scores, social behaviour, emotional well-being, or health.

- For the middle cohort, SSP had small positive effects on children's cognitive and school outcomes. On many other measures, program and control groups did not differ.

- For children in the older cohort, SSP may have increased minor delinquency and tobacco, alcohol, and drug use. The program did not affect many other outcomes that were examined.

In order to determine the costs and effects of providing job-search assistance in addition to SSP, a small group of randomly-selected New Brunswick participants were offered "SSP Plus" and compared both with controls receiving regular SSP, and with controls receiving no special programs. The additional impacts of SSP Plus were significant: more participants conducted active job searches, more found full-time jobs, and family incomes were higher (when compared with basic SSP) (Quets, Robins, Pan, Michalopoulos, and Card, 1999).

As with basic SSP, long-run costs and effects depend on participants remaining employed when the program ends.

Overall, Michalopoulos, Robins, and Card (1999) conclude that for applicants SSP "increased employment, earnings, and income for welfare recipients, while holding constant after-tax government transfer payments." Although SSP appears to be a cost-effective method for reducing the welfare dependence of families with children[3] and increasing family income, it has not yet shown beneficial impacts on the children, although this may well be a function of lack of opportunity to follow-up on long term impacts.

Lone Parenthood and Maintenance Payments by Absent Parents

In a policy context, lone parenthood is inseparable from child poverty. Half of all low-income families in BC are lone parent families,[4] and children in lone parent families are at higher risk of poor developmental outcomes. Because lone parenthood and low income are associated with many factors that might influence development outcomes, cause and effect are not well established. However, whatever the nature of the association, it is clear that there is unavoidable overlap between policies that address child poverty and those that relate to difficulties of one-parent families.

Dooley (1995) reports that the incidence of female lone parenthood in Canada has increased from 8% of all mothers in the early 1970s to 14% by the early 1990s. The 1996 census reveals that 18.8% of all Canadian children lived in one-parent families. (By contrast, the incidence of lone parent families in France and Germany is 9% and 7% respectively.)

Having a lone parent is often seen as a double disadvantage for children. First, lone parents are much more likely to be poor. Second, children of lone parents are almost twice as likely to have other problems. Lipman, Offord, and Dooley (1996) report that children in single-mother families are 1.7 times as likely (40.6% versus 23.6%) to have one or more problems such as hyperactivity, conduct or emotional disorders, or repeating a grade at school.[5] Even looking only at families above the LICO, higher rates of these disorders are seen for children in single-parent than in two-parent families (35.8% versus 22.6%). The authors conclude that, "Being the offspring of a single mother placed a child at increased risk of emotional or behavioural problems or academic or social difficulties whether the family was poor or not."

Despite the strong association between poor outcomes and living in a one-parent family, however, most children in single-parent families (as in two-parent families) grow up healthy. Ross, Roberts, and Scott (1998a) studied the variation in outcomes among children of one-parent families and concluded: "these results do not mean that lone-parenthood *per se* is the main factor; rather, there is most likely a constellation of factors strongly associated with lone parenthood." In a companion paper, Ross, Roberts, and Scott (1998b) suggest that assistance be targeted to specific problems, rather than directed at one-parent families in general. They recommend policies to support development of parenting skills for parents of young children, and to increase parental income and education.

Increasing the income of lone parents generally involves not only social assistance payments, but also maintenance payments from the absent parent (usually the father). It is well known that marital breakup affects the living standards of custodial and non-custodial parents differently. Comparing changes in the income-to-need ratio (INR)[6] after divorce using longitudinal data for 1982-86, Finnie, Betson, Kluge, and Zweibel (1994) have shown that non-custodial fathers experienced a gain of 30%, while custodial lone mothers and children experienced a loss of 48% (the INR falls to 52% of its pre-divorce level). With regard to poverty, 59% of custodial lone mothers fell below the LICO in the year after divorce, compared with 18% of non-custodial fathers.

Sharing family income more fairly after divorce seems a desirable goal, whether or not it has direct benefits for children's outcomes. Fortunately, this is an area in which society can have an influence, through policies that affect the level of child support that the non-custodial parent must pay, and/or the extent to which ordered child support payments are made. Various approaches have been tried.

Wisconsin began a series of pilots to test the effects of different approaches to child support payments in 1980. One pilot fixed child support orders as a percentage of income rather than as a specific dollar level. The goal was to have child support respond to changes in the absent parent's income without the custodial parent having to apply for a new court order to change the dollar amount. A non-custodial parent would not be able to avoid paying child support by quitting his job before the court date and seeking re-employment again afterwards. Child support staff in Wisconsin expressed reservations regarding percentage-expressed orders because of the difficulty in monitoring compliance (Meyer, Bartfeld, Garfinkel, and Brown, 1996). Nonetheless, Bartfeld and Garfinkel (1996) found that the pilot program was effective at increasing monthly payments relative to what would have occurred with fixed-dollar orders. By the third year, the mean for percentage-expressed orders was $131 higher per month than the mean for fixed order payments. Although mean monthly payments actually declined for both fixed orders and percentage-expressed orders, payments under percentage-expressed orders declined much less than payments under fixed orders. In 1991/92, 41% of child support orders in Wisconsin were expressed as a percentage of the absent parents' incomes.

Wisconsin also required routine withholding (garnisheeing) of child support payments. Meyer and colleagues (1996) report the results of a number of studies of its effect. They report that judges did use routine withholding in just over three-quarters of cases. All studies that they reviewed reported increased compliance,[7] and one (Danziger and Nichols-Casebolt, 1990) estimated that immediate withholding increased child support payments by $25 per month (over garnisheeing in response to delinquency).

Largely as a result of the Wisconsin studies, the American Congress required states to use guidelines for child support payments and to routinely garnishee non-custodial parents' incomes in the Family Support Act of 1988. But even in Wisconsin, which leads the country in child support enforcement, there are significant problems in collecting child support payments. Meyer and Bartfeld matched data from court records and the income tax system in Wisconsin for a sample of paternity and divorce cases from 1981 to 1989. They found overall compliance rates of 32% to 60% for paternity cases (Bartfeld and Meyer, 1994) and 55% to 72% for divorce cases (Meyer and Bartfeld, 1996). Nationally, the picture is worse. Sorensen (1996) analyzed 1990 data from the Survey of Income and Program Participation and concluded that non-custodial fathers could have paid as much as $34 to $48 billion more in child support if Wisconsin-type guidelines had been in effect nationwide and orders were fully paid. This is far beyond the $15 billion actually paid.

A consortium of private foundations, together with the US Department of Health and Human Services and the US Department of Labor, have launched the Parents' Fair Share project. It was intended to "help fathers: (1) find more stable and better-paying jobs; (2) assume an important and responsible parental role; and (3) pay child support on a consistent basis" (Berlin, 1998, p. 1). It was to achieve these goals using a combination of peer support, mediation, and employment and training services. Berlin reports that Parents' Fair Share did increase child support payments, even though it did not increase the employment or earnings of the participants, but he does not quantify the extent of the increase.

In some European countries government is directly involved. In Sweden, the government pays tax-free child support payments to lone parent families, and attempts to collect the payment back from the absent parent; in 1983, 38% of these payments were recovered in this way (Phipps, 1996, p. 108). The benefits of this system are the reliability of payments for custodial parents, and perhaps the reduced stigma attached to child support (versus welfare) payments. In addition, having a child support system separate from the welfare system would decrease the apparent welfare caseload, and might make it easier to tailor the requirements of the child support and welfare programs to the needs and obligations of the recipients. The disadvantage is that it would mean that lone parents would be eligible for different welfare benefits than others, which could lead to the public perception that the payment system rewards (and therefore encourages) marital breakup.

Based on experience in Canada and elsewhere, Finnie and colleagues (1994) recommended adoption of percentage-of-income guidelines in Canada. In 1997, the provinces, with the federal government, agreed to guidelines that judges must consider when determining the level of child support to be paid by the non-custodial parent. The guidelines set support payments in dollars (not percentages) based on income. In addition, BC and other provinces have set up family maintenance enforcement programs to enforce child support orders.

These programs go some way toward reducing the economic impact of divorce on children, but cannot eliminate the basic problem. As Finnie and colleagues (1994) note, "divorce necessarily results in declines in standards of living due to the loss of economies of scale associated with the breakup of the household," of the order of 20 to 25% for a family with two children (Finnie et al., 1994, pp. 111-112). Fairness in child support payments means sharing these losses equitably. Since the effectiveness of Canada's amended system in improving fairness has not yet been tested, further changes should probably await evaluation of the current system.

Teenage Childbearing

It is widely believed that teenage childbearing is an event with irreversible (negative) consequences for the teen mother's schooling and work, leading to prolonged dependence on public assistance. However, Hotz, McElroy, and Sanders (1999) recently re-estimated these impacts using USNLSY data on women who miscarried as teenagers compared to women who gave birth while teenagers. This study finds much smaller negative effects from teenage childbearing than have been estimated previously, and in fact reveals some positive effects (by age 28, teen mothers had more work experience, higher earnings, and were less likely to live in poverty or depend on public assistance than those who miscarried as teens). The authors suggest that "the negative consequences previously attributed to teenage childbearing are, in fact, the result of the many unobserved disadvantages not accounted for by observable background characteristics." As a group, teen mothers are likely to live in poverty, but this appears to be because of influences in their lives before they became teen mothers, not because of their early childbearing. A policy that sought to improve outcomes for these young women by encouraging them to delay their childbearing is not the answer; in fact, the study finds that total annual (US) expenditure on public assistance would actually *rise* by US $1.3 billion if all teenage mothers deferred their pregnancies, because of the reduction in work by these women.

This is an important study, which has used an innovative method to obtain better estimates of the true impact of teen parenthood than have been available before. However, it has not addressed all important questions; for instance, outcomes for the children of teen mothers were not examined. It would seem prudent to study the question with Canadian data, and perhaps not to expand existing programs aimed at preventing teen pregnancy until impacts are re-estimated.

School Readiness, Parenting Skills, and Early Childhood Interventions

Unequal achievement in school frequently has its origins before birth, or in early childhood. It is now recognized that young children experience key development stages before ever entering school. According to the Carnegie Task Force on Meeting the Needs of Young Children (Carnegie, 1994):

- Brain development before age one is more rapid and extensive than was previously realized. Although cell formation is virtually complete before birth, brain maturation continues after birth.

- Brain development is much more vulnerable to environmental influence than was suspected. Inadequate nutrition before birth and in the first years of life can seriously interfere with brain development and lead to such neurological and behavioral disorders as learning disabilities and mental retardation.

- The influence of early environment on brain development is long-lasting. There is considerable evidence showing that infants exposed to good nutrition, toys, and playmates had measurably better brain function at 12 years of age than those raised in a less stimulating environment.

- Early experiences are important partly because there are critical "windows" for brain development related to particular functions (e.g., vision, birth to six months; emotional development, birth to 18 months). Developmental opportunities missed at these critical times cannot always be made up later.

- Environment affects not only the number of brain cells and the number of connections among them, but also the way these connections are "wired." The process of eliminating excess neurons and synapses from the dense immature brain, which continues well into adolescence, is most dramatic in the early years of life, and it is guided to a large extent by the child's sensory experience of the outside world.

- Early stress can affect brain function, learning, and memory adversely and permanently. New research provides a scientific basis for the long recognized fact that children who experience extreme stress in their earliest years are at greater risk for developing a variety of cognitive, behavioral, and emotional difficulties later in life.

Material deprivation is not the only cause of poor outcomes. Even among stunted children in low-income neighbourhoods, in a low-income country,[8] stimulation without nutritional supplementation had larger impacts than nutritional supplementation without stimulation (Grantham-McGregor, Powell, Walker, and Himes, 1991). This finding is particularly relevant in the North American context. There is extensive evidence that children in low-income homes in the US and Canada live in an environment that is less stimulating for children. For example, Hanson, McLanahan, and Thomson (1997, pp. 191-192) report that "low income was related to low scores on the Home Observation for Measurement of the Environment (HOME) inventory, which accounts for 18-43 percent of the effects of persistent economic deprivation on children's welfare."

Clearly, difficulties in early childhood can have lasting effects. Since parents are the most important influence on young children, poor parenting skills are a serious risk factor for children. Because good parenting practices are only weakly associated with socioeconomic status, however, Chao and Willms (1998) assert that universal programs to improve parenting skills would be preferable to programs targeted at low-income or poorly-educated parents.

A study of refugees resettled in the US highlights the importance of parents, and reminds us that it is easy to over-emphasize the possibility of permanent harm from early experiences. Children are resilient, and in low-income households that provide appropriate stimulation, children can do very well even after suffering early adversity. Caplan, Choy, and Whitmore (1992) studied 536 school-age children from families of Indochinese boat people who settled in the US in the late 1970s and early 1980s. All of the children attended schools in low-income metropolitan areas, had little knowledge of English when they arrived, and had lost schooling time while in refugee camps. Despite these multiple handicaps, after an average of only 3½ years in the US, the children scored above average (54th percentile) on the California Achievement Test. Caplan and colleagues highlight the role of the family in achieving these remarkable results, saying: "Although some of our findings are culturally specific, others point overwhelmingly to the pivotal role of the family in the children's academic "success."

Child Day Care and Pre-School

Our growing awareness of the developmental importance of early childhood, and reports of highly effective intervention programs for children at risk, have combined to create new interest in public programs for young children (CIAR, 1999). Both child day care (full-day care, generally designed to permit parents to work) and preschool programs (partial-day programs aimed at providing enrichment for children) warrant additional attention in Canada (Cleveland and Krashinsky, 1998).

Many young children already attend day care, but the quality and type varies tremendously. In BC, generous child care subsidies are available to parents on welfare or at very low incomes, giving them good access to higher-quality care in licensed centres. Middle-income parents generally do not qualify for child care subsidies and consequently have difficulty affording licensed centre care, particularly for children under age three.[9] There is no consistency across Canada regarding subsidy policies, however. Given the shortage of licensed care spaces in most provinces, many families use unlicensed child care or licensed family care (operated in the caregiver's home).

The Cochrane Collaboration commissioned a review of child day care (Zoritch, Roberts, and Oakley, 2000) which concluded that day care is beneficial to both children and mothers.[10] Children showed improvements in intelligence, behavioural development, school achievement, and employment, and a reduction in teen pregnancy and criminality, and there were also positive effects on mothers' education, employment, and interaction with their children. Since all of the studies that met Cochrane inclusion criteria for rigour were conducted in the US with disadvantaged populations, these results are more likely to apply to disadvantaged children in Canada (rather than to all children).

The US experience with early childhood programs (including preschool as well as day care) was summarized in a RAND-sponsored review (Karoly et al., 1998). The RAND review examined a number of US studies in order to assess the likely costs and benefits of these programs, and their conclusions can be used in the design of new programs. The review found wide variation in the interventions themselves, and in the child outcomes evaluated. Not surprisingly, the review concludes that while early intervention programs have the potential to return benefits greater than program costs, these benefits are not always achieved in practice. The potential benefits include:

- improving high-risk children's chances of achieving economic self-sufficiency (and avoiding becoming chronic or violent criminals);
- improving high-risk mothers' chances of employment, and reducing their drug-dependency;
- reducing increases in government spending for welfare, special education, and corrections; and
- reducing losses due to crime in society generally.

The main element that helps programs return benefits that exceed costs to government is targeting, or delivering services to those who will benefit most. Evaluation and monitoring may be needed to determine who benefits most from a particular kind of program. Usually, more disadvantaged children have the potential for larger benefits, but some multiple-risk children require specialized services and are not well served by programs that would benefit less disadvantaged children. In order for evaluations to show benefits exceeding costs, it is important for the evaluation to recognize benefits to mothers as well as children, and to follow families for a long enough period (since the benefits of successful programs accrue for many years).

The review also determined that although there are a number of unanswered questions about how to design successful programs, it does appear that longer program duration, combining preschool and after-school programs, combining home visits and centre-based day care, and offering services to both children and parents (e.g., parenting training) are features that help programs produce lasting beneficial results.

Health

Children in low-income families are at higher risk of poor health for a variety of reasons. Some health risks related to early childhood were discussed above; this section discusses hazards related to smoking, substance abuse, and parental depression.

Smoking is a significant source of poor health for vulnerable children and youth in Canada. Overall, 23.5% of Canadians smoke (Statistics Canada, 1996/97), but smoking is nearly three times as prevalent in the lowest income quintile as in the highest (ACPH 1999, Exhibit 5.7), and the deaths and illnesses caused by smoking are distributed accordingly. Despite the known increased risk of miscarriage, premature birth, SIDS (see **Chapter 4**), and low birth weight, Connor and McIntyre (1998) report that nearly a quarter (23.7%) of Canadian women smoke during pregnancy, including more than 40% of teen mothers and a third of mothers aged 20-24; these rates are higher than the average (Statistics Canada data) for all Canadian women (21.3%), or for Canadian teens (16.6%), probably reflecting the lower income levels of young mothers. Low-income children are also much more likely than high income children to be exposed to environmental tobacco smoke (ETS) at home. ETS is a known risk factor for respiratory diseases including bronchitis, pneumonia, and asthma; and respiratory disease is the leading cause of hospitalizations for preschoolers. In addition, children whose parents smoke are more likely to smoke as teens and adults. Aboriginal children in BC are more likely to be exposed to daily tobacco smoke in their homes (27% versus 15%) and to take up smoking at younger ages (40% smoke by age 13 versus 20% overall in BC). Having physicians routinely ask whether patients smoke, and provide counselling and treatment to help smokers quit, has been judged cost-effective (10-15% quit). Continued expansion of programs to reduce smoking would provide important benefits to children and youth. Pregnant women, aboriginals, and youth are the most crucial targets for enhanced programs (PHO, 1998, pp. 46, 110-111.)

The expense of smoking tobacco magnifies its negative effects at low incomes. In BC, even a light smoker (3 to 4 packs of cigarettes a week) would spend $750-1,000 on smoking in a year, a substantial amount for a minimum-wage worker or a lone parent on social assistance. A moderate smoker (1 pack a day) would spend $1,800 per year. In this situation, smoking both worsens health (for the smoker and for children in the home), and significantly reduces available income. McIntyre, Connor, and Warren (2000) analyze data from the 1994 NLSCY, and report that among the 1.2% of families where the parent reported that their child had ever gone hungry because the family had run out of food, 49% of the responding parents smoked (versus 29.7% smokers among the 99% of families where children had never gone hungry). Among the 0.4% of families where a parent reported that their children frequently went hungry (almost all of these families have no income except social assistance), 72.2% of the responding parents smoked. Higher rates of asthma were seen among children of families that had experienced hunger, probably reflecting the higher prevalence of smoking in these homes. It is a testament to the addictiveness of tobacco that even at very low incomes, with themselves[11] and their children experiencing hunger, parents continue to spend money on smoking.

Whether or not the above numbers are accurate,[12] it is apparent that public policy directed at smoking prevention and medical treatment to assist in smoking cessation would confer significant health benefits on smokers (and their families) at all income levels, and would increase the funds available to low-income smokers for food and other necessities, without requiring any increase in social assistance payments. (Costs would be incurred for smoking cessation treatment, of course.) The Cochrane review on nicotine replacement therapy for smoking cessation (Silagy, Mant, Fowler, and Lancaster, 2000) reported that all available forms of nicotine replacement therapy (gum, patch, nasal spray, inhaler, sublingual tablets) were effective aids to smoking cessation, increasing quit rates by a factor of 1.5 to 2. Yet these effective aids are underused by low-income smokers in Canada because their cost is not generally covered under Medicare. The Cochrane Collaboration also reviewed programs to help pregnant smokers quit (Lumley, Oliver, and Waters, 2000), and reported that these programs are effective in reducing smoking, low birth weight, and pre-term birth. Yet targeted programs to help pregnant women quit smoking are not consistently offered or available across Canada.

Untreated parental depression and substance abuse are also serious risk factors for children and youth. Depressed parents are unable to respond appropriately to their children, and the NPHS (ACPH, 1999) reveals that depression is more prevalent at low incomes in Canada. For both men and women, the rate of depression is nearly three times as high in the lowest income quintile as in the highest (13% versus 5% for women, 11% versus 4% for men). A recent study in Canada (Byrne et al., 1998) used a standard assessment tool and determined that 45.4% of lone parents applying for income assistance in Ontario were depressed in the 12 months following their application. Of course, depression may be either a cause of low income (by reducing ability to work) or an effect (for instance of job loss). Mayer (1997, p. 118) concludes that the effect of income on parental depression (after adjustment for confounders) is small, meaning that improving income is not a promising avenue for reducing depression. But more consistently providing medical treatment for depression could be expected to benefit both parents and their children.

Substance abuse affects parents as well as youth; it includes prenatal alcohol consumption, injection drug use, and other substance abuse. As with smoking, aboriginal youth are at higher risk for substance abuse, and are more likely to begin substance abuse at younger ages. Injection drug users are now the highest-risk group for HIV infection in Canada, and account for 70% of hepatitis C cases (ACPH, 1999, pp. 19, 122-124). Better prevention and treatment programs for pregnant women, aboriginals, and injection drug users are a priority, although piloting and evaluation is essential to ensure effective programs. The Cochrane Review of programs for people with both mental illness and substance misuse (Ley, Jeffery, McLaren, and Siegfried, 2000) reported that the quality of research on these programs is poor (key outcomes are poorly measured or not measured) and that there is no clear evidence that these special programs offer any advantage over standard care.

IMPLEMENTATION ISSUES

Head Start (a large-scale preschool program for disadvantaged children) is the flagship of American anti-poverty programs, and studies from the High/Scope Perry Preschool of Ypsilanti, Michigan are frequently cited to demonstrate that Head Start is effective. Between 1962 and 1965, 58 children were randomly selected from a pool of 123 for participation in the Perry Preschool. It was a very expensive intervention, costing $12,356 per participant, but in follow-ups over the next 24 years program participants were found to be more likely to graduate from high school, be employed, have higher earnings, own their own home, and less likely to commit crimes or receive welfare. The cumulative result of all of these effects (by age 27) was a total return of $88,433, or $7.16 for each dollar spent, with the largest category of benefits being savings to the justice system ($12,796) and to crime victims ($57,585). By any measure, though, this pilot program was a good investment for taxpayers (Barnett, 1996, pp. xi, 11).

Schweinhart and colleagues (1993, pp. xi-xii) note that the High/Scope Perry Preschool had a major impact on public feeling about Head Start:

> *Knowledge of the High/Scope Perry Program's return on public investment has affected how US business leaders think about preschool programs....Furthermore, with bipartisan congressional support spearheaded first by President Bush and then by President Clinton, federal spending for Head Start increased from $1.2 billion in 1988 to $3.5 billion in 1995.*

The euphoria regarding Head Start is widespread:

> *In a time when publicly supported social programs face cutbacks, consolidation or even elimination, Head Start is an early childhood program for low-income families that has garnered widespread public and bipartisan support. Its unique status as a favored program for poor children has attracted attention and a well-publicized appraisal of its current operations and the quality of its programs* (Takanishi and DeLeon, 1994, p. 120).

Head Start is an excellent example of an attempt at evidence-based public policy. A random assignment study found significant benefits from a program and as a result it was implemented on a wide scale. Unfortunately, the example of Head Start also demonstrates how difficult it is to move from successful pilots to successful large-scale programs.

It is now clear that the High/Scope Perry Program's results are not generalizable to the Head Start program as a whole. The Perry Preschool was funded at a higher level and involved better-trained staff than typical Head Start programs, and numbers in the Perry study were small. Haskins (1989) reviewed studies of both Perry and Head Start, and found significant differences between outcome measures for "model programs" (like Perry) and Head Start; he noted that more than 80% of the taxpayer benefits from Perry "come from earnings increases, welfare reduction, and crime reduction, variables about which there is almost no information for Head Start." For Head Start as a whole, Currie and Thomas find that although "the results for white children suggest that the potential gains are much larger than the costs," "when viewed strictly in terms of lasting benefits provided to children, Head Start programs serving African-American children are not cost-effective" (Currie and Thomas, 1995, pp. 342-343, 361).

Zigler (1994, p.38) points to chronic problems with quality control:

> *Head Start's basic concept, methodology, and goals are sound....But the literature also shows that these services must be of high quality to achieve desired outcomes. There are almost 1,400 Head Start programs, and many of them are excellent. Others, however are mediocre, and some are downright poor. Quality problems have actually plagued Head Start since its hasty beginnings. In a matter of a few months, the program was transformed from an idea before the planning committee to a national summer preschool serving over one-half million children. Quality controls were left behind, and the program has been playing catch-up ever since. Although we now have performance standards and other safeguards, funds to train staff to implement them and to monitor centers for compliance have nearly disappeared. The best standards in the world are meaningless if they are not enforced. Years of inadequate funding have jeopardized quality in all of the services that define Head Start.*

Quality control in a decentralized program such as Head Start is always difficult, because the people who unambiguously benefit from a program (the contractors who provide services), will vigorously oppose any administrator who wants to evaluate or shut down an ineffective site. Normally the contractor will be armed with the success stories that come out of any program, whether it is a success or a failure.[13] In the case of Head Start, the contractor has another weapon that arises from ambiguity regarding the intended beneficiaries of the program. Although Head Start is presented to the public as a program for children, it also has some of the characteristics of an employment program. One third of employees of Head Start programs are themselves disadvantaged, being parents of current or former Head Start students. This is important because it gives the contractor the ability to paint an administrator who is shutting down an ineffective site as attacking disadvantaged employees.

The lesson from Head Start is clear: successful pilots don't always become successful programs. Potential benefits to children can fail to be realized if feelings of compassion for children spill over into compassion for the contractors and their employees. For this reason, the work of evidence-based policy does not end when pilot programs demonstrate successful approaches; it must continue throughout implementation and routine operation. Specifically, programs must be implemented over a number of years, participants must be selected randomly, and the outcomes for the children participating the program must be compared with the outcomes of the children who were not selected, in order to ensure that the program is achieving the same impact as the pilot. (Random selection does need not impair access, since many newly-created public programs cannot serve all potential clients immediately anyway. Wait lists provide natural control groups.)

Conclusions

The following initiatives have the potential to help vulnerable children achieve their full potential, whatever the underlying causal mechanisms, and are therefore good candidates for expansion in British Columbia and Canada:

- preschool programs for high-risk children that include services to children and parents;
- preschool-age child day care subsidies for middle income families currently not eligible for public subsidies;
- parenting training for parents at all income levels, perhaps in combination with routine prenatal care or prenatal education;
- appropriate in-kind assistance, based on identification of sub-populations where such assistance (food, shelter, clothing, services) would help meet the needs of children in low-income families;
- medical treatment for smoking cessation, including nicotine replacement therapy, particularly for pregnant women;
- programs to detect and treat depression, particularly for parents; and
- substance abuse prevention and treatment programs, particularly for parents.

In the area of improving standards of living for low-income children, the evidence reveals that:

- increases in welfare payments will be costlier to taxpayers and produce smaller gains in income to recipients than enhanced incentives to move from welfare to work; and
- policy can help ensure that family income is shared more fairly after family breakup.

The variation in results obtained elsewhere suggests it would be prudent to pilot programs with random assignment, monitor quality standards, and conduct ongoing evaluation of established programs in order to ensure that potential benefits become actual benefits.

Teen pregnancy prevention is a priority for research using Canadian data. It is important to determine the true impacts of teen pregnancy on mothers' future employment and welfare dependence, and on children's outcomes. Until the true impacts are known, further expansion of programs to prevent teen pregnancy should be lower in priority than programs to assist teen mothers to complete their education and become productive adults.

In-kind assistance is also a priority for Canadian research. Practical ways to identify sub-populations that might benefit are essential, as is rigourous evaluation of the effectiveness of both pilot and ongoing programs.

BC is well situated to launch a Head Start-type pilot program for children from families receiving welfare or known to Family Services, with the goal of reducing the intergenerational transmission of poverty. Children from these families are known to be more likely to become Children in Care, more likely to drop out of school before Grade 12, and (having dropped out) to be more likely to depend on welfare themselves as adults.[14] A large sample (5,000 or more) of children who would be candidates for a Head Start program could be identified from administrative records, and a quarter of those randomly selected for participation in the new program. Results from the pilot project could then be used to design a province-wide program, including specifying target groups and identifying crucial program features. A small start, with careful quality standards and monitoring built in from the beginning, would protect against the quality problems that have plagued the US programs. A pilot study is also important because the child care subsidies already available to low-income families in BC may reduce the benefits of providing a separate Head Start program here.

A pilot program to test the long-term costs and effects of enhanced preschool-age day care subsidies for middle-income parents would be a logical complement to a Head Start pilot in BC. As with preschool programs for low-income families, random assignment for the pilot project, and a small start and careful ongoing monitoring of new programs, would be essential.

REFERENCES

ACPH (Federal, Provincial and Territorial Advisory Committee on Population Health) (1999). *Toward a healthy future: Second report on the health of Canadians.* Ottawa: Government of Canada.

Barnett, W.S. (1996). *Lives in the balance: Age 27 benefit-cost analysis of the High/Scope Perry Preschool Program.* Monograph NR1056. Ypsilanti, MI: High/Scope Foundation.

Bartfeld, J., and Garfinkel, I. (1996). The impact of percentage-expressed child support orders on payments. *Journal of Human Resources*, 31(4), 794-815.

Berlin, G.L. (1998). Testimony of Gordon L. Berlin, Senior Vice President (Manpower Demonstration Research Corporation) before the Subcommittee on Human Resources, House Committee on Ways and Means, 1998. *http://www.mdrc.org/Speeches&Presentations/ pfstest.html*

Byrne, C., Browne, G., Roberts, J., Ewart, B., Schuster, M., Underwood, J., Flynn-Kingston, S., Rennick, K., Bell, B., Gafni, A., Watt, S., Ashford, Y., and Jamieson, E. (1998). Surviving social assistance: 12 month prevalence of depression in sole support parents receiving social assistance. *Canadian Medical Association Journal*, 158(7), 881-888.

Canadian Institute for Advanced Research (CIAR) (1999). Early years study: Final report. Co-Chairs M. McCain and J.F. Mustard. Toronto: CIAR.

Caplan, N., Choy, M.H., and Whitmore, J.K. (1992). Indochinese refugee families and academic achievement. *Scientific American*, February, 36-42.

Carnegie Corporation of New York (1994). Starting points: Meeting the needs of our youngest children. Waldorf, MD: Carnegie Corporation.

Chao, R.K., and Willms, J.D. (1998). The effects of parenting practices on children's outcomes, presented at HRDC conference *Investing in Children: A National Research Conference*, Ottawa, November 1998.

Cleveland, G., and Krashinsky, M. (1998). *The benefits and costs of good child care: The economic rationale for public investment in young children.* Scarborough, ON: University of Toronto, Department of Economics. View at *http://www.childcarecanada.org/resources/CRRUpubs/ benefits/bctoc.html* or download at *http://www.childcarecanada.org/download/download.html.*

Corak, M. (1998). How children get ahead in life: Does money matter? *Policy Options*, September, 18-23.

Currie, J. (1994). Welfare and the well-being of children: The relative effectiveness of cash and in-kind transfers. In J.M. Poterba (Ed.), *Tax policy and the economy*, Vol. 8. Cambridge: MIT Press.

Currie, J., and Thomas, D. (1995). Does Head Start make a difference? *American Economic Review*, 85(3), 341-364.

Danziger, S.K., and Nichols-Casebolt, A. (1990). Child support in paternity cases. *Social Service Review*, 64, 458-74.

Dooley, M.D. (1995). Lone-mother families and social assistance policy in Canada. In M.D. Dooley and R. Finnie (Eds.), *Family matters: New policies for divorce, lone mothers, and child poverty* (pp. 35-104). Ottawa: CD Howe Institute.

Feldstein, M., and Feenberg, D. (1995). *The effect of increased tax rates on taxable income and economic efficiency: A preliminary analysis of the 1993 tax rate increases.* NBER Working Paper No. W5370, November 1995.

Finnie, R., Betson, D.M., Kluge, E.B., and Zweibel, E.B. (1994). *Child support: The guideline options*. Montreal: Institute for Research on Public Policy.

Frenze, C. (1996). *The Reagan tax cuts: Lessons for tax reform* (Report of the Joint Economic Committee of the Congress of the United States). Washington, DC: Congress of the United States. *http://www.house.gov/jec/fiscal/tx-grwth/reagtxct/reagtxct.htm*.

Grantham-McGregor, S.M., Powell, C.A., Walker, S.P., and Himes, J.H. (1991). Nutritional supplementation, psychosocial stimulation, and mental development on stunted children: The Jamaican study. *Lancet*, 338:1-5.

Hanson, T.L., McLanahan, S., and Thomson, E. (1997). Economic resources, parental practices, and children's well-being. In G.J. Duncan and J. Brooks-Gunn (Eds.), *Consequences of growing up poor* (pp. 190-238). New York: Russell Sage Foundation.

Haskins, R. (1989). Beyond metaphor: The efficacy of early childhood education. *American Psychologist*, 44(2), 274-282.

Haveman, R., and Wolfe, B. (1995). The determinants of children's attainments: A review of methods and findings. *Journal of Economic Literature*, 33(Dec), 1829-1878.

Hotz, V.J., McElroy, S.W., and Sanders, S.G. (1999). Teenage childbearing and its life cycle consequences: Exploiting a natural experiment, NBER Working Paper 7397. Cambridge: National Bureau of Economic Research. *http://www.nber.org/papers/w7397*

Karoly, L.A., Greenwood, P.W., Everingham, S.S., Hoube, J., Kilburn, M.R., Rydell, C.P., Sanders, M., and Chiesa, J. (1998). *Investing in our children: What we know and don't know about the costs and benefits of early childhood interventions*. Santa Monica, CA: Rand.

Killingsworth, M.R. (1983). *Labor supply*. Cambridge: Cambridge University Press.

Kohen, D., and Hertzman, C. (1998). The importance of quality child care, presented at HRDC conference *Investing in Children: A National Research Conference*, Ottawa, November 1998.

Ley, A., Jeffery, D.P., McLaren, S., and Siegfried, N. (2000). Treatment programs for people with both severe mental illness and substance misuse (Cochrane Review). In *The Cochrane Library*, Issue 4, 2000. Oxford: Update Software.

Lin, W., Robins, P.K., Card, D., Harknett, K., Lui-Gurr, S., Pan, E.C., Mijanovich, T., Quets, G., and Villeneuve, P. (1998). When financial incentives encourage work: complete 18-month findings from the self-sufficiency project, Executive Summary. Ottawa: Social Research and Demonstration Corporation, 1998.

Lipman, E.L., Offord, D.R., and Dooley, M.D. (1996). What do we know about children from single-mother families in *Growing Up in Canada: National Longitudinal Survey of Children and Youth*. Ottawa: Human Resources Development Canada and Statistics Canada.

Lumley, J., Oliver, S., and Waters, E. (2000). Interventions for promoting smoking cessation during pregnancy (Cochrane Review). *The Cochrane Library*, 4. Oxford: Update Software.

McIntyre, L., Connor, S.K., and Warren, J. (2000). Child hunger in Canada: Results of the 1994 National Longitudinal Survey of Children and Youth. *Canadian Medical Association Journal*, 163(8), 961-965.

McLanahan, S., and Sandefur, G. (1994). *Growing up with a single parent: What hurts, what helps*. Cambridge: Harvard University Press.

Mankiw, N.G., Kneebone, R.D., McKenzie, K.J., and Rowe, N. (1999). *Principles of microeconomics: First Canadian edition*. Toronto: Harcourt Brace & Co.

Mayer, S.E. (1997). *What money can't buy*. Cambridge: Harvard University Press.

Meyer, D.R., and Bartfeld, J. (1996). Compliance with child support orders in divorce cases. *Journal of Marriage and the Family*, 58(1), 201-212.

Meyer, D.R., Bartfeld, J., Garfinkel, I., and Brown, P. (1996). Child support reform: Lessons from Wisconsin. IRP reprint #744. Madison, WI: University of Wisconsin, Institute for Research on Poverty, 1996, and *Family Relations*, 45(1), 11-18.

Michalopoulos, C., Robins, P.K., and Card, D. (1999). *When financial work incentives pay for themselves: Early findings from the self-sufficiency project's applicant study.* Ottawa: Social Research and Demonstration Corporation.

Moffitt, R. (1992). Incentive effects of the US welfare system: A review. *Journal of Economic Literature*, XXX(March), 1-6.

Morris, P., and Michalopoulos, C. (2000). *The self-sufficiency project at 36 months: Effects on children of a program that increased parental employment and income.* Ottawa: Social Research and Demonstration Corporation.

Phipps, S.A. (1996). Lessons from Europe: Policy options to enhance the economic security of Canadian families. *National Forum on Family Security, Family Security in Insecure Times* (2-3), 87-122. Ottawa: Canadian Council on Social Development.

PHO (BC Provincial Health Officer) (1998). *A report on the health of British Columbians, Annual Report 1997.* Victoria: Ministry of Health and Ministry Responsible for Seniors.

Quets, G., Robins, P.K., Pan, E.C., Michalopoulos, C., and Card, D. (1999). *Does SSP Plus increase employment? The effect of adding services to the self-sufficiency project's financial incentives.* Ottawa: Social Research and Demonstration Corporation.

Ross, D.P., Roberts, P.A., and Scott, K. (1998a). *Variations in child development outcomes among children living in lone-parent families, W-98-7E.* Ottawa: Applied Research Branch, Human Resources Development Canada.

Ross, D.P., Roberts, P.A., and Scott, K. (1998b). *Mediating factors in child development outcomes: Children in lone-parent families, W-98-8E.* Ottawa: Applied Research Branch, Human Resources Development Canada.

Ross, D.P., Scott, K., and Kelly, M. (1996). *Child poverty: What are the consequences?* Ottawa: Canadian Council on Social Development.

Schweinhart, L.J., Barnes, H.V., Weikart, D.P., Barnett, W.S., and Epstein, A.S. (1993). *Significant benefits: The High/Scope Perry Preschool study through age 27*, Monograph NR1034. Ypsilanti, MI: High/Scope Foundation.

Silagy, C., Mant, D., Fowler, G., and Lancaster, T. (2000). Nicotine replacement therapy for smoking cessation (Cochrane Review). In *The Cochrane Library*, Issue 4. Oxford: Update Software.

Sorensen, E. (1996). *A national profile of noncustodial fathers and their ability to pay child support.* Washington, DC: The Urban Institute. *http://www.urban.org/family/newprof.htm*

Takanishi, R., and DeLeon, P.H. (1994). A head start for the 21st century. *American Psychologist*, 49, 120-122.

Wilkins, R. (1995). Mortality by neighbourhood income in urban Canada, 1986-1991, conference presentation to *Canadian Society for Epidemiology and Biostatistics*, St. John's NF, August 1995.

Wilkins, R., Adams, O., and Brancker, A. (1989). Changes in mortality by income in urban Canada from 1971 to 1986. *Health Reports*, 1(2), 137-174.

Wilkinson, R.G. (1996). *Unhealthy societies: The afflictions of inequality*. London: Routledge.

Wilkinson, R.G. (1997). Health inequalities: Relative or absolute material standards? *British Medical Journal*, 314, 591-5.

Willms, J.D. (1996). Indicators of mathematics achievement in Canadian elementary schools. In *Growing Up in Canada: National Longitudinal Survey of Children and Youth* (pp. 69-82). Ottawa: Human Resources Development Canada and Statistics Canada.

Wolfe, B., Haveman, R., Ginther, D., and An, C.B. (1996). The 'window problem' in studies of children's attainments: A methodological exploration, Institute for Research on Poverty reprint #752. *Journal of the American Statistical Association*, 91(435), 970-982.

Zigler, E. (1994). Reshaping early childhood intervention to be a more effective weapon against poverty. *American Journal of Community Psychology*, 22(1), 37-47.

Zoritch, B., Roberts, I., and Oakley, A. (2000). Day care for pre-school children (Cochrane Review). In *The Cochrane Library*, Issue 4. Oxford: Update Software.

ENDNOTES

[1] Range during the late 1990s, from BC Ministry of Social Development and Economic Security data.

[2] Statistics Canada's Low-Income Cut Off (LICO) is currently the most widely-used measure of poverty in Canada. The LICO is a relative measure of poverty, and is not actually a "poverty line," although it is often referred to in this way. The LICO is based on the estimated percentage of income spent on food, shelter, and clothing from family expenditure survey data. The LICO is the income level at which a family would spend 20 percentage points more on basic necessities than the average family. The current LICOs (based on 1992 expenditure data) show the estimated income levels (for various family sizes) where food, shelter and clothing would consume 54.7% of income (since average families spent 34.7% of income on these necessities). Families at the LICO are therefore expected to have 45% of their income available to spend on non-necessities, while the average family would have 65% of income available to spend on non-necessities.

[3] The SSP included a study to determine whether the SSP supplements would draw people on to welfare by measuring the rate at which applicants for welfare left after they had been told that they would be eligible for the subsidy if they remained on welfare for a year. It concluded that the supplements would not increase welfare dependence. Concerns about the long term cost-effectiveness of SSP focus on the potential for additional people applying for welfare in order to receive the supplement.

[4] Using the Families micro data file for BC from the 1991 census, 49.8% of families with children that were below Statistics Canada's LICO were single parent families.

[5] The authors excluded lone fathers from the study "because there were so few of them (only 7.3% of single parents were fathers) and because single fathers' incomes are much closer to those of two-parent families."

[6] Comparisons are based on the income-to-need ratio (INR), the ratio of income to the LICO for that family type, before and after divorce, among parents not remarried. In the sample, 10.6% of fathers and 5% of mothers remarried in the year after divorce.

[7] The compliance rate is the amount paid divided by the amount due.

[8] Jamaica's GNP per capita was just 13% of Canada's in 1998. Source: GNP per capita 1998, adjusted for purchasing power parity, at: *http://www.worldbank.org/data/databytopic/databytopic.html#MACROECONOMICS AND GROWTH*

9 In BC the child to staff ratio is 4:1 in licensed infant and toddler centres (for children under age 3), resulting in higher costs than at preschool centres (for children aged 3-5), where the ratio is 8:1.

10 Effects on fathers have not been examined in rigourous studies.

11 34% of respondents whose children had ever been hungry reported that they themselves skipped meals when the family had run out of food.

12 Since only small numbers of survey respondents (1.2% or 0.4% of the total) indicated that their children had experienced hunger, the proportions for smokers within these groups may not be reliable.

13 45% of the Perry preschool *control* group graduated from high school, 32% were employed, 49% were never arrested, and 20% never received welfare. These success stories occurred without any intervention. If these individuals had attended a poorly-run Head Start program, the contractor could have claimed that some of this success was attributable to the program.

14 Administrative data, BC Ministry of Social Development and Economic Security and BC Ministry of Education.

Plate 4 The future learning from the past ▶

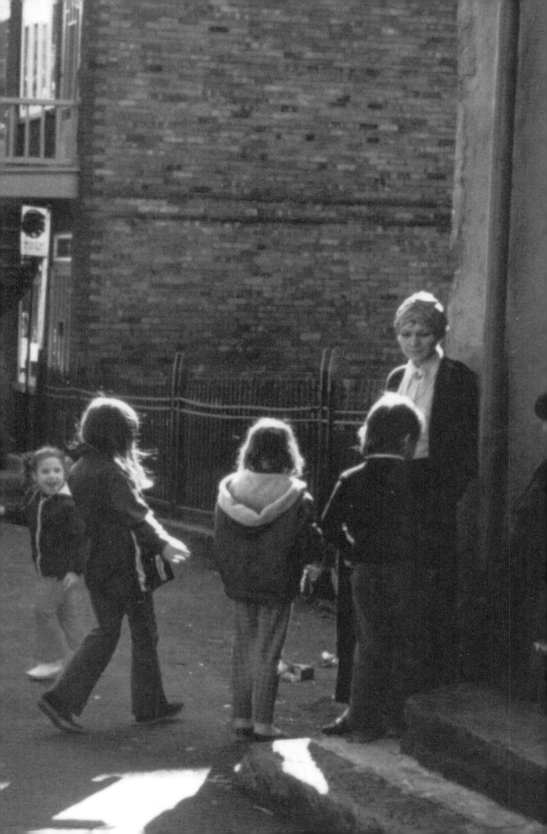

Knowing the Constituency: Youth—Their Health and Behaviour

10

Roger S. Tonkin and Aileen Murphy

McCreary Centre Society, Burnaby, BC

INTRODUCTION

Politicians, clothing and sports equipment manufacturers, film and music producers, and junk food distributors are constantly monitoring the changing nature and interests of our youth. Social marketers and policy makers may also try to understand the needs and wants of contemporary youth. Often these groups formulate their impressions from indirect sources such as the media, supply and demand in the marketplace, or small scale opinion polls or market research. Sometimes the information is merely imported from other jurisdictions or cultures, for example, Europe or the US. Rarely is there a systematic, scientifically based, large scale approach to youth themselves.

Service delivery organizations such as hospitals, child protection services, and mental heath programs may or may not offer youth-specific services. All too often these services count clients and report utilization rates without offering much more information on them than age and gender. There is no profile of their adolescent client population, nor do they tell us much about the needs of those youth who don't pass through their doors. Rarely are the youth who come to these services asked to provide feedback. Nor are youth in the broader community likely to be polled about their views of the accessibility or appropriateness of services available to them.

Within the youth community there are many sub-populations. These include obvious groups such as street and homeless youth, aboriginal youth, youth in custody, those in care or from disadvantaged families, high risk youth, and youth from multicultural or refugee backgrounds. Often these youth are known because they are potential clients of case workers and youth workers. Sometimes they are known targets of society's predators, such as pimps and sexual offenders. However, there are other important subgroups worthy of our special focus. For example, those with chronic health conditions, youth who look older than their stated age, and youth living in rural or northern settings.

This chapter is about our community's youth: what we know about them, how they are doing developmentally, and what tasks or issues some of the various subgroups face. It is about listening to our youth and indirectly makes the case for a more systematic approach to knowing about our youth constituency.

BACKGROUND

In BC we are fortunate to have excellent vital statistics and service utilization data bases that include information on youth health status and health care utilization patterns (BC Provincial Health Officer, 1998; BC Ministry for Children and Families, 1997). In addition, we have had a number of initiatives, both provincial and federal, designed to gather information from youth on such things as their smoking habits, alcohol and drug use, sexuality, health attitudes and behaviours, etc. (King, Boyce, and King, 1999; Federal, Provincial and Territorial Advisory Committee on Population Health, 1999; Hanvey et al., 1994). This chapter will not focus on these excellent data sets except to indicate that among their shortcomings is that they report on yesterday's youth (who are now young adults). In addition, the data are not reported as consistent age or grade groupings and are not regionally representative. They are often unidimensional (i.e., do not cover the broad range of correlated adolescent behaviours) and focus on an isolated problem such as smoking or drug use.

In order to address some of these shortcomings in our knowledge base the McCreary Centre Society (MCS) has worked, since the late 1980s, to create a new, large scale data set on the health status and risky behaviours of grades 7 through 12 students in all regions of BC. In 1992, and again in 1998, the Adolescent Health Survey was administered to BC students in each region of the province (MCS, 1993; MCS, 1999a). To date, over 41,000 students have been surveyed. This body of work provides a rich data set that is at once contemporary, credible, regionally representative, and capable of informing youth, their families and communities, and the province's service providers. In addition, the survey questionnaire has been modified and administered to small convenience samples from special focus, out-of-school populations such as street youth, young sex trade workers, youth in custody, and aboriginal youth (MCS, 1994; MCS 1999b; MCS, 1999c; MCS, 2000). When combined, these data sets provide unique and invaluable information on the common concerns of our youth constituency. This chapter will focus on the analysis and interpretation of three specific aspects of the data: adolescent development in BC; determinants of adolescent health; and special subgroups, including aboriginal, out-of-school, gay and lesbian, and inner city and rural youth.

METHODOLOGY

With the exception of cited references, the data referred to in this chapter is derived from the MCS's Adolescent Health Surveys (AHS I and AHS II conducted in 1992 and 1998 respectively). This section briefly describes the methodology. The Adolescent Health Survey uses a self-complete, anonymous questionnaire to gather information about the current health status of young people, and about factors that can influence health during adolescence and in later life. AHS II provides information about youth in school, representing 88% of all youth in the study age group.

The survey sample was drawn to be representative of all youth enrolled in grades 7 through 12 in BC schools. In total, the survey was conducted in 1,490 different classrooms in 407 different schools. About 8% of the 316,000 students in grades 7 through 12 across the province completed a questionnaire. Only about 1% of questionnaires were eliminated because the student provided frivolous or contradictory answers, or failed to complete more than 50% of questions. Nearly 16,000 BC students in grades 7 through 12 participated in the first school-based Adolescent Health Survey, conducted in 1992.

AHS II was designed to track trends showing how adolescent health and behaviour had changed since 1992, and to identify new issues facing youth today. In all, 25,838 students completed the survey in the spring or fall of 1998. Trained administrators, mostly public health nurses, conducted the survey in the students' classrooms. Students completed the anonymous, pencil and paper questionnaire in about 45 minutes. Participation in the survey was voluntary, and parents' consent was arranged through each school district. In all, 43 of BC's 59 school districts agreed to participate in the 1998 survey.

The AHS II questionnaire included 127 items on health status, health-promoting practices, and risky behaviours. Questions were chosen to identify factors that influence both present and future health and well-being. Most health problems during the teenage years are caused by preventable actions, such as drinking and driving or unprotected sexual activity. Adolescence also is the time when individuals often establish lifelong attitudes and habits, such as smoking, diet, and exercise. The survey also looked at factors such as gender, cultural background, family income, and connectedness to family and school, that affect health in a broader sense.

ADOLESCENT DEVELOPMENT

For many, adolescence is seen and interpreted in stereotypical fashion. Often that interpretation is negative and explained away as a normal period of "storm and stress." We would challenge those negative stereotypes by stating that, by and large, today's adolescents are an impressive, healthy group with positive, stable behaviours and traditional hopes and dreams (MCS, 1999a). Certainly the McCreary data support that notion (Table 10.1).

Adolescent development is a complex functional process rather than a simple, chronologically defined part of the life cycle (Figure 10.1). The onset of puberty, the beginning of a growth spurt, and the development of secondary sex characteristics vary considerably between genders, within genders, and across various ethnic and socioeconomic subgroups. Factors such as temperament, family coping styles, delayed/early onset of puberty, presence of a chronic condition, or educational/vocational goals may influence the progress

Table 10.1   Positive, stable behaviours of BC students (%)

Good/excellent health status	87
Not emotionally distressed	93
Plans to attend post-secondary	74
Medium/high family connectedness	85
Medium/high school connectedness	87
Volunteer activities	81
Extra-curricular activities	72
Like school (some, quite a bit, much)	74

of adolescent development and affect the timing of the eventual entry into a functioning adulthood. Sometimes it is useful to think of the adolescent population as falling into and moving between the various cells of a matrix. Such a matrix can assist us with program planning by making us aware of how heterogeneous the members of this developmental group are.

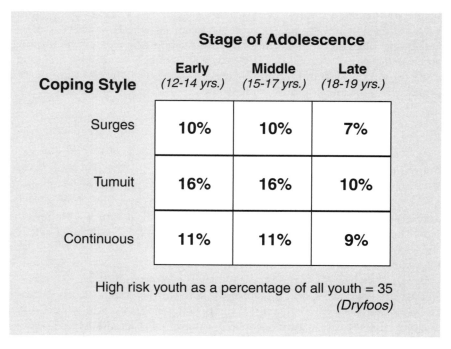

Figure 10.1 A developmental framework of adolescent populations

Adolescent behaviours are often thought of as problems, especially by adults and service providers. Admittedly, adolescents may experiment with various risky behaviours that have serious negative outcomes. However, from a prevention or health promotion perspective it becomes important to understand, in a positive sense, the significance to youth of what they know to be a potentially risky behaviour such as smoking cigarettes or driving too fast. Both are excellent examples of risky adolescent activities whose prevalence has changed little over the past two decades. This despite our best efforts to have an influence on the behaviour.

Adolescent health specialists recognize that what adults see as problems, adolescents often see as solutions. For example, we may not like to accept it, but adolescent smoking may be normative. However, the adolescent who engages in smoking at a younger age than his or her peers may be signalling more significant problems. Indeed, Jessor and Jessor describe the meaning of this early onset phenomenon in their concept of adolescent "Problem Behaviors" (Jessor and Jessor, 1997). Within this context the challenge becomes that of understanding what the adolescent is trying to solve. Is the youth who is a regular smoker trying to look cool, control her weight, deal with her social anxieties, or just enjoying the pleasures of a frowned upon activity? Furthermore, does she know (care?) about the important correlations or crossovers between many risky adolescent behaviours? The data indicate that the adolescent who smokes cigarettes commonly engages in other risky behaviours (Table 10.2). From a clinical and a program planning perspective it also becomes important to be able to differentiate between the large group of adolescents who engage in a single risky behaviour and those in the smaller, more elusive group for whom that behaviour is a prelude to a dangerous mix of multiple, riskier behaviour patterns.

Table 10.2 Comparison of smoking and non-smoking students

	Nonsmoker (%)	Smoker (%)
Skips school	17	65
Rode with a drinking driver in past month	12	51
Attempted suicide	3	17
Engaged in physical fights in past year	23	47
Binge drank in past month (of users)	23	76
Used marijuana 40+ times in life (of users)	14	57
Used harder drugs	14	72
Ever had sexual intercourse	9	67
First had sex at age 14 or younger	37	53

Determinants

Another way of thinking about our youth constituency is by using a population based, determinants of health approach. Applying this concept to adolescents involves looking at the influence of such things as gender, ethnicity or race, education level and literacy, poverty, etc. on their present and future health.

Gender

All adolescents worry about their appearance (Table 10.3). Skin, hair, and shape are their primary concerns, and their gender influences what they do about it. Females exercise because they want to lose weight, whereas males do so to gain weight. These concerns are not trivial or without risks. Adolescents see them as having little to do with long term concerns about obesity, cardiovascular disease, or even more immediate risks such as susceptibility to eating disorders. While being an adolescent female introduces obvious biologic risks such as pregnancy and problems with menstruation, the modern adolescent girl must also confront other, non-biologic but gender-related risks such as dealing with sexual harassment and abuse, or confronting suicidal ideations. For adolescent males injuries and violence are issues.

Table 10.3   Gender differences among BC students

	Males (%)	Females (%)
Want to lose weight	19	52
Want to gain weight	27	4
Regular smoker	9	12
Have been sexually abused	3	15
Considered suicide in past year	10	18
Physically assaulted at school in past year	17	6

Socioeconomic Status and Ethnicity

Perceived socioeconomic status and ethnicity has a powerful influence on the lives of adolescents. Youth from lower income families are less likely than higher income family youth to plan to attend post-secondary schooling and more likely to report less than excellent health status. Educational expectations, age of onset of sexual intercourse, and safe sex practices (and risk of pregnancy or sexually transmitted diseases [STDs]) vary according to the ethnic group to which adolescents identify themselves as belonging (Table 10.4). Poor and aboriginal students have lower academic expectations and earlier age of onset of sexual intercourse than do other students. By comparison, other subgroups such as urban Asian adolescents have higher academic expectations and engage in fewer risky behaviours. Adolescents also report that they experience discrimination, harassment and even assault that is based on who they are or are seen to be.

Table 10.4 Comparison of Aboriginal, Chinese, South Asian, and British students' behaviours (%)

	Aboriginal	Chinese	South Asian	British
Plan to attend post-secondary	61	83	80	75
Ever had sexual intercourse	39	11	18	25
Used birth control pills last sex	32	20	20	38
Discriminated against due to race/colour	17	21	37	5
Physically assaulted school past year	12	9	11	12

Age and Grade

Adolescence is a developmental stage that embraces at least seven school grade levels and includes from 5 to 10 or more years of the life span. Onset is clearly marked by physiological events, but its conclusion is variably marked by laws (e.g., legal purchase of alcohol) and conventions (e.g., age of consent to sex). The Adolescent Health Survey shows that there is a progression in behaviours, feelings of connectedness to family and school, and changes in emotional health that are naturally occurring developmental phenomena (Table 10.5).

Table 10.5 Comparison of student behaviours at 13, 15, 17 years of age (%)

	13 years	15 years	17 years
High level of family connectedness	17	10	9
Never smoked	59	38	32
Ever used marijuana	22	48	59
Ever had sexual intercourse	9	23	42
Emotional distress (severe)	5	8	9

The data also demonstrate that appearing older than you are is associated with premature onset of certain risky behaviours such as sexual activity and substance use and the increased risk of experiencing negative outcomes such as sexual assault. This reflects the fact that, while not all adolescents enter puberty at the same age (some are early maturers and others quite late), adults respond to them on the basis of their physical appearance. This can place adolescents at risk since they do not progress through their developmental tasks at the same pace as their physical development. As a result, some early maturers move or are forced to move faster than their age mates while others, such as those with chronic illness, may be allowed to extend their adolescent development into their adult years.

Residence

Where adolescents live and go to school has a considerable influence on their lifestyle and opportunities. In BC there is a well recognized north-south gradient in access to services and in mortality and morbidity rates. For example, infant mortality is higher in the north than in the lower mainland, while Caesarian section rates and immunization levels are higher in major urban settings (Tonkin, 1981). The same holds true for what adolescents tell us about their health and their behaviour (Table 10.6). Adolescents living in northern and more rural communities are more likely to smoke cigarettes, to drink and drive, and to engage in fighting than are adolescents in the urban areas of the lower mainland of BC.

Table 10.6   Region of residence: Comparison of students in two regions *(%)*

	NorthWest	*Greater Vancouver*
Occasional/regular smoker	23	12
Ridden with drinking driver	27	19
Involved in physical fights	33	28
Sustained an injury	43	34
Always feel safe at school	50	45

The reasons behind these differences are complex but, like the differences in Caesarian rates, may have more to do with the setting than with intrinsic differences between the adolescents. Drinking and driving rates may be influenced by lack of access to public transport and reduced recreational opportunities. Stricter bans on smoking in public places, restaurants, and bars have been more common in urban settings and may reduce adolescent smoking rates in those communities, while living in the "big city" is commonly seen as a major risk factor, especially for young people. Numerically, more bad things happen where the population is densest. However, the rates for negative, risky adolescent behaviours are generally higher outside the major urban centres. These differences are not just due to the benefits of the urban environment, such as educational or recreational opportunities, but may also reflect the family values, academic expectations, and ethnic mix in the different settings (Table 10.7). Studying the differences between living in an urban vs a rural setting may help us identify the factors most protective for adolescents during their development.

Table 10.7   Selected characteristics of urban vs rural students

	Urban (%)	Rural (%)
Aboriginal ethnicity	3	8
Speak other than English at home	23	5
Mother attended college/university/vocational	53	49
Always feel safe at night in neighbourhood	28	42
Had sexual intercourse	19	27

Time Period

Adolescents are greatly influenced by the attitudes, fads and fashions, and lifestyles of their time. The Adolescent Heath survey studied students in 1992 and in 1998. While these are two very different cohorts of adolescents (most of the 1992 study population are no longer in school) the results show an impressive degree of stability in the health status and risky behaviours of the students over time. The 1998 group are just as healthy, just as hopeful, just as positive as those in 1992. This despite the prevailing negative, sometimes stressful climate prevalent in BC communities and families at the end of the millennium. Both cohorts are also just as likely to smoke, drink and drive, engage in physical fights, attempt suicide, and engage in unsafe sex practices (Table 10.8).

Table 10.8   Trends in student behaviour: 1992 vs 1998

	1992 (%)	1998 (%)
Smoked cigarettes in past 30 days (of users)	25	25
Involved in a physical fight in past year	33	29
Attempted suicide in past year	7	7
Females who have had sexual intercourse	28	23
Females who have been sexually abused	21	15
Females who had sex at 14 years or less	62	44

Some things seem to never change, while others have changed. For example, more adolescent females are choosing to delay onset of sexual intercourse, fewer are being sexually abused, and fewer are sexually active. Another major change has been in the prevalence of marijuana use among adolescents. The age of onset, frequency of use, and number of both male and female users has increased substantially between 1992 and 1998. The data must be interpreted in context. Other jurisdictions in Canada and the US have reported similar trends (Addiction Research Foundation, 1997; Nova Scotia Department of Health and Dalhousie University, 1998; Centers for Disease Control and Prevention, 1999).

While some have argued that marijuana is a benign product and should be legalized, the impact of marijuana on adolescent development, especially among vulnerable or marginalized youth, is never benign. The increased accessibility of marijuana and other illegal substances is a factor in the increase in the frequency of use and the numbers of adolescent users, but it does not adequately explain the younger age of onset of use. This shift is worrisome because it presages experimentation with other drugs and problems with multiple drug use among highly susceptible early adolescents. The potential for the appearance of marijuana use related behaviours such as skipping school, weapon carrying, and conflict with family in early adolescents is a substantial concern.

Being Connected

In the adolescent literature there is a growing interest in the concepts of resiliency and the capacity of adolescents to overcome obstacles to their healthy development. Factors that promote resiliency include caring, connected families, stable school and community environments, experiencing positive relationships with non-family adults, and opportunities to become engaged in meaningful activities such as work (Blum, 1998). The 1998 Adolescent Health Survey explored the concept of connectedness as a measure of resiliency. It discovered that most students felt connected to family and school (MCS, 1999). The degree of connectedness predicted health status and risky behaviour, and connectedness levels decreased with increasing age and grade (Figure 10.2). It also discovered that, when in need of help, rather than seeking out professionals, adolescents turn to parents or peers. The nature of the problem and the adolescent's gender influenced which issue they would take to whom. We found that, with the exception of reproductive health issues, adolescents rarely saw professionals (including teachers) as their primary source of advice or help. This information argues for strengthening the roles and the helping skills of parents, peers, and schools in the lives of adolescents. Providing current, credible, understandable information on what adolescents say and really do is an important component in any such process.

Percent

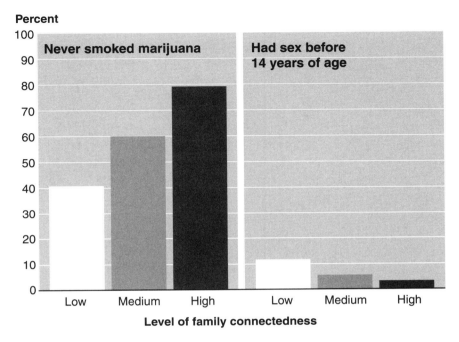

Figure 10.2 Level of family connectedness and risk behaviours in students

Special Focus

While the determinants of health impact all adolescents, the extent to which a specific adolescent develops a problem during adolescence is a function of resilience, opportunities for change, and luck. For example, car crashes are not uncommon incidents in the lives of adolescents. They are the most common cause of death and hospitalization among adolescent males in BC (Tonkin, 1981). Multiple factors influence these occurrences and their outcome. They include: road conditions, driver experience, use of safety belts, driver impairment, and excessive speed. Sometimes the difference between an incident and a near miss is measured in fractions of a second and something the adolescent involved (driver or passenger) is too inexperienced to do much about. Sometimes the difference in final outcome is due to after the event circumstances such as prompt medical care, excellent rehabilitation, and supportive peers, families, and schools.

Detailed reviews of individual car crashes will usually identify most of the various contributing factors listed above. When collected together these same analyses can contribute to a significantly different picture—a picture of a subgroup of adolescents who are "accidents waiting to happen." This subgroup may have behavioural or emotional problems, or come from families in which violence, alcohol and substance abuse, and neglect are the norm. All too often they are "system kids." They have a pattern of school truancy, conflict with the law, being victimized or neglected at home, and being in and out of government care. They are a special subset of which we need to be aware. Many of them are not included in our school-based data simply because they are not in school. The lives of these adolescents warrants a special focus. Efforts need to be made to engage them in both quantitative and qualitative research.

There are many identifiable adolescent subgroups that might be deserving of a special focus. The list includes: aboriginal youth, youth in custody, out-of-school youth, gay and lesbian youth, inner city and rural youth, street and homeless youth, just to mention a few of the obvious, easily identifiable high risk groups. The McCreary Centre Society has conducted research on the health status and risky behaviours of some of these groups (MCS, 1994; MCS, 1999b; MCS, 1999c; MCS, 2000). While the results are quite different (worse) from that of mainstream, in-school adolescents, it is important to avoid stereotyping. For example, in-school aboriginal adolescents are not substantially different from non-aboriginals, but out-of-school aboriginal adolescents are quite different from both.

There are groups of adolescents whose needs are often overlooked when youth policies are being set. Sometimes this is because the focus is on high risk youth, but in other cases it is because we are unaware of the needs of a particular group or we assume that society is already addressing their needs and protecting them. For example, the MCS data on students with chronic medical conditions found that those youth with chronic conditions sufficient to limit their activity or compromise school attendance have lower academic expectations, more physical and emotional complaints, are more likely to have been abused, and more likely to engage in risky behaviours such as alcohol and substance abuse and unsafe sex (Table 10.9).

Table 10.9   Comparison of students with chronic health conditions with all other students

	Chronics (%)	All others (%)
Plan to attend post-secondary	69	75
2+ health problems at least/week	60	34
Ever been sexually abused	17	8
Ever been physically abused	28	15
Regular/occasional smoker	21	14
3+ sexual partners in lifetime	40	32

The Road Ahead

Just knowing more about our youth constituency is not enough. Calling for additional research should not become an excuse for delays in placing youth issues on national and provincial agendas. Fortunately, BC has begun to move in more youth friendly, youth empowering directions (Cargo and Tonkin, 1998; BC Ministry for Children and Families, 1999). Progress should be informed by what the Adolescent Health Surveys have discovered and public attention should be focused on the following messages obtained from listening to BC's adolescents.

They appreciated being asked and took seriously their part in answering the questionnaire. Less than 1% of questionnaires had to be rejected for too many incomplete or nonsensical responses. They expressed interest in the results and certainly did not use being asked sensitive questions as an excuse to "go out and do it"—the "it" being becoming more sexually active, consuming more alcohol, or attempting suicide. In fact the prevalence of these behaviours declined or remained the same between 1992 and 1998.

The results show the stability of most adolescents' health and behaviour. In instances such as smoking cigarettes and drinking-driving these are discouraging findings. They should force us to re-evaluate school-based health promotion strategies and high profile media campaigns. At the same time, some things have changed. We need to apply ourselves to understand the reasons behind these shifts.

The results also show the important influence of feeling connected to one's family and school. What parents and schools do makes a difference and can have a positive impact on an adolescent's physical, emotional, and social health and can reduce the likelihood of their engaging in risky behaviours. Today's adolescents are more resilient, more involved in their community or school, and more likely to volunteer their time when they feel safe, cared for, have opportunities to experience life in a positive manner, and have the sense that they are being listened to by caring, respectful adults.

Finally, the results help to identify those groups of adolescents, especially the early tumultuous adolescents, who might benefit from more targeted early intervention programs. Some of these adolescents are already recognized as being at high risk, but others have often remain overlooked. This may be because we see them as already being protected. It may be that they are less visible by virtue of living in less well served parts of the province or because we have stereotypical views or biases about them. Whatever the reason, our future lies in knowing more about all of our constituents.

REFERENCES

Addiction Research Foundation (1997). *Ontario student drug survey, 1997: Executive summary.* Toronto: Addiction Research Foundation.

BC Ministry for Children and Families (1997). *Measuring our success: A framework for evaluating population outcomes.* Victoria: BC Ministry for Children and Families.

BC Ministry for Children and Families (1999). Business plan 1999-2001 (*http://www.mcf.gov.bc.ca/business_plan/index_1.htm*).

BC Provincial Health Officer (1998). *A report on the health of British Columbians: Provincial Health Officer's Annual Report 1997.* Victoria: BC Ministry of Health and Ministry Responsible for Seniors.

Blum, R.W.M. (1998). Healthy youth development as a model for youth health promotion. *Journal of Adolescent Health,* 22, 368-375.

Cargo, M., and Tonkin, R.S. (1998). Youth involvement: Beyond informed consent. *British Columbia Medical Journal,* 40(1), 21-22.

Centers for Disease Control and Prevention (1999). *Fact Sheet: Youth risk behavior trends: From CDC's 1991, 1993, 1995, and 1997 youth risk behavior surveys.* Silver Spring, Maryland: National Center for Chronic Disease Prevention and Health Promotion, Division of Adolescent and School Health (*http://www. cdc.gov/nccdphp/dash/yrbs/trend.htm*).

Federal, Provincial and Territorial Advisory Committee on Population Health (1999). *Toward a healthy future: Second report on the health of Canadians* (prepared by the Federal, Provincial and Territorial Advisory Committee on Population Health for the meeting of Ministers of Health, Charlottetown, PEI, September 1999). Ottawa: The Committee.

Hanvey, L., Avard, D., Graham, I., Underwood, K., Campbell, J., and Kelly, C. (1994). *The health of Canada's children: A CICH profile* (2nd ed.). Ottawa: Canadian Institute of Child Health.

Jessor, R., and Jessor, S. (1997). *Problem behavior and psychosocial development: A longitudinal study of youth.* New York: Academic Press.

King, A.J.C., Boyce, W.F., and King, M.A. (1999). *Trends in the health of Canadian youth.* Ottawa: Health Canada.

McCreary Centre Society (1993). *Adolescent health survey: Province of British Columbia.* Burnaby, BC: McCreary Centre Society.

McCreary Centre Society (1999). *Healthy connections: Listening to BC youth: Highlights from the Adolescent Health Survey II.* Burnaby, BC: McCreary Centre Society.

McCreary Centre Society (1994). *Adolescent health survey: Street youth in Vancouver.* Burnaby, BC: McCreary Centre Society.

McCreary Centre Society (1999). *Our kids too: Sexually exploited youth in British Columbia: An adolescent health survey.* Burnaby, BC: McCreary Centre Society.

McCreary Centre Society (1999). *Being out: Lesbian, gay, bisexual and transgendered youth in BC: An adolescent health survey.* Burnaby, BC: McCreary Centre Society.

McCreary Centre Society (2000). Silk Road to health: A journey to understanding Chinese youth in BC. Burnaby, BC: McCreary Centre Society.

Nova Scotia Department of Health and Dalhousie University (1998). *NovaScotia student drug use, 1998: Technical report.* Halifax: NS Department of Health and Dalhousie University.

Tonkin, R.S. (1981). *Child health profile: Birth events and infant outcome: British Columbia 1981.* Vancouver: University of British Columbia, Department of Pediatrics.

Tonkin, R.S. (1981). *Child health profile: Violence in adolescence: British Columbia 1981.* Vancouver: University of British Columbia, Department of Pediatrics.

Youth at Risk: Systemic Intervention from an Attachment Perspective

11

Marlene M. Moretti
Department of Psychology, Simon Fraser University

Roy Holland
Maples Adolescent Centre, Ministry for Children and Families

Ken Moore
Secure Care Implementation, Ministry for Children and Families

INTRODUCTION

In all communities, there are children for whom our social service and mental health programs have failed. These children typically have a longstanding history of severe emotional and behavioural problems and are usually identified because of high levels of socially unacceptable, delinquent, and/or aggressive behaviour. Their families are frequently burdened by a multitude of risk factors, including poverty, poor education, mental health problems, and substance use disorders which compromise their capacity to provide care for their children. Maltreatment, including physical and sexual abuse, and neglect may occur. Temporary, and sometimes permanent removal from the home becomes part of life experience for these children. Schools and community programs struggle to manage their behavioural problems but often, in frustration or fear, expel them from educational programs and ban them from recreational facilities.

Over time the adversity that these children experience compounds and expands such that by the time they reach adolescence they are extremely socially marginalized and burdened by a host of mental health problems. Often they find others like themselves who share their life experience and provide solace, if only in the sense that they are not alone in their experience. Together they cling for support and survival, and disenfranchised from society and adults they decide on their own rules and standards regarding what constitutes socially acceptable behaviour. Sometimes they end up living on and off our streets, victims of exploitation through involvement in the sex and/or drug trades. They are easy targets for involvement in organized gangs, become involved in criminal behaviour and often end up in the juvenile justice system.

Those of us with experience in social services and mental-health know these children well. Despite our best intentions, and as much as we may not want to admit it, these are the children and the families we sometimes refer to as 'treatment resistant' or 'nonresponders,' the ones who repeatedly reappear on case loads and require emergency intervention. Yet nothing seems to change —their lives become increasingly disorganized and opportunities for productive change seem more and more restricted as they move toward adulthood. Why have we failed in meeting the needs of these children? In this chapter we address the need for an integrated understanding of the life conditions and psychological development of these children, an understanding that brings together our knowledge of the impact of ecological context with our knowledge of child development. We begin with a brief discussion of risk factors that have a prospective relationship with the development of risk. Next we present a rationale for a transactional-ecological model of development and argue that attachment theory provides such a framework. Implications for intervention are discussed and two model programs in use in BC are presented. These programs utilize attachment theory as a framework for understanding the dynamic interplay between exposure to adversity and the organization of internalized regulatory mechanisms and ecological contexts. These programs do not provide solutions to the challenge of providing care to high-risk youth, but rather are points of departure for innovative programming. In this chapter we focus on high-risk adolescents, although much of our discussion can be extrapolated to preventative programming and remedial interventions for younger high-risk children.

THE DEVELOPMENT OF RISK: A MULTILEVEL ECOLOGICAL PERSPECTIVE

The term 'high-risk youth' is often used to describe adolescents who are involved in behaviours that are believed to place them and/or those around them in socially unacceptable and/or potentially dangerous circumstances. Unfortunately the term 'high risk youth' suggests that risk resides within individuals. Our discussion here will show, however, that risk is distributed within the ecology and occurs in *transaction* with youth. The term ecology is used here to capture the diverse range of social contexts in which child development is embedded, from the broad cultural context to the immediate family and caregiver context (Sameroff, 1995). Transactions include all dynamic, reciprocal interactions between an individual and his or her ecology (Cicchetti and Lynch, 1993).

The vast majority of youth who fall under the category 'high risk' are identified clinically and in research as either severely conduct disordered or delinquent. Although these two populations are not identical, they are sufficiently similar in terms of risk profiles and associated conditions (Loeber and Stouthamer-Loeber, 1998) to be considered together for the purpose of this discussion. Other relevant samples of high-risk youth include those children exposed to maltreatment and trauma. Conduct disorder (CD) is the most chronic of all childhood psychological disorders affecting from 2 to 10% of the adolescent population (Kazdin, 1997). Both CD and delinquency are associated with a host of other psychosocial functioning problems including family and peer relationship disruption, school and vocational problems, attention deficit disorder, and substance use disorder (Loeber and Keenan, 1994; Loeber and Stouthamer-Loeber, 1998; Nottelman and Jensen, 1995). Boys diagnosed with CD before the age of 10—early onset CD—have a higher likelihood of persisting in antisocial activities to adulthood than do boys diagnosed in adolescence (Loeber and Stouthamer-Loeber, 1998; Moffitt, 1993; Tremblay, 2000). Adolescent onset of CD in girls, however, is linked with persistence in antisocial behaviour, aggression, and criminality into adulthood (Silverthorn and Frick, 1999). These girls are also likely to have a multitude of mental health problems in adulthood, including substance dependence, involvement in abusive relationships, antisocial personality disorder, and social welfare dependence (Bardone, Moffitt, Caspi, and Dickson, 1996; Robins, 1986; Silverthorn and Frick, 1999).

A broad range of risk factors is associated with the development of CD, delinquency, and other 'high risk' behaviours. One way to understand the complexity of factors that are linked with the emergence of high-risk status is to consider the 'multilevel ecology' in which child development unfolds (Bronfenbrenner, 1977; Cicchetti and Lynch, 1993). From this perspective, influences can be conceptualized as existing at the level of the macrosystem (e.g., broad cultural or subcultural ideology, laws, and customs), exosystem (e.g., neighbourhoods, informal social networks, support groups, socioeconomic climate), and microsystem (e.g., relations between the child and immediate environment including family members, sibling relationships, peer relationships). In general, individual factors exert only small 'main effects.' No single risk factor alone is believed to cause subsequent severe adjustment problems. Risk factors typically exert influences in combination with each other.

For example, it is well established that poverty is associated with increased risk for behavioural problems (see, for example, Offord and Lipman, 1996). Children who grow up in poor families, with relatively few middle class neighbours and high social disorganization, are at increased risk for involvement in delinquent behaviour and multiple mental health problems (Peeples and Loeber, 1994). However the impact of poverty on child development is partially due to other factors common in low socio-economic scale families—low family support and high family stress (Dodge, Pettit, and Bates, 1994). In turn, mothers who raise children in poverty tend to be harsh and controlling, parenting practices that have consistently been found to increase child aggression and non-compliance stress (Dodge et al., 1994).

The question of whether socio-economic conditions, family, and parenting factors have direct, mediated, or moderated effects on the development of child problems is a complex and hotly debated issue (Deater-Deckard and Dodge, 1997). It is clear, however, that the accumulation of risk factors exponentially increases risk for multiple problems in child adjustment (Coie et al., 1993; Furstenberg, Cook, Eccles, Elder, and Sameroff, 1999). In a study of children growing up in poverty, Sameroff, Seefer, and Bartko (1997) found that children in homes with two risk factors (e.g., minority status, large family size, low maternal education, or parental mental disorder) were four times more likely to experience adjustment problems than children in homes with only one risk factor. The presence of four risk factors escalated the level of risk 10-fold. Similar findings have been reported by Herrenkohl and colleagues (Herrenkohl, Maguin, Hill, Hawkins, Abbott, and Catalano, 2000) in predicting risk for youth violence. Unfortunately, risk factors often cluster together and children in high-risk ecologies typically contend with a broad range of adverse conditions.

Poverty is also linked with higher rates of child maltreatment (e.g., Connelly and Straus, 1992; Gelles, 1992; Foster and Martin, this volume) and occurs disproportionately in neighbourhoods with few social resources (Garbarino and Crouter, 1978; Garbarino and Sherman, 1980). In turn, multiple child adjustment problems have been linked with a history of child maltreatment. For example, higher rates of physical abuse have been found in adolescents with aggressive and violent behaviour (Lewis, Mallough, and Webb, 1989; Maxfield and Widom, 1996), substance use problems, and suicidality (Cavaiola and Schiff, 1988). Studies of incarcerated youth show that physical and sexual victimization is common, particularly among girls (Bergsmann, 1989; Chesney-Lind and Sheldon, 1998; Crawford, 1988; Lewis, Yeager, Cobham-Portorreal, Klein, Showater, and Anthony, 1991; Rosenbaum, 1989; Warren and Rosenbaum, 1986). For example, in a study of 110 incarcerated girls in BC, Corrado, Odgers, and Cohen (2000) found that 70% of youth reported exposure to physical abuse. Family dysfunction was very common among these girls: 70% had a family member with a criminal record, 76% had a family member with a significant substance abuse problem, and 78% reported that a family member had been physically abused. The majority of these girls had either left home or been 'kicked out.'

Prospectively, however, only a minority (30%) of children exposed to maltreatment subsequently show mental health problems in later childhood or adulthood (Trupin, Tarico, Low, Jemelka, and McClellan, 1993). This is not surprising if we consider that the impact of maltreatment depends on transactional patterns within the child's ecology. If the ecology—for example, the cultural context, social system, and family climate—is responsive to the trauma of child maltreatment, this will likely diminish the effect of maltreatment on development and reduce the likelihood of chronic victimization over time. In contrast, an ecology characterized by disorganization, impoverished resources, and attitudes that fail to recognize the trauma of child maltreatment will exacerbate the impact of maltreatment and increase the probability of maladaptive development over time. Consistent with this view, the deleterious developmental impacts of maltreatment become increasingly clear as children get older (Crittenden, Claussen, and Sugarman, 1994).

Peer relationships are another source of influence on the development of high-risk behaviour. For example, both longitudinal and cross-sectional studies have shown that affiliation with peers who engage in substance use is one of the most powerful predictors of adolescent drug use (Catalano and Hawkins, 1996; Jessor, Van Den Bos, Vanderryn, Costa, and Turbin, 1995). Youth who have low expectations of success and a sense of hopelessness are most drawn to substance use as a means of boosting self-image and gaining status in peer groups (Maggs and Galambos, 1993). The likelihood of involvement with delinquent peers is elevated in economically disadvantaged neighbourhoods where engagement in drug trafficking and gang related activities may be viewed as the only way out of poverty (Feigelman, Stanton, and Ricardo, 1993).

It is clear that factors that characterize the child—including genetic influences, intelligence, and temperament—also play a role in the likelihood that youth will become involved in high-risk behaviour. For example, children who are of below average intelligence are at increased risk for negative outcomes associated with exposure to adversity (Werner and Smith, 1992). Similarly, children who show an undercontrolled, difficult temperament early in development (age 3) are more likely to be aggressive later in life (Newman, Caspi, Moffitt, and Silva, 1997). Yet not all children with low intelligence or difficult temperament go on to develop aggressive behaviour problems. As with other risk factors, the relationship between individual differences in intelligence and temperament to the development of adjustment problems depends on other characteristics of the child's ecology, including family socio-economic status and parenting style (McMahon and Estes, 1997).

In sum, a wide spectrum of risk factors has been linked prospectively with development of adjustment problems in children and adolescents. Different factors influence adjustment at different points in time; for example, family factors tend to have greater impact on adjustment in early childhood while peer influences most strongly affect adjustment in adolescence. In addition, risk factors operate at multiple levels of the ecology—from the broad cultural context at the macrosystem level to the immediate child-parent relationship at the microsystem level. The impact of any particular risk or protective factor can not be understood in isolation. Risk factors cluster both within and across levels of the ecology, thereby increasing their impact exponentially synergistically.

DEVELOPMENT NESTED WITHIN ECOLOGY: TRANSACTIONAL-ECOLOGICAL MODELS OF RISK

As the preceding discussion illustrates, progress in understanding the relation between risk factors and the development of psychopathology has made static single factor or symptom-focused models of maladaptive development increasingly untenable (Jensen and Hoagwood, 1997; Moretti and Odgers, in press). It is true that some researchers persist in the belief that specific risk factors—

for example, psychopathy (Lynam, 1996)—are relatively immutable, reside predominantly within children, and account almost entirely for their movement toward antisocial or high-risk behaviour. Yet these 'models' can often be reduced to nothing more than superficial descriptions of what are essentially symptoms. There are two fundamental problems with static single-factor models of risk development. First, such models are inconsistent with the fact that very few factors have a 'sledgehammer effect' on development, even those for which there is substantial genetic heritability (Rende and Plomin, 1995). There is a growing consensus that the impact of risk factors and the relative immunity provided by protective factors is a function of a sequence of complex moderating factors over the course of a child's life. This means that although two children may begin life with highly similar profiles of risk and protective factors, the likelihood that developmental outcomes will be similar in adolescence or adulthood is actually quite low.

Second, static models of risk fail to capture the fact that development is *transactional*. As individuals adapt to new experiences within their ecology, they alter the way that they initiate and respond to events within their ecology, thus changing the likelihood of particular outcomes (Cicchetti and Tucker, 1994). The dynamic interplay between the ecology and child development requires that we move beyond simple cause-effect models. Indeed, Marvin and Stewart (1990) claim that "the notion of causality has probably done more to hamper progress within the field of developmental psychology than any single concept...in the search for these simple causal relationships, the field has largely abandoned its descriptive phase and has ignored the fact that 'effects' often feed back and become their own 'cause'"(Cicchetti and Tucker, 1994, p. 55).

In contrast to simple cause-effect models, transactional-ecological models assume that development is recursive. It is widely accepted that experience affects the development of self-regulatory mechanisms at multiple levels of functioning: neurological, cognitive, behavioural, and affective (Posner and Rothbart, 2000). As self-regulatory systems become organized, they alter the effects of new experiences often by narrowing the impact of novel experiences that deviate from past experience (Marvin, 1977). In this way, one's history of experience leads to changes in the likelihood that new experiences will be identified, encoded, interpreted, and responded to in particular ways. Certain experiences may have profound impacts on the organization of development. For example, traumatic experience is associated with such extreme arousal and risk for survival that exposure to such experiences is now believed to powerfully impact the organization of the self-regulatory system at multiple levels of functioning (Glaser, 2000). At a practical level, the implication of this concept is that youth who have experienced *chronic* stressful or traumatic experiences in their relationships with caregivers, particularly during critical periods of development, may have difficulty *not* responding (i.e., inhibiting old response patterns) to new caregivers with similar patterns of physiological arousal, cognitive beliefs, feelings of mistrust, and behavioural displays.

Although the recursive nature of development tends to increase the propensity toward continuity along particular developmental trajectories, this does not mean that once patterns are established they are immutable. In the same way that development is skewed by the presence of risk factors, it may be set back on course by the presence of new opportunities for adaptive growth. Yet, as previously noted, risk factors tend to cluster. Thus, children born into poverty are more commonly parented by single parents with limited education, low social support, and high family stress than are children born into more affluent families (see **Chapter 9**). The clustering of risk factors concurrently and over time reduces the probability of new opportunities for change. In other words, children who live in poverty and disorganized neighbourhoods with limited community resources are simply unlikely to encounter life-enriching experiences. Over time their impoverished life experience limits their skill set development so that they are restricted in their capacity to take advantage of whatever limited opportunities may become available.

Attachment Theory:
A Transactional-Ecological Model of Development

The concept of individual-ecology transactions and systemic adaptation (Marvin and Stewart, 1990) is neither new nor restricted to any particular field of psychology or science. Yet few theories of development are solidly based on the assumptions of such a view. Attachment theory is distinctive in this regard. This model of human development embraces the view that children and their caregivers form units or systems that are mutually regulating within the larger ecological context. At the core of attachment theory is the assumption that child-caregiver transactions and the development of self-regulatory systems are driven by a fundamental human need that is essential for survival—the need for human connectedness or attachment (Baumeister and Leary, 1995; Bowlby, 1969; 1973; 1980).

Attachment theory (Bowlby, 1969; 1973; 1980) accounts for social and emotional development across the lifespan based on the premise that the tendency for infants to seek proximity to caregivers is biologically based and essential for survival. Bowlby (1969, 1973) proposed that the quality of infant-caregiver transactions becomes consolidated into expectancies and beliefs reflecting the degree to which infants can rely on caregivers to provide proximity and companionship, a safe haven in the face of threat or anxiety, and a secure base from which to explore (Ainsworth, Blehar, Waters, and Wall, 1978). Over time, children's attachment experiences are integrated into internal "working models" of self, other, and self-in-relation-to-other with respect to attachment. These working models have recursive effects on development because they guide cognitive, affective, and behavioural processes, through which they affect adjustment and continuity in developmental trajectories. Expectations and attributions about close relationships (Youngblade, Park, and Belsky, 1993), the ability to regulate emotion (Kobak, Cole, Ferenz-Gillies, and Fleming, 1993), and behaviour (Putallaz and Heflin, 1990) are influenced by attachment representations at each developmental phase. Development of secure attachment emerges from transactions in which the child's signals of distress are effectively identified by caregivers and responded to in such a way that ensures safety and well-being, while at the same time promoting healthy exploration and autonomous development. In contrast, development of insecure attachment has been linked to either oversensitivity or undersensitivity to signals of distress, the failure to provide safe haven in times of distress, and overprotection or excessive control of healthy exploration and autonomous development.

Several sources of research show a link between insecure attachment patterns (avoidant, ambivalent, disorganized patterns) in infancy and behavioural problems in early childhood. Compared to secure children, insecurely attached children are more aggressive and confrontational with their mothers (Main and Weston, 1981), and more aggressive, hostile, and distant with their peers (Erickson, Sroufe, and Egeland, 1985; Sroufe, 1983; Lyons-Ruth, Repacholi, McLeod, and Silva, 1991; Wartner, Grossmann, Fremmer-Bombik, and Suess, 1994). Similar findings emerge from studies on the relation between attachment patterns in adolescence and adjustment. In normative population studies, adolescents who are classified as securely attached are rated by their peers as less anxious, less hostile, and more able to successfully regulate their feelings (i.e., more ego resilient) compared to insecurely attached adolescents (Kobak and Sceery, 1988). Adolescents who report a secure attachment with their parents, and who feel comfortable turning to them for support, have been found to have a greater sense of mastery of their worlds (Paterson, Pryor, and Field, 1995) and to experience less loneliness (Kerns and Stevens, 1996). More positive attachment with parents among 15 year olds is also associated with fewer mental health problems such as anxiety, depression, inattention, conduct problems (Nada-Raja, McGee, and Stanton, 1992), less experimentation with drugs, and less frequent substance use (Cooper, Shaver, and Collins, 1998). Security of attachment is also related to more positive attitudes about safe-sex and for girls, lower rates of risky sexual behaviour, and fewer past pregnancies compared to insecurely attached girls (Cooper et al., 1998).

Research in high-risk contexts confirms findings based on normative samples: high-risk adolescents with insecure attachment patterns are more likely than securely attached adolescents to experience a range of mental health problems (Allen, Hauser, and Borman-Spurrell, 1996), including suicidality (Lessard and Moretti, 1998), drug use (Lessard, 1994), and aggressive and antisocial behaviour (Fonagy et al., 1997; Moore, Moretti, and Holland, 1998; Reimer, Overton, Steidl, Rosenstein, and Horowitz, 1996; Rosenstein and Horowitz, 1996). For example, in a sample of male adolescent in-patients, Rosenstein and Horowitz (1996) found that youth with severe conduct problems were likely to be insecurely attached to their parents. In our own research, we have found that multiproblem youth characterized by aggressive and antisocial behaviour are almost uniformly insecurely attached to caregivers and have pronounced difficulty relying on caregivers to provide direction and care for their needs (Moretti, Lessard, Scarfe, and Holland, 1999).

Although similar patterns of results are present in normative and clinical samples (e.g., Allen and Hauser, 1996), the relation between attachment and adjustment is stronger among children in high-risk (e.g., poverty, low social support, parental psychopathology) than low-risk contexts (Lyons-Ruth et al., 1991). Extrapolating from this research suggests that adolescents who grow up in conditions of adversity and inadequate access to resources may not suffer from psychopathology if they share secure attachment relationships with their parents.

In sum, attachment theory provides a comprehensive understanding of the recursive relationship between child-ecology transactions and development; an understanding that highlights the fundamental motivational importance of human connectedness as guiding development. The emergence of internal working models are adaptive to all children in the sense that they provide predictability about the likelihood that particular types of transactions will transpire in relation with their caregiver and significant others in their lives. The securely attached child anticipates that others will be responsive and supportive; in turn, they are likely to approach adults for support and direction when needed. Unfortunately, children exposed to chronic conditions of adversity and maltreatment also develop internal working models. In contrast to securely attached children, the internal models of insecurely attached children lead them to anticipate disinterest, rejection, or harm. As a result, these youth move increasingly beyond the reach of opportunities for growth and change because they anticipate similar transactions to those they have previously experienced.

Systemic Perspectives on Intervention

What are the implications of transactional-ecological models for developing and delivering interventions with high-risk youth? First, this approach highlights the importance of understanding risk as a complex transactional process —not as an additive function of exposure to one or more risk factors. The factors that account for risk behaviour are complex and distributed both within the ecology and within transactions between youth and their ecology. As children develop, the scope of their ecology increases. Whereas the lives of young children are dominated by their primary caregivers, adolescents interact within a wide range of contexts (e.g., peer group, school system, vocational activities), each of which is important in challenging or supporting their adaptive adjustment. Furthermore, as children mature into adolescence, attachment patterns presumably become increasingly generalized (Allen and Land, 1999) and self-other representations become more complex and important in self-regulation

(Moretti and Higgins, 1999; Moretti, Holland, and McKay, 2001; Moretti and Wiebe, 1999).

Clearly as children move outside of their families, other influences, including peer relations and school functioning, become increasingly salient in contributing to the development and maintenance of risk behaviours. As the scope of contexts that contribute to and are recursively influenced by risk behaviour broadens so must the scope of intervention strategies. The recognition that children develop in dynamic relation to their ecology has prompted fundamental shifts in the delivery of mental health and other services to children and families. This shift is reflected in a 1994 American Psychological Association statement of consensus regarding innovative models of mental health service delivery (Henggeler, 1994). The principles derived from this task force underscore the importance of providing comprehensive, integrated, and individualized services to children and their families within their ecology. Reorganization of the service delivery system to facilitate ongoing organization and integration of services over time was also emphasized.

The emergence of systems-based thinking in understanding the needs of youth at risk has given rise to a number of intervention programs including multi-systemic treatment (MST) (Henggeler, 1991), multidimensional treatment foster care (Fisher and Chamberlain, 2000), and other 'wrap around services' (US Surgeon General, 2001). The commonality among these programs is that they are systemically conceptualized, individualized programs that integrate a variety of interventions (e.g., family interventions, cognitive-behavioural interventions, peer intervention strategies, and school interventions) to respond to the broad range of ecological factors that have been shown to contribute to risk behaviour (Henggeler, 1991; Henggeler, Schoenwald, Borduin, Rowland, and Cunningham, 1998). The programs deliver interventions within the context of the adolescent's family, school, and community environment rather than within institutions to ensure ecological validity.

In terms of MST, several trials have confirmed its efficacy with adolescent juvenile delinquents as compared to individual counselling or community programming. Specifically, MST has been shown to reduce delinquency, improve the quality of family relationships and reduce criminal behaviour for periods of up to 5 years after treatment (Henggeler et al., 1998). Cost estimates for MST are one-fifth that of more conventional interventions such as institutionalization (Henggeler et al., 1998). The integration of multiple interventions within an ecological context is without question the most promising new strategy to emerge in the treatment of severe adolescent behaviour problems. Similar levels of cost effectiveness have been reported for other forms of systemic intervention (US Surgeon General, 2001).

What might attachment theory offer beyond a systemic perspective? Like other systemic models, attachment theory does not prescribe or prohibit any particular set of reasonable interventions. Unlike other systemic models, however, attachment theory encompasses an understanding of how transactions between children and their ecologies lead to the development of *internal* regulatory mechanisms including organized patterns of experiencing the self in the world. From an attachment perspective interventions need to be individually tailored with an appreciation of the attachment dynamics that underlie the transactions between youths and their ecologies. In this way, an attachment perspective provides a guiding structure of individualizing intervention at *both* the level of the ecology and the individual (Doyle and Moretti, 2000). For example, some children who display high-risk behaviour refuse to rely on the guidance of caregivers or other adults in their lives because they fear further rejection and punishment from them (fearful avoidance stance); others dismiss adults as insignificant to their well-being and inept in their ability to provide help (dismissing avoidance stance). The profiles of these two young people may be identical in a number of ways—their failure to conform to social standards and expectations, their engagement in behaviours that place them at risk for harm, and the range of contributing factors within their ecologies. Yet these two youth may respond quite differently to attempts to engage them in intervention. The fearful-avoidant youth may be reluctant, but interested, if coaxed slowly and with encouragement, to trust that their needs will be acknowledged and responded to with benevolence. In contrast, the dismissing-avoidant youth may be simply unwilling to engage at a personal level; strategies that assist him/her in developing adaptive independent living skills (i.e., vocational training) may be best suited to his/her needs.

An attachment perspective also speaks to the importance of changing the ecology in the service of providing optimal conditions for altering the internal working models of attachment and internalization of coping strategies. Changing the ecology not only changes the relative level of risk in the ecology —it can also provide a context that facilitates a shift toward greater attachment security and internalization of effective coping strategies. This is most likely to occur when ecological support is pervasive enough and long enough to ensure increased development of competence. Changes at this level help to support youth in reaching more autonomous functioning in society.

In BC, two programs have been developed that are based on an attachment model of risk—the Response Program (Holland, Moretti, Verlann, and Peterson, 1993; Moretti, Holland, and Peterson, 1994) and the Orinoco Program (Moore et al., 1998), both based out of the Maples Adolescent Centre. These programs strive to provide support for youth in BC between the ages of 11 to 17 years with severe behavioural problems including aggression, violence, family and peer relations problems, school problems, and substance use. The majority of youth referred to these programs suffer from multiple mental health problems. Based on diagnostic interviewing, Moretti and colleagues (Moretti, Lessard, Weibe, and Reebye, 2000) found that only 16% of boys referred to these programs were diagnosed with CD alone; 80% were diagnosed with from one to three additional disorders, most notably attention deficit disorder, depression, and substance use disorder. For girls, 37% met criteria for from one to three additional disorders and a further 63% were diagnosed with four or more additional disorders. Substance use disorders were exceedingly common in girls. Maltreatment experiences including physical abuse, emotional abuse, and, in girls, sexual abuse are commonly reported (Reebye, Moretti, Wiebe, and Lessard, 2000). Not surprisingly, many youth, particularly girls, are diagnosed with post-traumatic stress disorder. These profiles confirm that youth referred to these programs constitute some of the most severely compromised and high-risk adolescents in the province.

The impetus for developing innovative programming for high-risk youth in BC was clinical, fiscal, and political. Prior to the mid-1980s, youth were held in secure (locked down) long-term treatment facilities at the Maples Centre; treatment was primarily behavioural and pharmacological. It was increasingly clear, both at the Maples and in other programs across North America, that the use of institutionalized long-term treatment was neither clinically effective nor financially feasible (Henggeler and Santos, 1997). So great was the failure of intervention to produce positive change that researchers and clinicians began to conclude that 'nothing works' (Shamsie, 1981). Not only were residential programs ineffective, but they were enormously expensive because only a handful of youth could be housed at any one time and they typically stayed in 'treatment' for up to 2 years. The nail in the coffin of residential care for youth in BC came with the review of the *Mental Health Act* in 1989 which disallowed the detention of youth in secure (locked) units on the basis of guardian consent. Since it was no longer legal to lock up troubled youth, it was necessary to develop another model of care.

The development of new programs at the Maples was founded on the recognition that intervention needed to be ecologically embedded and supportive of the integration of youth within their communities. The role of attachment in development was also a cornerstone of program development. The Response Program was the first to be developed—a 1-month program that accepted youth from across the province based on referrals from communities (for a detailed description of the program see Moretti et al., 1994; Moretti et al., 1997). The goals of the program are to provide an in-depth, comprehensive understanding of the dynamic relationships between factors leading to the development and maintenance of problems in child adjustment, taking into consideration transactions at various levels of the ecology and the underlying importance of attachment as an organizing principle. To achieve this goal, a multidisciplinary team works with each youth and his or her family—both on site and in the community—to gather information at each level of the ecology (cultural, community, family, and individual). The participation of the community in this process is inclusive rather than exclusive—all individuals who have a relevant interest and commitment to the child's well being are invited to participate. The process is collaborative and dynamic, building on the expertise of community players in understanding and participating in the development of a consolidated view of the situation. To guide this process, the program and each discipline has an established focus of investigation and procedures that are uniformly applied to ensure a comprehensive and replicable process.

At the end of the first 3 weeks of the program, the multidisciplinary team, community, family, and the youth come together to share information and develop a 'care plan' which provides an understanding of the attachment dynamics of the youth within his or her ecology, the relative strengths and weaknesses of the ecology, and the strategies that are most likely to support adaptive functioning within the home community. Outreach staff work with community teams to support the implementation of the care plan with the youth's home community. Respite care for up to 2 weeks can be accessed by the youth, his or her community, or caregivers to ensure that systems of care remain intact over time. Both outreach support and respite care are provided to youth, their caregivers, and their communities until age 18.

Consistent with research supporting the efficacy of systemic intervention, evaluation of the Response Program has shown reductions in problem behaviour (e.g., aggressive and delinquent behaviour, anxiety, depression) from both caregiver and youth perspectives for up to 18-months follow-up (Moretti et al., 1994). These reductions were noted for even the most highly aggressive youth included in the evaluation. The pattern of change found in the evaluations is revealing: results showed that caregivers were first to shift in their perception of youth problem behaviour; youth reported fewer problems months later. One interpretation of these findings is that by shifting caregivers understanding of the ecology and attachment dynamics underlying problem behaviour, the caregiver-youth dyad changes and this permits change in youth behaviour.

The Orinoco program is an extension of the Response Program (Moore et al., 1998). This program admits both youth and their caregivers into an intensive 3-month multi-modal program that focuses on increasing the family capacity for constructive problem solving and mutual support in moving toward individual life goals. Services are delivered within the context of each youth's unique ecology with an emphasis on maintaining and enhancing existing attachment relationships. The program is an integrated community program with Monday to Friday residential capacity coupled with ongoing involvement of caregivers and other community members. The final 2 weeks of the program take place entirely in the community and respite services are provided for up to 2 weeks for youth until age 18. Respite care supports youth and family in bridging stressful times and preserves attachments and placements by providing brief periods of restabilization.

REALIGNING SERVICES TO A SYSTEMS PERSPECTIVE

In the past decade there has been a shift from 'one size fits all,' highly focused, behavioural programs to individualized, wrap-around, systemic approaches. This shift corresponds with our growing appreciation of the fact that child development is embedded within a complex multilevelled ecology. Unfortu-nately, the implementation of innovative intervention strategies rarely depends on scientific progress or treatment efficacy but is determined by whether or not strategies coincide with political agendas of the day. In some provinces, like BC, government initiatives to bring care closer to home have provided the necessary impetus and opportunity for change and reorganization.

Good structural organization is essential to the delivery of systemic pro-grams that cut across domains (e.g., family services, mental health, education) which traditionally have been represented by separate ministries or govern-ment agencies. When services are not integrated with a common goal, a common paradigm for understanding social problems, a common language, and a shared agreement of how to work together, families and children fall prey to fragmented services and interagency debates about mandates and responsibilities. Strong conceptual frameworks, such as attachment theory, are useful in conveying the complexity of transactional impacts of ecological risk on development and thus help to create a common language for different service providers.

Creating an integrated yet ecologically sensitive system of care is chal-lenging because it requires both structural integrity and flexibility to cultural, community, and individual needs. The geographical configuration and popu-lation distribution of BC presents unique challenges in this regard as mental health services and expertise tend to become concentrated in the south-west-ern region of the province. This makes it difficult to ensure that services are available and tailored to unique situations in less central areas of the province. Maintaining the balance between structural integrity, a shared vision of a model of practice and the goals of intervention, and sensitivity to the uniqueness of each community needs to be at the forefront of reorganization.

Unfortunately the balance of services in the province remains focused on remedial intervention rather than preventative and maintenance measures. Children are often identified as 'at-risk' early on in their lives, yet service pro-vision is based on an 'acute needs' model. That is, children and their families must reach a 'threshold' of severity in order to access services, and once crises have subsided their files are closed. An alternate view is that families who are 'at-risk' require long-term support in order to maintain healthy functioning in much the same way that individuals with chronic health conditions require long-term intervention to ensure health. Some may argue that proactive pro-vision of services is too costly, yet evidence shows that early intervention strat-egies are typically more effective and less costly than interventions for 'at-risk' adolescents (see **Chapter 8**).

Beyond the cost savings associated with preventative interventions, there is the issue of reducing the burden of suffering in this generation and in gen-erations to follow. Intergenerational transmission of risk is well documented; for a variety of reasons, individuals who have suffered through adversity and maltreatment as children are at greater risk for revisiting these burdens upon their own children despite their best intentions to prevent this from occurring. Preventative interventions offer savings both fiscally and in terms of reducing the burden of human suffering both in the immediate and distant future. Why are the gains of preventative intervention so difficult for governments and communities to appreciate? Unfortunately, mental health interventions are often a function of short-term political agendas that are intent on appearing to solve current problems rather than on preventing future ones. However this is not the only or the most significant obstacle. Far greater is the pervasive societal view that the welfare of children is the primary responsibility of parents. Often this leads to resistance or to a lack of support for interventions to high-risk families; the opposition argues that parents are to blame for their children's problems and they should be held responsible. Until the rights of children— independent from their parents—are fully appreciated and consolidated in society they remain at the whims of political and social values which often do little to promote their welfare in the long term.

What directions need to be pursued to improve the quality and efficacy of care for all children in BC? First, continued efforts must be made to encourage systemic integration and ecological embeddedness of programs. Despite efforts to realign and integrate services for children and families, we are far from this goal (see **Chapter 8**). The integration of services requires more than simply realigning ministries; integration requires a common view of the challenges and solutions for ensuring care for children in our province. Second, preventative initiatives and long-term support programs must be established. Finally, on the political front, mental health providers need to find avenues to exert more influence on government policy. Perhaps the best route to achieve this outcome is by developing demand within communities for integrated services for youth at risk and preventative programs for young children. Until we are all convinced of the value of a systemic and integrated strategy to ensure the welfare of our children, we will continue to fail in meeting the needs of those children who most require our support.

REFERENCES

Ainsworth, M.S., Blehar, M.C., Waters, E., and Wall, S. (1978). *Patterns of attachment: A psychological study of the strange situation.* Potomac, MD: Lawrence Erlbaum.

Allen, J.P., and Hauser, S.T. (1996). Autonomy and relatedness in adolescent-family interactions as predictors of young adults' states of mind regarding attachment. *Development and Psychopathology*, 8, 793-809.

Allen, J.P., Hauser, S.T., and Borman-Spurrell, E. (1996). Attachment theory as a framework for understanding sequelae of severe adolescent psychopathology: An 11-year follow-up study. *Journal of Consulting and Clinical Psychology*, 64, 254-263.

Allen, J. P., and Land, D. (1999). Attachment in adolescence. In J. Cassidy and P.R. Shaver (Eds.), *Handbook of attachment: Theory, research, and clinical applications* (pp. 319-335). New York: Guilford Press.

Bardone, A.M., Moffitt, T., Caspi, A., and Dickson, N. (1996). Adult mental health and social outcomes of adolescent girls with depression and conduct disorder. *Development and Psychopathology*, 8, 811-829.

Baumeister, R.F., and Leary, M.R. (1995). The need to belong: Desire for interpersonal attachments as a fundamental human motivation. *Psychological Bulletin*, 117, 497-529.

Bergsmann, I.R. (1989). The forgotten few: Juvenile female offenders. *Federal Probation*, 53, 73-78.

Bowlby, J. (1969). *Attachment and loss: Vol. 1. Attachment.* New York: Hogarth Press.

Bowlby, J. (1973). *Attachment and loss: Vol. 2. Separation.* New York: Basic.

Bowlby, J. (1980). *Attachment and loss. Vol. 3 Loss, sadness and depression.* New York: Basic Books.

Bronfenbrenner, U. (1977). Toward an experimental ecology of human development. *American Psychologist*, 32, 513-531.

Catalano, R.F., and Hawkins, J.D. (1996). The social development model: A theory of antisocial behavior. In J.D. Hawkins (Ed.), *Delinquency and crime: Current theories. Cambridge criminology series* (pp. 149-197). New York: Cambridge University Press.

Cavaiola, A.A., and Schiff, M. (1988). Behavioral sequelae of physical and/or sexual abuse in adolescents. *Child Abuse and Neglect*, 12, 181-188.

Chesney-Lind, M., and Sheldon, R. (1998). *Girls, delinquency, and juvenile justice* (2nd ed.). Pacific Grove, CA: Brooks/Cole.

Cicchetti, D., and Lynch, M. (1993). Toward an ecological/transbactional model of community violence and child maltreatment: Consequences for children's development psychiatry. *Interpersonal and Biological Processes*, 56, 96-118.

Cicchetti, D., and Tucker, D. (1994). Development and self-regulatory structures of the mind. *Development and Psychopathology*, 6, 533-549.

Coie, J.D., Watt, N.F., West, S.G., Hawkins, J.D., Asarnow, J.R., Markman, H.J., Ramey, S.L., Shure, M.N., and Long, B. (1993). The science of prevention: A conceptual framework and some directions for a national research program. *American Psychologist*, 48, 1013-1022.

Connelly, C.D., and Straus, M.A. (1992). Mother's age and risk for physical abuse. *Child Abuse and Neglect*, 16, 703-712.

Cooper, M.L., Shaver, P.R., and Collins, N.L. (1998). Attachment styles, emotion regulation, and adjustment in adolescence. *Journal of Personality and Social Psychology*, 74, 1380-1397.

Corrado, R., Odgers, C., and Cohen, I. (2000). The use of incarceration for female youth: Protection for whom? *Canadian Journal of Criminology*, 42, 189-206.

Crawford, J. (1988). *Tabulation of nationwide survey of female inmates.* Phoenix, AZ: Research Advisory Services.

Crittenden, P., Claussen, A.H., and Sugarman, D.B. (1994). Physical and psychological maltreatment in middle childhood and adolescence. *Development and Psychopathology*, 6, 145-164.

Deater-Deckard, K., and Dodge, K.A. (1997). Externalizing behavior problems and discipline revisited: Nonlinear effects and variation by culture, context, and gender. *Psychological Inquiry*, 8, 161-175.

Dodge, K.A., Petit, G.S., and Bates, J.E. (1994). Effects of physical maltreatment on the development of peer relations. *Development and Psychopathology*, 6, 43-55.

Doyle, A.B., and Moretti, M.M. (2000). *Attachment to parents and adjustment to adolescence: Literature review and policy implications* (File number 032ss.H5219-9-CYH7/001/SS). Ottawa: Health Canada, Child and Family Division.

Erickson, M.F., Sroufe, L.A., and Egeland, B. (1985). The relationship between quality of attachment and behavior problems in preschool in a high-risk sample. *Monographs of the Society for Research in Child Development*, 50, 147-166.

Feigelman, S., Stanton, B.F., and Ricardo, I. (1993). Perceptions of drug selling and drug use among urban youths. *Journal of Early Adolescence*, 13, 267-284.

Fisher, P.A., and Chamberlain, P. (2000). Multidimensional treatment foster care: A program for intensive parenting, family support, and skill building. *Journal of Emotional and Behavioral Disorders*, 8, 155-164.

Fonagy, P., Target, M., Steele, M., Steele, H., Leigh, T., Levinson, A., and Kennedy, R. (1997). Morality, disruptive behavior, borderline personality disorder, crime and their relationship to security of attachment. In L. Atkinson and K.J. Zucker (Eds.), *Attachment and psychopathology* (pp. 223-274). New York, NY: The Guilford.

Furstenberg, F.F., Cook, T.D., Eccles, J., Elder, G.H., and Sameroff, A. (1999). *Managing to make it: Urban families and adolescent success*. Chicago: University of Chicago Press.

Garbarino, J., and Crouter, A. (1978). Defining the community context for parent-child relations: The correlates of child maltreatment. *Child Development*, 49, 604-616.

Garbarino, J., and Sherman, D. (1980). High-risk neighborhoods and high-risk families: The human ecology of child maltreatment. *Child Development*, 51, 188-198.

Gelles, R.J. (1992). Poverty and violence toward children. *American Behavioral Scientist*, 35, 258-274.

Glaser, D. (2000). Child abuse and neglect and the brain—A review. *Journal of Child Psychology and Psychiatry and Allied Disciplines*, 41, 97-116.

Henggeler, S.W. (1991). Multidimensional causal models of delinquent behavior and their implications for treatment. In R. Cohen and A. Siegel (Eds.), *Context and development* (pp. 211-231). Hillsdale, NJ: Erlbaum.

Henggeler, S.W. (1994). A consensus: Conclusions of the APA task force report on innovative models of mental health services for children, adolescents, and their families. *Journal of Clinical Child Psychology*, 23, 3-6.

Henggeler, S.W., and Santos, A.B. (Eds.) (1997). *Innovative approaches for difficult-to-treat populations*. Washington, DC: American Psychiatric Press, Inc.

Henggeler, S.W., Schoenwald, S.K., Borduin, C.M., Rowland, M.D., and Cunningham, P.B. (1998). *Multisystemic treatment of antisocial behavior in children and adolescents*. New York: The Guilford Press.

Herrenkohl, T.L., Maguin, E., Hill, K.G., Hawkins, J.D., Abbott, R.D., and Catalano, R.F. (2000). Developmental risk factors for youth violence. *Journal of Adolescent Health*, 26, 176-186.

Holland, R., Moretti, M.M., Verlaan, V., and Petersen, S. (1993). Attachment and conduct disorder: The response program. *Canadian Journal of Psychiatry*, 38, 420-431.

Jensen, P.S., and Hoagwood, K. (1997). The book of names: DSM-IV in context. *Development and Psychopathology*, 9, 231-249.

Jessor, R., Van Den Bos, J., Vanderryn, J., Costa, F.M., and Turbin, M.S. (1995). Protective factors in adolescent problem behavior: Moderate effects and developmental change. *Developmental Psychology*, 31, 923-933.

Kazdin, A.E. (1997). Conduct disorder across the lifespan. In S.S. Luthar, J.A. Burak, D. Cicchetti, and J.R. Weisz (Eds.), *Developmental psychopathology: Perspectives on adjustment, risk, and disorder* (pp. 248-272). Cambridge: Cambridge University Press.

Kerns, K.A., and Stevens, A. (1996). Parent-child attachment in late adolescence: Links to social relations and personality. *Journal of Youth and Adolescence*, 25, 323-342.

Kobak, R.R., Cole, H.E., Ferenz-Gillies, R., and Fleming, W.S. (1993). Attachment and emotion regulation during mother-teen problem solving: A control theory analysis. *Child Development*, 64, 231-245.

Kobak, R.R., and Sceery, A. (1988). Attachment in late adolescence: Working models, affect regulation, and representations of self and others. *Child Development*, 59,135-146.

Lessard, J.C. (1994). *The role of psychological distress and attachment in adolescent substance use.* Unpublished master's thesis. Simon Fraser University.

Lessard, J.C., and Moretti, M.M. (1998). Suicidal ideation in an adolescent clinical sample: Attachment patterns and clinical implications. *Journal of Adolescence*, 21, 383-395.

Lewis, D.O., Mallough, C., and Webb, V. (1989). Child abuse, delinquency and violent criminality. In D. Cicchetti and V. Carlson (Eds.), *Child maltreatment: Theory and research on the causes and consequences of child abuse and neglect* (pp. 707-721). New York: Cambridge University Press.

Lewis, D.O., Yeager, C.A., Cobham-Portorreal, C.S., Klein, N., Showater, C., and Anthony, A. (1991). A follow-up of female delinquents: Maternal contributions to the perpetuation of deviance. *Journal of the American Academy of Child and Adolescent Psychiatry*, 30, 197-201.

Loeber, R., and Keenan, K. (1994). Interaction between conduct disorder and its comorbid conditions: Effects of age and gender. *Clinical Psychology Review*, 14, 497-523.

Loeber, R., and Stouthamer-Loeber, M. (1998). Development of juvenile aggression and violence: Some common misconceptions and controversies. *American Psychologist*, 53, 242-259.

Lynam, D.R. (1996). Early identification of chronic offenders: Who is the fledgling psychopath? *Psychological Bulletin*, 120, 2, 209-234.

Lyons-Ruth, K., Repacholi, B., McLeod, S., and Silva, E. (1991). Disorganized attachment behavior in infancy: Short-term stability, maternal and infant correlates, and risk-related subtypes. *Development and Psychopathology*, 3, 377-396.

Maggs, J.L., and Galambos, N.L. (1993). Alternative structural models for understanding adolescent problem behavior in two-earner families. *Journal of Early Adolescence*, 13, 79-101.

Main, M., and Weston, D.R. (1981). The quality of the toddler's relationship to mother and to father: Related to conflict behavior and the readiness to establish new relationships. *Child Development*, 52, 932-940.

Marvin, R.S. (1977). An ethological-cognitive model for the attenuation of mother-child attachment behavior. In T. Alloway, L. Krames, and P. Pliner (Eds.), *Advances in the study of communication and affect, Vol. 3: Attachment behavior* (pp. 25-60). New York: Plenum.

Marvin, R.S., and Stewart, R.B. (1990). A family systems framework for the study of attachment. In M.T. Greenberg, D. Cicchetti, and E.M. Cummings (Eds.), *Attachment in the preschool years: Theory, research and intervention* (pp. 51-86). Chicago: University of Chicago Press.

Maxfield, M.G., and Widom, C.S. (1996). The cycle of violence: Revisited 6 years later. *Archives of Pediatric and Adolescent Medicine*, 150, 390-395.

McMahon, R.J., and Estes, A.M. (1997). Conduct problems. In E.J. Mash and L.G. Terdal (Eds.), *Assessment of childhood disorders*, 3rd ed. (pp. 130-193). New York: The Guilford.

Moffitt, T.E. (1993). Adolescence-limited and life-course-persistent antisocial behavior: A developmental taxonomy. *Psychological Review*, 100, 674-701.

Moore, K., Moretti, M.M., and Holland, R. (1998). A new perspective on youth care programs: Using attachment theory to guide interventions for troubled youth. *Residential Treatment for Children and Youth*, 15, 1-24.

Moretti, M.M., Emmrys, C., Grizenko, N., Holland, R., Moore, K., Shamsie, J., and Hamilton, H. (1997). The treatment of conduct disorder: Perspectives from across Canada. *Canadian Journal of Psychiatry*, 42, 637-648.

Moretti, M.M., and Higgins, E.T. (1999). Own versus other standpoints in self-regulation: Developmental antecedents and functional consequences. *Review of General Psychology*, 3, 188-223.

Moretti, M.M., Holland, R., and Peterson, S. (1994). Long-term outcome of an attachment-based program for conduct disorder. *Canadian Journal of Psychiatry*, 39, 360-370.

Moretti, M.M., Holland, R., and McKay, S. (2001). Self-other representations and relational and overt aggression in adolescent girls and boys. *Behavioral Sciences and the Law*, 19, 109-126.

Moretti, M.M., Lessard, J.C., Wiebe, V.J., and Reebye, P. (2000). *Comorbidity in adolescents with conduct disorder: The gender paradox.* Unpublished manuscript, Simon Fraser University, Burnaby, BC.

Moretti, M.M., Lessard, J.C., Scarfe, E., and Holland, R. (1999). *Attachment and conduct disorder in adolescence: The importance of differentiating fearful from dismissing patterns.* Unpublished manuscript, Simon Fraser University, Burnaby, BC.

Moretti, M.M., and Odgers, C. (in press). Aggressive and violent girls: Prevalence, profiles and contributing factors. In R. Corrado, R. Roesch, and S. Hart (Eds.), *Multi-problem and violent youth: A foundation for comparative research.* Amsterdam: IOS Press.

Moretti, M.M., and Wiebe, V. J. (1999). Self-discrepancy in adolescence: Own and parental standpoints on the self. *Merrill-Palmer-Quarterly*, 45, 624-649.

Nada-Raja, S., McGee, R., and Stanton, W.R. (1992). Perceived attachments to parents and peers and psychological well-being in adolescence. *Journal of Youth and Adolescence*, 21, 471-485.

Newman, D.L., Caspi, A., Moffitt, T.E., and Silva, P.A. (1997). Antecedents of adult interpersonal functioning: Effects of individual differences in age 3 temperament. *Developmental Psychology*, 33, 206-217.

Nottelman, E.D., and Jensen, P.S. (1995). Comorbidity of disorder in children and adolescents: Developmental perspectives. In T.H. Ollendick and R.J. Prinz (Eds.), *Advances in clinical child psychology*, Vol. 17 (pp. 109-155). New York: Plenum.

Offord, D.R., and Lipman, E.L. (1996). Emotional and behavioural problems. In *Growing up in Canada: National longitudinal survey of children and youth*, pp. 119-126. Ottawa: Human Resources Development Canada and Statistics Canada.

Paterson, J., Pryor, J., and Field, J. (1995). Adolescent attachment to parents and friends in relation to aspects of self-esteem. *Journal of Youth and Adolescence*, 24, 365-376.

Peeples, F., and Loeber, R. (1994). Do individual factors and neighborhood context explain ethnic differences in juvenile delinquency? *Journal of Quantitative Criminology*, 10, 141-157.

Posner, M.I., and Rothbart, M.K. (2000). Developing mechanisms of self-regulation. *Development and Psychopathology*, 12, 427-441.

Putallaz, M., and Heflin, A.H. (1990). Parent-child interaction. In S.R. Asher and J. Coie (Eds.), *Peer rejection in childhood.* New York: Cambridge University Press.

Reebye, P., Moretti, M.M., Wiebe, V. J., and Lessard, J.C. (2000). Symptoms of posttraumatic stress disorder in adolescents with conduct disorder: Sex differences and onset patterns. *Canadian Journal of Psychiatry*, 45, 746-751.

Reimer, M.S., Overton, W.F., Steidl, J.H., Rosenstein, D.S., and Horowitz, H. (1996). Familial responsiveness and behavioral control: Influences on adolescent psychopathology, attachment, and cognition. *Journal of Research on Adolescence*, 6, 87-112.

Rende, R., and Plomin, R. (1995). Nature, nurture, and the development of psychopathology. In D. Cicchetti and D.J. Cohen (Eds.), *Developmental psychopathology (Vol. 1): Theory and methods* (pp. 291-314). New York: Wiley.

Robins, L.N. (1986). The consequences of conduct disorder in girls. In D. Olweus, J. Block, and M. Radke-Yarrow (Eds.), *The development of antisocial and prosocial behavior: Research, theories and issues* (pp. 385-414). Orlando, FL: Academic Press.

Rosenbaum, J.L. (1989). Family dysfunction and female delinquency. *Crime and Delinquency,* 35, 31-44.

Rosenstein, D.S., and Horowitz, H.A. (1996). Adolescent attachment and psychopathology. *Journal of Consulting and Clinical Psychology,* 64, 244-253.

Sameroff, A.J. (1995). General systems theories and developmental psychopathology. In D. Cicchetti and D.J. Cohen (Eds.), *Developmental Psychopathology, Vol. 1: Theory and Methods. Wiley Series on Personality Processes* (pp. 659-695). New York: John Wiley & Sons.

Sameroff, A.J., Seifer, R., and Bartko, W.T. (1997). Environmental perspectives on adaptation during childhood and adolescence. In S.S. Luthar, J.A. Burack, D. Cicchetti, and J.R. Weisz (Eds.), *Developmental psychopathology: Perspectives on adjustment, risk, and disorder* (pp. 277-307). New York: John Wiley & Sons.

Seidman, E., Yoshikawa, H., Roberts, A., Chesir-Teran, D., Allen, L., Friedman, J.L., and Aber, J.L. (1998). Structural and experiential neighbourhood contexts, developmental stage, and antisocial behavior among urban adolescents in poverty. *Development and Psychopathology,* 10, 259-281.

Shamsie, S.J. (1981). Antisocial adolescents: Our treatments do not work—Where do we go from here? *Canadian Journal of Psychiatry,* 26, 357-364.

Silverthorn, P., and Frick, P. (1999). Developmental pathways to antisocial behavior: The delayed-onset pathway in girls. *Development and Psychopathology,* 11, 101-126.

Sroufe, L.A. (1983). Infant-caregiver attachment and patterns of adaptation in preschool: The roots of maladaptation and competence. In M. Perlutter (Ed.), *Minnesota symposium in child psychology, Vol. 16* (pp. 41-83). Hillsdale, NJ: Erlbaum.

US Surgeon General (2001). Youth violence: A report of the surgeon general. *http://www. surgeongeneral.gov/library/youthviolence.*

Tremblay, R.E. (2000). The development of aggressive behaviour during childhood: What have we learned in the past century? *International Journal of Behavioral Development,* 24, 129-141.

Trupin, E.W., Tarico, V.S., Low, B.P., and Jemelka, R., and McClellan, J. (1993). Children on child protective service caseloads: Prevalence and nature of serious emotional disturbance. *Child Abuse and Neglect,* 17, 345-355.

Warren, M.Q., and Rosenbaum, J.L. (1986). Criminal careers of female offenders. *Criminal Justice and Behavior,* 13, 393-418.

Wartner, U.G., Grossmann, K., Fremmer-Bombik, E., and Suess, G. (1994). Attachment patterns at age six in south Germany: Predictability from infancy and implications for preschool behavior. *Child Development,* 65, 1014-1027.

Werner, E.E., and Smith, R.S. (1992). *Overcoming the odds: High risk children from birth to adulthood.* Ithaca, NY: Cornell University Press.

Youngblade, L.M., Park, K.A., and Belsky, J. (1993). Measurement of young children's close friendship: A comparison of two independent assessment systems and their associations with attachment security. *International Journal of Behavioral Development,* 16, 563-587.

Family Dynamics, Labour Market Attachment, and "At-Risk" Children

12

Joseph H. Michalski
Trent University

INTRODUCTION

Maintaining the health and well-being of Canadians has direct implications for the country's future prosperity and security. The traditional "medical" or "disease" model of health encourages the belief that the most appropriate and effective response to health problems consists of spending more for the provision of health care. Yet there are limits to the proportion of resources that any society can commit to health services. In 1991, Canada was second to the US in health expenditures, with 10% of the gross domestic product devoted to health care. Nearly half (48.9%) of these expenditures were for hospital care (Nair and Karim, 1993). The research indicates, however, that the expansion of health services and increased spending for health care have a progressively smaller impact upon the health status of the population (Mustard and Frank, 1991).

In contrast, a population health perspective emphasizes the social, economic, and environmental determinants of health, which can be modelled to include the relative impacts of genetic endowments and stages of the life cycle, to help explain and even predict health-related outcomes (Evans, Barer, and Marmor, 1994; Premier's Council on Health, Well-Being and Social Justice, 1993; Renaud, 1994). The focus on the determinants of health in the early 1990s contributed to the development of an innovative framework for understanding health (Boothroyd and Eberle, 1990; Premier's Council on Health Strategy, 1991; Renaud, 1993). Apart from the role of genetics and biological endowments (Nair and Karim, 1993), the evidence consistently has pointed to the significance of the social, psychological, economic, and environmental correlates of health (Mustard and Frank, 1991; Premier's Council on Health, 1993; Renaud, 1994; Evans and Stoddart, 1990; Marmot, Kogevinas, and Elston, 1987). For example, researchers generally accept that poverty or socioeconomic inequality can help to account for significant variations in the exposure to health risks, mortality rates, and access to health services (Blane, Brunner, and Wilkinson, 1996; Smith, Bartley, and Blane, 1990; National Council on Welfare, 1990; Wilkinson, 1986). Other research has highlighted the importance of job-related factors such as status inequality in work hierarchies, autonomy, social support in the workplace, and unemployment in affecting the health of the individual (Premier's Council on Health Strategy, 1991; Wilkinson, 1986).

The importance of the population health perspective has garnered wide-spread support among academicians and policymakers alike (Evans et al., 1994; Hayes and Dunn, 1998). A great many stakeholders increasingly recognize that health encompasses a much broader state of being than simply the absence of illness. Factors such as safe and comfortable work environments, the quality of living conditions, community structures, and informal support networks appear to be important determinants of health. In short, traditional views of health have led to a separation of the health issues of individuals from the families and the communities in which they live. Thus the current chapter focuses on the family context of the health and well-being of children. The analysis concentrates on the significance of family characteristics, health outcomes and family functioning, labour market attachment, resiliency, and the implications for identifying "at risk" children.

STUDY CONTEXT

In 1996, a research team from the Canadian Policy Research Networks conducted an exploratory study of how families exchange resources both within their households and with key individuals, organizations, and institutions external to their households (Michalski and Wason, 1998). The main purpose of this study was to examine families across the full range of labour market attachments and the "transactions" in which they engaged to help reconcile the often conflicting demands of work and family life (Peters, 1996). The researchers conducted a series of in-depth interviews and focus groups with a sample of 25 families who were living in Surrey, BC at the time of the study. The Government of BC assisted both by providing partial funding for the study and through the recommendation of the lower mainland city as the potential research site. There were several reasons for selecting Surrey, including the large size and relative heterogeneity of the population, diverse economic bases, and higher rates of income assistance and employment insurance recipients than in comparison with the general population of BC. The assumption was that such an environment would be more conducive to testing ideas and assumptions about resiliency, family dynamics, and labour market attachment.

The sample of study participants included both lone parent families (one adult caregiver co-residing with one or more children) and two parent families (two adult caregivers co-residing with one or more children). Several of the families had experienced recent changes in their labour market situations, especially unemployment, while others had no employment changes. Building on work done in other countries (such as Finch and Mason, 1993), the interviews systematically traced the interactions between all family members aged 6 and older, asking them to identify key exchanges and the processes by which they took place. The research team also collected detailed employment histories and information on coping with stress and times of change. The full range of data collection methods included a questionnaire, individual interviews, family interviews, and focus groups of similar families.

Apart from the requirement of having children, the key inclusion criterion for selecting participants was *labour market attachment*. There were four categories selected at the outset to reflect their experiences of the previous 18 months: 1) no employment disruption (NED); 2) employment lost and regained (JOBFOUND); 3) employment lost and not recovered (JOBLOST); and 4) continuous unemployment (CU). The research team selected these employment categories because of the desire to create more diversity in employment situations to study a small group of families, to utilize parameters that would resonate with policy concerns, and to examine both lone-parent and two-parent families. The purposive sample eventually yielded a total of 25 families who participated fully in the study, split nearly evenly among the four categories.

The results presented here focus on the demographic characteristics of the participants and their self-reported quality of life and health issues obtained through the questionnaires. The interviews generated rich, detailed information about the key family transactions in which these families engaged and contained a series of questions aimed at assessing the "resiliency" of these families. The combination of these two sources of data permits an overarching assessment of which children might be considered "at risk" for significant developmental problems or maladaptive outcomes in the longer term.

FAMILY CHARACTERISTICS

As shown in Table 12.1, there were 11 lone-parent families (4 single/never married, 4 separated, and 3 divorced parents) and 14 two-parent families (11 married and 3 common-law arrangements) in the final sample. The average age for parents, whether in lone-parent or two-parent families, was about 34 years. The sample contained 5 families where there had been continuous unemployment (CU), 6 where jobs were lost and not recovered (JOBLOST), 7 where jobs were lost but recovered (JOBFOUND), and 7 where there had been no employment disruption (NED). Most of the 25 families had either one or two children, although 6 families had three or more children. More than two-thirds of the families had either pre-school children only or at least one child aged 6 or younger currently in their care; only four families (16%) had children exclusively 12 years of age or older. Roughly half of all families in the study had received income assistance within the past year, while two others had received unemployment insurance. The lone-parent families were clearly struggling more financially, as 7 of 11 had total family incomes of less than $20,000 for the preceding 12 months and none earned more than $40,000. In contrast, of the 10 two-parent families reporting family income, only 2 fell below $10,000, while 4 earned between $30,000-$60,000 and 3 received at least $80,000 or more in the last year.

Table 12.1   Demographic characteristics of 25 families in BC

LONE-PARENT FAMILIES

Marital status	Age	Employment status	Children (ages)	Income assistance	Family income
Divorced female	32	CU	3 (1,6,7)	Yes	$30,000-39,999
Single female	22	CU	1 (5)	Yes	Less than $10,000
Single female	19	CU	1 (1)	Yes	Less than $10,000
Separated female	42	CU	1 (10)	Yes	$10,000-19,999
Separated female	39	JOBLOST	2 (7,11)	Yes	$10,000-19,999
Single female	21	JOBLOST	1 (1)	Yes	$10,000-19,999
Single female	26	JOBFOUND	2 (2,6)	Yes	$10,000-19,999
Divorced male	48	JOBFOUND	2 (12,13)	No	$10,000-19,999
Separated male	32	JOBFOUND	2 (4,7)	Yes	$30,000-39,999
Divorced female	40	NED	3 (12,14,17)	Yes	$20,000-29,999
Separated female	42	NED	2 (10,15)	No	$20,000-29,999

TWO-PARENT FAMILIES

Marital status	Ages (M, F)	Employment status	Children (ages)	Income assistance	Family income
Common-Law	33, 27	CU	6 (1,1,2,3,5,6)	Yes	$20,000-29,999
Married (Blended)	39, 43	JOBLOST	3 (6,7,15)	UI	$50,000-59,999
Common-Law	24, 20	JOBLOST	1 (1)	Yes	$20,000-59,999
Common (Blended)	34, 23	JOBLOST	2 (6,7)	UI	$30,000-39,999
Married	24, 24	JOBLOST	1 (1)	Yes	$10,000-19,999
Married	32, 25	JOBFOUND	1 (1)	No	Unknown
Married (Blended)	37, 37	JOBFOUND	3 (12,15,15)	No	$80,000-89,999
Married	29, 24	JOBFOUND	2 (2,3)	No	$30,000-39,999
Married	37, 33	JOBFOUND	2 (5,16)	No	$10,000-19,999
Married	40, 37	NED	2 (6,8)	No	$110,000-119,999
Married	34, 29	NED	1 (3)	No	$40,000-49,999
Married	40, 43	NED	4 (9,12,14,16)	No	$150,000-199,999
Married	55, 51	NED	2 (15,19)	No	Unknown
Married	40, 34	NED	2 (6,8)	No	$20,000-29,999

Health-Related Outcomes for Families

Although the focus of the study was primarily on family dynamics and resiliency in relation to labour market attachments, the research team delved into a number of quality of life and health-related issues through the questionnaires that parents (*n* = 39) and their teenaged children (*n* = 14) completed. While each parent in the lone-parent and two-parent families responded, it should be noted that nearly all of the older children lived in families where one or more parent worked in the paid labour force (for example, there were teenaged children present in families experiencing "continuous unemployment"). The specific health-related outcomes examined in the current analysis include the following: 1) satisfaction with life in general; 2) overall stress in one's life; and 3) self-appraisal of one's health.

The small number of cases obviously precludes more sophisticated multivariate modelling, although several factors from a population health perspective can be correlated with the above outcomes. These include the following: 1) family structure (lone-parent vs two-parent); 2) gender; 3) income assistance status; 4) presence of young children; 5) recent crises; and 6) available supports.

Life Satisfaction

One question inquired about overall satisfaction with life: "Are you satisfied or dissatisfied with your life in general?". The results are presented in Table 12.2, which includes both the percentages within each category evaluated and the total number of participants or cases for each category (see the column "Total N"). In the aggregate, 8 of 39 parents (20.5%) indicated that they were "very satisfied," while 20 responded "somewhat satisfied" (51.3%), and the remainder were either "somewhat dissatisfied" (7 parents) or "very dissatisfied" (4 parents). The older children who responded to the question expressed more satisfaction, as 7 out of 12 (58.3%) were very satisfied, 4 were somewhat satisfied, and only 1 responded "somewhat dissatisfied."

In terms of correlates of life satisfaction, the parents in two-parent families (8 of 28) were more likely to state "very satisfied" compared to lone-parents (0 of 11) and less likely to express dissatisfaction (6 of 28 vs 5 of 11). A higher percentage of those *not* currently receiving income assistance were very satisfied compared to those receiving income assistance. Although the samples were quite small, a chi-square test indicated that neither gender nor presence of young children was associated with general life satisfaction.

The most powerful correlates, however, were the number of crises experienced in the past 12 months and the availability of informal supports. Those who had not experienced *any* recent crises or traumatic events (for example, bankruptcy, separation or divorce, death or serious illness, etc.) were generally more satisfied. Those who had experienced two or more traumatic events within the past 12 months were clearly much more dissatisfied with life at the present moment. Moreover, those who responded positively to two questions regarding the availability of informal supports (to help with crisis situations or to turn to for advice) were generally more satisfied than those who expressed having only one or no such supports.

Table 12.2   Correlates of life satisfaction in general

Variables	Very satisfied (%)	Somewhat satisfied (%)	Dissatisfied (%)	Total N
Family structure				
Lone-parent	0.0	54.5	45.5	11
Two parents	28.6	50.0	21.4	28
Children	58.3	33.3	8.3	12
Gender				
Female	21.7	47.8	30.4	23
Male	18.8	56.3	25.0	16
Income assistance (IA)				
Receiving IA	7.7	69.2	23.1	13
Not receiving IA	26.9	42.3	30.8	26
Young children				
No children under 6	9.1	54.5	27.3	11
One child under 6	27.3	45.5	13.6	22
Two or more under 6	16.7	66.7	16.7	6
Number of crises				
None	40.0	60.0	0.0	10
One	20.0	60.0	20.0	15
Two or more	7.1	35.7	57.1	14
Informal supports				
One or fewer	0.0	45.5	54.5	11
Two or more	28.6	53.6	17.9	28

Life Stress

The next issue concerns the extent to which the study participants described their lives as stressful or not. Among the current sample, 12 of 39 parents (30.9%) responded that their lives were "very stressful," while another 18 (or 46.2%) described their lives as "somewhat stressful," and the remaining 9 (23.1%) stated "not very stressful" or "not at all stressful." The older children who responded, as with the question about life satisfaction, expressed a more positive view than their parents, such that 4 of 12 described their lives as "not very stressful" and the other 8 reported "somewhat stressful" (see Table 12.3). Once more, the older children (with one exception) were found only within those families that had experienced no employment disruption or where a parent had lost a job but subsequently found a new one.

Table 12.3   Correlates with stress in life

Variables	Very stressful (%)	Somewhat stressful (%)	Not very stressful (%)	Total N
Family structure				
Lone-parent	36.4	45.5	18.2	11
Two parents	28.6	46.4	25.0	28
Children	0.0	66.7	33.3	12
Gender				
Female	34.8	43.5	21.7	23
Male	25.0	50.0	25.0	16
Income assistance (IA)				
Receiving IA	23.1	46.2	30.8	13
Not receiving IA	34.6	46.2	19.2	26
Young children				
No children under 6	36.4	54.5	9.1	11
One child under 6	31.8	45.5	22.7	22
Two or more under 6	16.7	22.7	50.0	6
Number of crises				
None	0.0	50.0	50.0	10
One	40.0	40.0	20.0	15
Two or more	42.9	50.0	7.1	14
Informal supports				
One or fewer	72.7	27.3	0.0	11
Two or more	14.3	53.6	32.1	28

Most of the factors examined were not correlated significantly with life stress in a formal statistical sense, including family structure, gender, income assistance, and presence of young children. However, slightly higher percentages of lone-parents, females, those *not* receiving income assistance, and those with fewer young children viewed their lives as "very stressful" compared to others in the study.

As with general life satisfaction, the key correlates were the number of recent crises and presence of informal supports. Five of the 10 participants who had *not* experienced any recent traumatic events reported their lives were "not very stressful" (none responded "very stressful"). In comparison, 3 of 15 (20.0%) of those who had one recent crisis and only 1 in 14 (7.1%) of those who had suffered at least two traumatic events responded "not very stressful." In addition, those responding positively to questions about the availability of two types of informal support were far less likely to describe their lives as "very stressful" compared to those with one or fewer such supports (4 in 28 vs 8 in 11).

Self-Reported Health

One of the classic questions to assess health status involves a subjective self-appraisal to a question such as the following from the General Social Survey (and used in the current study): "Compared to other people your age, how would you describe your state of health? Would you say it is...excellent, very good, good, fair, or poor?" The raw results indicate that among parents, the distribution was as follows: excellent (4 or 10.5%), very good (12 or 31.6%), good (15 or 39.5%), fair (6 or 15.8%), and poor (1 or 2.6%). The older children in the sample were much more likely to describe their health as very good or excellent (10 of 12, or 83.3%), with only one response each in the "good" and the "fair" categories.

As with the previous analyses, the correlates of self-reported health status were next examined through chi-square tests, the results of which are summarized in Table 12.4. The statistically significant correlates among this sample of families included gender and income assistance: male parents were far more likely than female parents to describe their health as "very good" or "excellent" (62.5% vs 27.3%), while those who were *not* receiving income assistance were more likely to report being healthier. Those with two or more children under 6 years old reported somewhat poorer health, as did those who had recently experienced two or more crises, though these differences were not statistically significant due to the small numbers of respondents. Finally, the presence of informal support was not correlated significantly with health status.

What are the implications of these results for the children and youth of these families? There appear to be certain demographic characteristics weakly associated with *parents'* life satisfaction, stress, and general health, but are the *children* living with "less healthy" parents themselves less healthy? These exploratory results seem to indicate that, on balance, no: the older children within these families reported much higher levels of satisfaction, less stress, and better health than their parents. The fact that parents might be somewhat dissatisfied, stressed out, or otherwise unhealthy does not necessarily translate into directly negative health effects on their children. What may matter more, though, are the availability of informal supports and the impact of traumatic events, both of which appear to have much more saliency to the quality of life for the families in the current study. Moreover, the question of whether children are growing up in "healthy functioning families" merits further attention as well, especially if one has an interest in determining the long-term prospects of children living in different family circumstances. That dimension receives attention in the next section.

Table 12.4   Correlates with self-reported health

Variables	Very good or excellent (%)	Good (%)	Fair or poor (%)	Total N
Family structure				
Lone-parent	36.4	45.5	18.2	11
Two parents	44.4	37.0	18.5	27
Children	83.3	8.3	8.3	12
Gender				
Female	27.3	45.5	27.3	22
Male	62.5	31.3	6.3	16
Income assistance (IA)				
Receiving IA	23.1	61.5	15.4	13
Not receiving IA	52.0	28.0	20.0	25
Young children				
No children under 6	45.0	45.0	9.1	11
One child under 6	47.6	33.3	19.0	21
Two or more under 6	16.7	50.0	33.3	6
Number of crises				
None	40.0	50.0	10.0	10
One	46.7	40.0	13.3	15
Two or more	38.5	30.8	30.8	13
Informal supports				
One or fewer	40.0	50.0	10.0	10
Two or more	42.9	35.7	21.4	28

Healthy Family Functioning

The scaled results of family functioning among these families may be an indicator of potential risk for growing up in an "unhealthy environment." The 12-item General Functioning Subscale (GFS) of the McMaster Family Assessment Device was administered to help determine family functioning in these families. The GFS contains a series of statements, to which the respondent indicates "strongly agree," "agree," "disagree," and "strongly disagree." The items are then scored from one to four, which thereby generates a minimum possible score of 12 and a maximum possible score of 48. The basic logic of the scale suggests that the higher the score, the higher the level of family dysfunction.

Previous research has confirmed both the reliability and validity of the GFS and the measure has been included in the National Longitudinal Survey of Children and Youth (NLSCY) and the Ontario Child Health Survey. The mean scores for the population tend to be between 19 and 20 (with a standard deviation [sd] of slightly greater than 5). These figures can be used to provide a baseline comparison for the current sample. In other studies, scores of 27 or higher are used to classify families as "dysfunctional," though a common practice with clinical measures consists of classifying those scoring at least one standard deviation above or below the mean as "at risk." In fact, evidence from a recent national study of 1,455 individuals and families accessing family service agencies (that is, those in crisis or seeking supportive services of some type) determined that the average GFS score was 27.3, which exceeds the somewhat arbitrary "dysfunctional" cutoff (Michalski, 1998). Hence the previously established norms of healthy family functioning receive further validation in this context.

The results indicate that these families were not markedly different from the general population, as GFS scores among parents averaged 21.8 (sd = 6.0). The lone-parents had a mean score of 22.9, while the adults in two-parent families averaged 21.4. Interestingly, the children's scaled results were nearly identical to that of the parents (mean = 21.5, sd = 6.3), suggesting that they tended to have similar views about the overall level of function or dysfunction within their families (confirmed by a case by case analysis comparing parents' and children's responses as well).

If one averages the scaled results of the two-parent families to produce one score, then the distribution breaks down 4:1 in terms of families within the "healthy functioning" range compared to those in the "dysfunctional" range. Stated differently, 20 of the families (80%) had GFS scores of 26 or less, while the other 5 (or 20%) scored 28 or higher.

While factors such as gender, family structure, income assistance, and presence of young children were *not* correlated with family functioning, once more the situational factors, such as recent crises and the availability of informal supports, proved significant. For example, those families where there were no traumatic events in the past 12 months averaged GFS scores of 18.1, while those experiencing one or more crises averaged 5 points higher toward the dysfunctional end of the scale. Similarly, those who responded in the affirmative to both questions pertaining to the availability of informal supports were more than 4 points better off than those lacking in either or both types of informal supports identified.

As with the previous analyses, the most important considerations appear to be related to the sources of support and the response to recent crises. Some families clearly have more—and more *effective*—external supports at their disposal than others. Perhaps less obvious, though, are the relative effects of different families' capacities to cope with crises, or the potentially devastating impact that traumatic events may have upon some families which are not as pronounced among other families. These latter considerations lead naturally to a discussion of family strengths and resiliency.

Family Strengths and Resiliency

A central purpose of the current study was to examine the strengths that families possessed and their relevance to dealing with the challenges with which they were confronted. The concept of resiliency, or the ability to bounce back after adversity, is currently a popular concept among psychologists, social workers, educators, family scholars, and organizational behaviourists. The Atlantic Health Promotion Research Centre (1994) of Dalhousie University provides a useful general definition of resiliency:

> *Resilience is the capability of individuals and systems (families, groups and communities) to cope successfully in the face of significant adversity or risk. This capability develops and changes over time, is enhanced by protective factors within the individual/ system and the environment, and contributes to the maintenance or enhancement of health* (page 1).

A growing body of literature and research on resiliency has developed in recent years. "What factors develop and support this capability for resiliency in individuals, families, organizations, and communities?" is the key question with which researchers struggle. At present, the majority of family resilience research still focuses on defining the characteristics of resilient children and families, understanding the risk and protective factors, and proposing strategies aimed at educators and therapists rather than policy makers (Barnard, 1994; Saleeby, 1996; Smith and Carlson, 1997).

In this snapshot of 25 families, data on the characteristics of families were collected that may contribute to an understanding of the nature of resiliency. It was not possible in a short- term, in-depth interview study to evaluate resiliency properly, which by definition requires a longitudinal analysis to assess the responses of individuals and families to crises over time. The research nevertheless generated information on the relative strengths and liabilities of families by using attributes identified in the resiliency literature, coupled with an analysis of additional processes and outcomes. Most of the 25 families in this study indicated that they had experienced a recent crisis or significant events such as illness, recent immigration to Canada, bankruptcy, birth of a child, male partner going to prison, finding employment, losing employment, or coming together as a blended family. Hence these families were especially important to examine, since crisis or change are the key periods during which the capacity for resiliency is most tested.

The growing body of resiliency literature identifies numerous characteristics of family resiliency, or common attributes and processes that appear most often among resilient, healthy, or functional families. These include: clear, open, and consistent communication; adaptability; problem-solving skills; confidence; cooperation; understanding; and acceptance. In the current study, an analysis of the interview transcripts resulted in the identification of those families where members agreed that their families tended to share the attributes identified previously. This group also included those families that believed themselves to be resilient (had bounced back from a crisis and/or were confident in their ability to weather crises in the future). Next, the families were examined for other similarities, or the extent to which they shared a cluster of processes such as an acceptance of the prevailing styles of negotiation, problem-solving, and decision-making.

The identification of families with similar clusters of attributes and processes facilitated the creation of a strengths-liabilities continuum. The families in the study were rated as having more or fewer of the strengths and liabilities. A variety of attributes and processes appeared to be strengths or protective factors among the families in the sample, particularly in establishing agreement or congruence among family members. The strengths of these families derived not from a hierarchical division of tasks considered appropriate by members of one cultural group or on a democratic decision-making structure prevalent in another. Such transactions may be considered appropriate or desirable for other reasons, but they did not have a direct relationship to family placements along the strengths-liabilities continuum. Instead, the families were ranked in terms of the prevailing attributes and processes identified, which have been summarized in Table 12.5.

Table 12.5   Characteristics of resilient families

Attributes	1.	Shared optimism and positive outlook
	2.	Shared goals and priorities
	3.	Sense of being a family and commitment to the family
	4.	Sense of control
Processes	1.	Accepted negotiation, problem-solving, and decision-making processes
	2.	Acceptance of role within the household
	3.	Flexibility and adaptability of roles to meet agreed-upon goals and priorities
	4.	Open, clear, consistent, frequent communication
	5.	Consistent contact with external friends, relatives, or community
Corollaries	1.	Health
	2.	Well-being

In brief, the presence of a greater number and more intensely experienced set of these attributes and processes served as a proxy to indicate a greater capacity for resiliency. An important consideration, however, was the degree to which individuals in the family's households truly possessed the attributes and accepted the processes specified. If one member openly agreed with a transactions process, but secretly was in disagreement, the capacity for resiliency was undermined and that family would appear less likely to be able to sustain resilience over time. Stated more succinctly, the degree to which each member of the family unit possessed an attribute such as "shared optimism and positive outlook" provided an operational measure of one dimension along the strengths-liabilities continuum. Finally, it should be noted that there is no single agreed-upon criterion in the literature of successful or unsuccessful adaptation to change. Hence the possession of a series of attributes and processes was cross-checked with other corollaries—the self-reported health and well-being of study participants—to help verify placement of each family along the strengths-liabilities continuum.

Table 12.6 then places the families (pseudonyms are used in all cases) in the study on a continuum ranging from the possession of more strengths to more liabilities, broken down further by family status (lone-parent vs two-parent) and type of labour force attachment (to be explained). The continuum has been divided into three groups: thriving, surviving, and struggling. These serve as a preliminary description of the family's capacity for resiliency, since no formal scale or measure of resiliency has been previously validated. The placement has been further cross-referenced with self-reported health and well-being.

Table 12.6 Strengths-liabilities continuum and labour market attachment

		Category 1 Standard attachment	Category 2 Non-standard attachment	Category 3 Transitional attachment	Category 4 Deferred attachment
Thriving	Two-parent	Suarez Pinto Singh Young Stevenson			
	Lone-parent			Bradshaw	Wilson
Surviving	Two-parent	Jefferson/Jones Longchamp Quentin	England/ Edwards	Fairholme Demasse/	Bolton
	Lone-parent	Ironhand Gauthier	Mason	Brown Andersen	
Struggling	Two-parent		King Campbell/Collins		
	Lone-parent	Octavia			Adams

"Thriving" families considered themselves to have successfully overcome crises in the past and exhibited most, if not all, of the attributes and processes identified previously. These families reflected family situations that were typically viewed quite positively by the members, as well as where health and well-being were highly correlated. Life might not be "perfect" in every sense of the term, but these families' strengths far outweighed their liabilities.

Families that were "surviving" featured fewer of the attributes and processes, or a mixture of strengths and liabilities (typically from four to six). These were households wherein the families generally viewed themselves as doing reasonably well, though by no means were they functioning at their optimal level. These households were coping well in some areas, but having difficulty with others. The members could identify certain strengths which helped to provide some anchors in their lives, but at the same time were quick to point out liabilities or problem areas that created a sense of vulnerability or negatively affected their health and well-being.

The "struggling" families by definition were experiencing a high degree of vulnerability to crisis and change. These were families that appeared to possess only one or two of the attributes and processes that cumulatively were the pillars of strength in other families. Their liabilities clearly and pervasively outweighed their strengths. The families could be characterized as "vulnerable" or "at risk" by most standard definitions, with relatively lower levels of self-reported health and well-being.

A second look at the employment patterns of those families in the study that had achieved labour market attachment demonstrates that the mere fact of labour attachment in and of itself was an insufficient indicator of the success and the capacity of resiliency of a family and its members. There was a range of attachments to the labour market. Among those families in which one or more adults were employed, there was considerable difference in their form of attachment to the labour market. Category 1 includes families in which there was a strong *standard labour market attachment*. This meant that adults in the household held at least one full-time continuous job, often with benefits. In many two-parent families, the mother remained at home full-time or part-time to care for the children. There were eight two-parent families and three lone-parent families in this category. Category 2 includes families in which there was weak, compromised, or *non-standard labour market attachment*. In these families there was at least one part-time or short-term employment situation, generally with low pay and no benefits. Often one person was less than satisfactorily employed and the other was looking for work while doing childcare. There were three two-parent families and one lone-parent family in this category. There are two categories of families with no current attachment to the labour market. Some of these were placed in Category 3, or *transitional labour market attachment*. The adults in these families had no current employment but were actively focused on the goal of becoming employed in the near future. In these families, there were either one or more adults undertaking training or education, preparing to do so in the short-term, job hunting, or planning their own home business. Childcare was a priority against which these plans were offset: the ability and/or inclination of an unemployed person or family to undertake transitional activities were directly affected by childcare responsibilities. This category included two of the two-parent families, and three of the lone-parent families. All of these families received income assistance. The final group of families has been placed in Category 4, or *deferred labour market attachment*. The attitude toward gaining employment was passive in the short-term. More specifically, there was no attempt being made to attach to the labour market, either through looking for work or through education and training. In these families, the main activity of the adults was childcare. This did not necessarily indicate a sense of failure or defeat, although it did in some cases. It did indicate that these households had found that they could not achieve a positive balance between income and the cost of childcare, or that they had deliberately chosen to look after their children and not seek employment. Two-parent families clearly had more options in making this choice than lone-parent families. In this category, there were four lone-parent families and one two-parent family, all receiving income assistance.

Health and Well-Being Correlates of Resiliency

As explained earlier, health and well-being served as indices to be correlated with their placement on the strengths-liabilities continuum, or the "capacity for resiliency" among these families. Thus when asked to compare their health to others their age, half (50%) of the respondents in the more resilient families indicated that their health was very good or excellent. Just over a third (37.6%) of the respondents in the more vulnerable families indicated the same. Approximately the same number of individuals in both groups of families said that their physical health was the same or better than 12 months ago, but 26.7% of the individuals in vulnerable families said that their physical health was worse, compared to 5.3% in the more resilient families. When asked to compare their emotional and mental health or state at the time of the interview compared to 12 months previously, there was no difference between respondents in the more resilient and more vulnerable families. However, when asked about specific behavioural indicators there was indeed a difference. More individuals in the vulnerable families reported an increase in medication use, more changes in sleeping behaviour, increased feelings of nervousness and anxiousness, less feeling of calmness and peace, and greater feeling of sadness or depression. This was corroborated during in-depth interviews that showed a pattern of some members of less resilient families identifying stress-related illnesses and depression.

In addition, as a proxy measure of well-being, 9 out of 10 individuals in more resilient families were somewhat satisfied or very satisfied with their lives. By the same token, only 5 in 10 members of more vulnerable families were satisfied, whereas 52.9% of those individuals were somewhat dissatisfied or very dissatisfied. A high percentage of individuals (52.9%) in more vulnerable families described their lives as very stressful compared to 12.5% of those in families with a greater capacity for resilience.

There was a strong relationship between family capacity for resilience and certain kinds of attributes and processes (including family dynamics and informal external support). The "thriving" families exhibited a package of different strengths, which correlated positively with health and well-being. As a final consideration, the GFS scales results of family functioning correlated moderately with the placement on the continuum. For example, none of the families classified as "thriving" fell within the "dysfunctional" range; indeed, their average scores (about 19) were just slightly less than the population mean. The "surviving" families averaged about 22, while those in the "struggling" category had a mean of 24.

Labour Market Attachment and Family Well-Being

Several finer points emerge from an analysis of the results of Table 12.6. First, the evidence indicates that one can find families from each of the different types of labour market attachment across most of the possible categories. For example, one observes two-parent families with standard labour market attachments who are thriving, as well as other two-parent families with non-standard attachments who are struggling. While 3 in 10 families receiving income assistance were "struggling," others were actually "thriving" by the measure developed for this study. Yet there were some notable patterns to emerge as well.

For example, clearly two-parent families on average were more likely to have standard labour market attachments *and* were more likely to be thriving, or at least "surviving." Although admittedly small in number, none of those families with "non-standard" labour market attachments could be found in the "thriving" category. In fact, the only two-parent families identified as "struggling" both relied upon non-standard attachments. The results further show that the families classified as having "transitional attachments" were in somewhat better shape than those in the "deferred attachment" category. Although each of these families received income assistance, the family dynamics differed such that those in transitional category exhibited more of the positive attributes and processes identified than those with deferred attachments. Finally, while three families were "struggling" as lone-parent families with dim prospects for securing employment, there were other families with deferred attachments who were coping more successfully.

IMPLICATIONS FOR THE HEALTH AND WELL-BEING OF CHILDREN

The various analyses conducted reveal a complex mosaic of possible factors relating to demographic characteristics, life circumstances, family dynamics, and labour force attachments that may be related both to the immediate family circumstances and long-term prospects for children. If one examines potential "risk" and "protective" factors for children, some of the families examined might be characterized as less resilient and less likely to be able to foster positive developments for children who are immersed in the situations. The seminal longitudinal work of Werner and Smith (Werner and Smith, 1981; Werner and Smith, 1992), for example, highlights the significance of a variety of major risk factors for children: chronic poverty; mothers without much education; moderate to severe perinatal complications; developmental delays or irregularities; genetic abnormalities; and parental psychopathology. Additional sources of stress in childhood and adolescence include (among other factors): prolonged separation from primary caregiver during first year; birth of younger siblings within two years after the another child's birth; serious or repeated child illnesses; chronic parental illness or mental illness; sibling with handicap, learning, or behavioral problem; chronic family discord; absent fathers; loss of job or sporadic employment; divorce of parents; change of residence or schools; remarriage and entry of step-parent; and the departure or death of older sibling or close friends.

By these measures, a number of the families studied are providing less than optimal situations for their children particularly in regard to instability of family situations and labour market attachments. Some families have already encountered or experienced both of these factors as well as a number of the factors cited above, including chronic low-income situations, parents with lower education, serious illnesses, family discord, and entry of step-parents into the family. Perhaps most distressing were the situations wherein families had experienced a number of these conditions and yet remained relatively isolated or without access to other types of supports. For example, there are a number of "protective" factors for the children that might be "missing" as well from some of these families: mothers who have some steady employment outside of the household; readily available additional caretakers beside mothers; availability of kin and neighbours; shared values and a sense of coherence; availability of counsel by teachers or ministers; and access to special services.

Yet, perhaps most remarkably, the children in the current study appeared to be incredibly resilient. Among the older children, the self-reported health and well-being measures were consistently higher than those of the adults. By the same token, their assessments of family functioning were quite realistic, at least as measured by their similar responses to those of their parents. These youngsters were firmly rooted in the realities of their situations, which for many meant providing baby-sitting or securing part-time employment to help out financially, or assuming more responsibilities—albeit reluctantly in many cases—for housework. At least in the short-term, the children appeared to be able to cope quite well with their circumstances.

The long-term impact of a number of these factors remains to be seen. Some of the evidence from other research suggests that factors such as low-income or income derived only from "earning" rather than from "assets" may have long-term negative effects on labour market earnings in the future. The relatively lower education of some of the mothers, non-standard employment or possibly deferred labour market attachments, and the impacts of such factors as divorce or being in a blended family mean that some children *statistically* are more likely to be at risk. The results from research such as *Canada's Population Health Survey* and the *National Longitudinal Survey of Children and Youth* should provide some of the more definitive answers. For example, some preliminary results from the NLSCY suggest that higher incomes, depressed parents, parents lacking in social supports, and poor family functioning are correlated with increased vulnerability among children or vulnerability to "poor or unhealthy development" (Ross, Roberts, and Scott, 1998).

In the interim, there are a number of factors that can buffer the impact of these events or other sources of stress, many of which were not measured in this study. Even factors such as a parent's willingness and ability to read to his or her child can make a difference (Schlesinger, 1998). For those without other means, the availability of supporting counselling, particularly in crisis situations, can be of critical importance to long-term well-being. A range of other parenting supports (both to assist parents for their benefit *and* in their capacities to "practice" as parents) may help a number of families, especially where "natural" support networks are less available or accessible. A key factor that deserves further investigation appears to be the nature of the labour market attachment that parents enjoy, particularly in light of the fact that those families with "nonstandard" attachments appear to be in a somewhat more precarious position. If labour markets continue to evolve in the direction of an increase in such employment, then supportive policies to mitigate some of the negative aspects of such insecurity may reap longer-term benefits in terms of healthier children.

Finally, the children themselves appear to have broad, albeit varying, capacities for resilience. The limited evidence indicated that the vast majority of children in the present study were coping quite well, despite some of the indignities they suffered as a result of their circumstances. One youngster complained, for instance, of being teased for not having the trendiest clothes because of his family's economic situation. The *family* struggles, especially for the *parents,* as yet did not generally translate into poor health or otherwise compromise the short-term well-being of the children.

Perhaps the long-term objective of current dialogue should be the development of innovative models of health promotion, maintenance, and delivery, which logically should be rooted in the realities of current individual lifestyles, family environments, and community-based structures and supports. These domains cannot be separated from the social organization of work and industry, which not only impacts on the quality of life, but in turn stands to benefit directly from conditions that promote healthier children, families, and communities. While children should not be used as pawns to simply or naively argue for or against specific health or economic policies, the importance of understanding family dynamics and contexts and the nature of labour market attachments are critical to enhancing the prospects of nurturing healthy child development.

REFERENCES

Barnard, C.P. (1994). Resiliency: A shift in our perception? *The American Journal of Family Therapy*, 22(2), 135-144.

Blane, D., Brunner, E., and Wilkinson, R. (Eds.) (1996). *Health and social organization: Towards a health policy for the Twenty-First Century*. London: Routledge.

Boothroyd, P., and Eberle, M. (1990). *Healthy communities: What they are, how they're made*. Vancouver: UBC Centre for Human Settlements.

Davey Smith, G., Bartley, M., and Blane, D. (1990). The Black report on socioeconomic in-equalities on health ten years on. *British Medical Journal*, 301, 373-377.

Evans, R.G., Barer, M.L., and Marmor, T.R. (Eds.) (1994). *Why are some people healthy and others not? The determinants of health of populations*. New York: Aldine De Gruyter.

Evans, R.G., and Stoddart, G.L. (1990). Producing health, consuming health care. *Population Health Working Paper No. 6*. Toronto: Canadian Institute for Advanced Research.

Finch, J., and Mason, J. (1993). *Negotiating family responsibilities*. New York: Tavistock.

Hayes, M.V., and Dunn, J.R. (1998). *Population health in Canada: A systematic review* (CPRN Study No. HJO 1). Ottawa: Canadian Policy Research Networks, Inc.

Marmot, M.G., Kogevinas, M.A., and Elston, M. (1987). Social/economic status and disease. *Annual Review of Public Health*, 8, 111-135.

Michalski, J.H. (1998). *The strengths of Canadian families, 1997: Family Service Canada's national survey of clients accessing family service agencies*. Toronto: Canadian Policy Research Net-works, Inc.

Michalski, J.H., and Wason, M-J. (1998). *Family transactions, resiliency, and labour market at-tachment: An in-depth study of families in British Columbia*. Ottawa: Canadian Policy Re-search Networks, Inc.

Mustard, J. F., and Frank, J. (1991). *The determinants of health*. Toronto: Canadian Institute for Advanced Research.

Nair, C., and Karim, R. (1993). An overview of health care systems: Canada and selected OECD countries. *Health Reports*, 5(3), 259-279.

National Council on Welfare (1990). *Health, health care and Medicare*. Ottawa: Minister of Supply and Services Canada.

Peters, S. (1996). *Examining the concept of transactions as the basis for studying the social and economic dynamics of families* (CPRN Study No. FI01). Ottawa: Canadian Policy Research Networks, Inc.

Premier's Council on Health Strategy (1991). *Nurturing health: A framework on the determi-nants of health*. Toronto: Queen's Printer for Ontario.

Premier's Council on Health, Well-Being and Social Justice (1993). *Our environment, our health*. Toronto: Queen's Printer for Ontario.

Renaud, M. (1993). Social sciences and medicine: Hygeia versus Panakeia. *Health and Cana-dian Society*, 1(1), 229-247.

Renaud, M., avec la collaboration de L. Bouchard (1994). Expliquer l'inexplique: L'envi-ronnement social comme facteur cle de la sante. *Interface*, 15(2), 14-35.

Ross, D.P., Roberts, P.A., and Scott, K. (1998). Comparing children in lone-parent families: Differences and similarities. Paper presented at *Investing in children: A national research conference* (Applied Research Branch, Human Resources Development Canada), Ottawa, October 27-29.

Saleeby, D. (1996). The strengths perspective in social work practice: Extensions and cautions. *Social Work,* 41(3), 296-305.

Schlesinger, B. (1998). *Strengths in families: Accentuating the positive.* Nepean: The Vanier Institute of the Family.

Smith, C., and Carlson, B.E. (1997). Stress, coping, and resilience in children and youth. *Social Service Review,* 33(3), 231-256.

Werner, E.E., and Smith, R.S. (1981). *Vulnerable, but invincible: A longitudinal study of resilient children and youth.* New York: McGraw-Hill.

Werner, E.E., and Smith, R.S. (1992). *Overcoming the odds: High risk children from birth to adulthood.* Ithaca, New York: Cornell University Press.

Wilkinson, R. (Ed.) (1986). *Class and health.* London: Tavistock.

Wilkinson, R. (1996). *Unhealthy societies: The afflictions of inequality.* London: Routledge.

Epilogue[1]

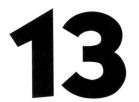

Michael V. Hayes

Institute for Health Research and Education, Simon Fraser University

Many changes in public policies and programs (Government of British Columbia, 2002) announced at the time this volume was going to press, part of the 'New Era' agenda of the Liberal government elected in May 2001, appear to be inconsistent with the perspective and some of the evidence reported in this volume, and the related policy documents that stimulated this book. It is disheartening to witness the extent to which what appears to be an ideological commitment to financial factors can outweigh some of the empirical evidence regarding fundamental influences upon life chances and health status. These policies, proclaimed in the name of eliminating dependency and improving economic efficiency, may actually make both worse. The fact that these changes came at the same time that the government was locked in a bitter dispute with the province's doctors about how to allocate an additional $392 million (to the point of withdrawn services and threatened strikes) has many confused, as politicians decry the unsustainable cost of providing publicly funded health care while at the same time promoting the very conditions that so often are the cause of poorest health and fewest life chances (thereby impacting education, justice, employment, and other programs in addition to health). The government chose tax cuts that differentially benefit relatively more affluent and secure people over providing and strengthening services to the most vulnerable. For many families, increases in Medical Services Plan premiums and sales taxes, combined with eliminated benefits (de-listing of chiropractic and massage therapy, for example), will more than offset the reduced taxes. In the face of an economic downturn, and with reduced funds available as a consequence of income tax cuts, the government will meet the shortfall by cutting further services and incomes going to some of the poorest of children and families.

As indicated in Chapter 6 by Foster and Wright, two thirds of children taken into care come from families on Income Assistance (IA). In December, 2001, the Social Planning and Research Council of BC estimated that incomes of people living on IA only met 45-65% of the minimum monthly costs for food, shelter, clothing, transportation, child care, and other basic needs (Day and Brodsky, 2002). Yet as of April 1, 2002, the basic living allowance of single parent families was cut by $50, while for employable couples it was cut by $100. Support for 'employable' IA recipients between ages 55-64 was cut by $47-$98 per month. To be eligible for IA, total family assets have been reduced from $5,500 to $2,500 (including $250 maximum in cash). Crisis grants for food, shelter and clothing have been reduced to $20 per month for food, $100 per year for clothing and one month's rent for shelter. Prior to April 1, recipients of IA were able to keep support payments from estranged spouses of up to $100 and/or earnings up to $100 without reduction in their monthly payments. Both exemptions have been eliminated. Time limits have been imposed upon periods of IA support. Employable persons will be limited to 24 months cumulative eligibility for IA within a 60 month (5 year) period starting April 1, 2002. Employable single parents (90% of whom are women) are expected to seek work when their youngest child turns 3 years of age. If the 2 year limit is reached, IA payments will be reduced by $100 per month for single parents, $100 per month for two-parent families where one parent is at the time limit, and $200 per month for two-parent families where both parents are at the time limit. The goal of the new policies is to reduce the number of people on IA from 240,000 to about 200,000 people while attempting to find jobs for those displaced (Goldberg and Long, 2001; Ministry of Human Resources, 2002; Reitsma-Street, 2002).

The Minister of Human Resources, previously a registered social worker, has been censured by the Board of Registered Social Workers of BC for not upholding the social work code of ethics and standards of practice in relation to these changes. The Minister has been condemned for introducing legislation 'that constitutes a broad social experiment based on little data, no formal research testing and no public consultation process' (Lavoie, 2002, p.A4; see also University of Northern British Columbia, 2002).

Reductions in income to people without work must be viewed against reductions in minimum wage from $8 to $6 under the new training wage initiative introduced by the new government. Many people who make the transition from IA to work will have to work longer hours to make the same wage they would have made a year ago.

At the same time as these reductions in income have been introduced, some subsidies for childcare have been eliminated. Ball, Pence, and Benner discussed the importance of quality childcare upon the health and development of children in Chapter 5. The new government revoked legislation enacted by the previous government (but never fully implemented) that sought to give families access to childcare for $5 per child per day. The income exemption that determines a parent's eligibility has been reduced by $235. Previously, single parents of one child earning up to about $35,000 were eligible for a small subsidy. Now, single parents with one child earning in excess of $28,400 are ineligible for a subsidy. Subsidies for single parents with one child have been reduced for parents earning over $17,000. Single parents with two children earning between $20,000-37,000 have also had subsidies reduced.

Further, Paul Pallan, in his final report as the Children's Commissioner for BC has indicated concern that these changes will seriously affect children and youth (McLintock, 2002). Pallan is also worried about the plans to cut 23% from the budget of the Ministry of Children and Family Development

(Pallan, 2002). These concerns are also echoed by Laverne MacFadden, in her final annual report of the Office of the Child, Youth and Family Advocate Legislature. MacFadden "strongly urges the government to rethink the impact to income assistance for children, youth and families" which is to experience a 30% reduction over 3 years (MacFadden, 2002, p.29). Both the Children's Commission and the Child, Youth and Family Advocate offices are being dismantled, and will be replaced by a single, much pared-down office. As a result, oversight of children's programs is being substantially diminished.

Extended families of children in care will be called upon to care for these children with some assistance from government. Given the concentration of children in care among families receiving IA, and the often familial nature of social exclusion, poor families will be stretched even further by the increased responsibilities. Yet the objective of the New Era agenda is to reduce the number of children in care and caseloads have indeed fallen dramatically over the past 12 months. The experiences documented by Morton in Chapter 8 appear to be inconsistent with this double-pronged approach of placing children with little support in the homes of extended family members and reducing the number of children in need of protection. The number of children at some risk of harm may actually increase, although government is investing more money in family support programs and passing through federal dollars for early childhood development and supports. The freezing of education budgets will force class sizes to increase and reduce support for those with highest needs. The hardest hit will likely be those schools in the poorest neighbourhoods. Special programs for children living in inner-city neighbourhoods are being kept afloat, but are vulnerable to elimination in 2003.

Under an agreement between the federal and provincial governments, BC will receive $88.7 million over the next 5 years to create affordable housing. In a reorganization of seniors housing, the government has decided to earmark $62.5 million of this funding (73.8%) for Assisted Living for seniors and persons with physical and mental disabilities. The remaining $26.2 million will be directed at all other housing programs—for families, singles, independent seniors, and homeless at risk. In addition to the disruption the concurrent decision to close extended and long term care beds has caused seniors currently in facilities, and the longer wait for housing for seniors in need, this policy (in effect, a supplement to the health care budget) leaves low income singles and families who are marginally housed on wait lists for subsidized housing.

Legal aid for poverty-related cases involving support and/or custody has been eliminated, and a number of courthouses have been closed or slated for closure, robbing those least able to afford transport (not to mention entire municipalities) of local access. The Attorney General has been censured by the Law Society of BC for these cuts/closures, and has reputedly lost the confidence of BC's Supreme Court judges. Of course, the correlation between criminality, poor health, and poverty needs no further explication.

Clearly, the combined effects of these changes go against the strategies outlined by Guralnick in Chapter 3, and ignore the many child protection issues and recommendations identified in chapters by Foster, Kierans, and Macdonald (4), Weller and Wharf (7), Morton (8), the Warburtons (9), and Moretti, Holland, and Moore (11). The resilience discussed by Michalski in Chapter 12, and risk behaviours discussed by Tonkin and Murphy in Chapter 10 are respectively threatened and facilitated by the New Era agenda.

The Human Right's Commission and the Human Rights Advisory Council are being disbanded (Bill 53, Human Rights Amendment Act), making BC the only province in Canada without a Human Rights Commissioner. The effects of the new policy upon the rights of poor children and their families goes counter to the discussion in Chapter 2 by Cook. Concern has also prompted a coalition of non-governmental organizations to petition the United Nations committee overseeing the International Covenant on Economic, Social, and Cultural Rights (ICESCR Committee) (Day and Brodsky, 2002).

Ultimately, the most disturbing aspect of the New Era agenda is the attitude toward others it embodies. The assumption made by the powerful people making public policy appears to be that everyone has basically the same life chances, and therefore is entitled only to minimal assistance from the public purse. Poverty, in this view, appears to be simply the consequence of bad life choices. Disparities in life chances are underplayed, ignored, or used for their iconic value—overcoming the odds of poverty is presented as the norm of hard work and successful entrepreneurialship, not the minor miracle that it is.

It is not surprising that elected representatives have little experience with what life is like on the social and economic margins of society. People on IA or who have lived in foster care or who have not been successful in finding and holding a job rarely, if ever, get elected to public office. Only one elected MLA from the governing party, an ordained minister, voted against the policies outlined above fearing the impact these policies will have upon the poor people he has served. The people who will live with the consequences of these decisions are Ignatieff's 'distant strangers' whose needs are neither understood nor addressed in the day-to-day life of powerful people (Ignatieff, 1984). And so, children in BC, especially the most vulnerable, remain too small to see. When the consequences become too big to ignore, who will pay the price? Only time will tell.

REFERENCES

Day, S., and Brodsky, G. (2002). Poverty and human rights submission to the United Nations ICESCR Committee. February 11. Available at *http://www.povnet.org/ICESCR.htm*.

Goldberg, M., and Long, A. (2001). *Falling behind: A comparison of living costs and Income Assistance rates (BC Benefits) in British Columbia*. Vancouver: Social Planning and Research Council of British Columbia.

Government of British Columbia (2002). *http://www.gov.bc.ca/prem/popt/corereview/default.asp*.

Ignatieff, M. (1984). *The needs of strangers*. London: Hogarth Press.

Lavoie, J. (2002). Social workers condemn Coell's stewardship. *Times Colonist*, June 14, p A4. Victoria, BC.

MacFadden, L. (2002). *Rethink the reductions: Children and youth need more*. 2001 Annual Report, Office of the Child, Youth and Family Advocate. Victoria, BC.

McLintock, B. (2002). Don't ever forget Matthew, warns children's officer. *The Province*, June 26, p. A8. Vancouver, BC.

Ministry of Human Resources (2002). *http://www.mhr.gov.bc.ca/factsheets*.

Pallan, P. (2002). *Looking back, looking ahead: BC's child and youth services in transition*. The Children's Commission Annual Report, 2001. Victoria, BC.

Reitsma-Street, M. (2002). A policy analysis of the proposed BC employment and assistance law. Available at *http://web.uvic.ca/spp/Views&News/WelfarePolicyAnalysis.htm*.

University of Northern British Columbia (2002). Programs statement. School of Social Work, UNBC, *http://www.bcwhistleblower.ca*.

ENDNOTE

1 The opinions expressed in this chapter are solely those of the author.

Plate 5 Future looking back ❯

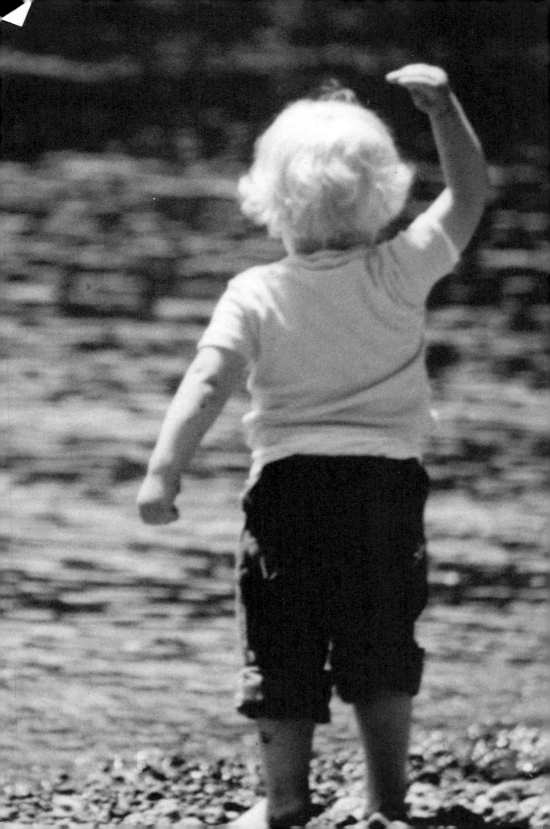